The Royal Society of Medicine
ENCYCLOPEDIA OF CHILD HEALTH

The Royal Society of Medicine

Encyclopedia of

CHILD

HEALTH

DR ROBERT YOUNGSON

BLOOMSBURY

First published 1996
by Bloomsbury Publishing Plc,
2 Soho Square,
London W1V 6HB

A copy of the CIP entry for this book is available
from the British Library

ISBN 0 7475 2753 9

10 9 8 7 6 5 4 3 2 1
Designed by Hugh Adams, AB3
Typeset by Hewer Text Composition Services, Edinburgh
Printed in Great Britain by Clays Ltd, St Ives plc

Contents

INTRODUCTION

To say that the child is father of the man is neither sexist nor paradoxical: every child is the model on which the future adult is based. And it is the physical and mental health of that model, to a large extent, which determines the health of the future adult. Many of the major but avoidable diseases of middle age have their roots in childhood. For instance, doctors are only now beginning to point out that the dangerous arterial disease, atherosclerosis, which is the single largest cause of premature death in adults, has its origins in childhood. And the behavioural patterns and habits formed in childhood have a major bearing on the future physical, mental and social health of the individual.

Genetics, of course, plays a large part in determining the characteristics of the child, and the genetic basis of a great many disorders is now understood. A basic understanding of this important subject, which this book aims to give you, will help you make informed choices about the upbringing of your children, by realistically anticipating certain disorders, possibly even in the choice of a partner. Genetics is currently in an explosive phase, and there will be a great deal more about it in the media in the future.

But what happens to the child between birth and late adolescence is at least as important as the inherited features. It is these aspects with which this book is primarily concerned – the massively influential factors that operate on the results of heredity to produce the final result. One of the most important elements of the total environment of the child, in the widest sense of the term, certainly includes the degree and application of parental knowledge. The future physical and psychological well-being of our children depends, in a very real sense, on how we behave towards them. And that, of course, depends on how much we know.

To help you access that knowledge as easily as possible, I have, where appropriate, extensively cross-referenced entries to other relevant articles. But for the fullest possible coverage of any subject, the secret is to consult the index. This is really the key to the whole work. Unless you use it, you are likely to miss at least some aspects of the subject in which you are interested. You will find that a large number of the index entries are couched in non-medical language. The index also contains many entries describing symptoms and signs. These are intended to lead to the range of conditions which will contain the one you are interested in.

First aid for children is so important that I have included a complete section on this. Well aware of the problems involved in a panic emergency scramble through a book of this kind, I have also, very briefly, covered the essential points of the more urgent items under their own headings. This is to increase the ease with which these can be found. In such cases, the entry is also cross-referenced to the main First Aid section at the beginning of the book.

Throughout history, the elders of the tribe have always been despairingly concerned over the behaviour of the young. Fortunately, most of the young end up as elders, at which point they begin to see what their parents were getting at. This trend is perennial and you will find evidence of it in this book. For this reason I must hasten to add that the opinions expressed in this book are my own and not necessarily those of my long-suffering publishers.

Dr RM Youngson

CHILD DEVELOPMENT

—

Note: words shown in small capitals are cross-references directing you to entries in the main text of the encyclopedia.

The early years of a child's life, especially the first, are critically important because nearly everything that happens during these years colours and conditions the rest of that child's life. Early impressions go deep and, especially if they are traumatic, may have a life-long effect. Indeed, many psychologists believe that early environmental influences play a major part in determining the whole future personality. It is probably more realistic, however, to take the view – a view held by the majority of biologist, incidentally – that the outcome is the result of the action of environmental forces on the genetically-programmed child. For these reasons this introductory section lays considerably more emphasis on the first year of life than on any other stage of development.

Growth and development are much more than a simple increase in the size of the body. The most important internal changes are in the brain and nervous system – changes that make it possible for the child to register and store information, to acquire social skills, and to mature emotionally. Above all, the maturing of the nervous system allows the child progressively greater degrees of freedom to interact with the environment so as to obtain more information.

Indeed, the child's brain can only develop if there *is* input of information. Unless the brain receives the normal rich input of data from all the sense organs, it will inevitably fail to develop properly. Such information is very complex and covers a wide range. It is known as sensory input and comes from the mouth, nose, hands, eyes, ears and the whole surface of the skin. Anything that can be experienced through these portals of the senses – taste, smell, texture, shape, colour, speech, sounds and music – constitutes sensory input. Sensory deprivation is at least as damaging as deprivation of food. Well-fed babies who are deprived of human relationships and contact soon fall behind their more fortunate contemporaries both in terms of mental and physical development.

Because most of the growth of the brain has already occurred before birth, a newborn baby's head is about three quarters of its eventual adult size and a quarter of its total body length. An adult's head is only about one eighth of the body length. Even though brain growth and development continue at a rapid rate, half of the life-time growth of the brain has been completed by the end of the first year of life. Thereafter, most of the growth is in new nerve fibres and in complicated connections, known as synapses. These new connections are formed largely as a result of the effect of sensory input – in other words, as a result of experience. Most physiologists believe that these synaptic connections are the basis of memory. There is a considerable difference between the physical complexity of the brain of a well-educated child and one that has been deprived of sensory input. In some extreme cases these differences can even be seen on microscopic examination after death.

As the nervous system develops, so the bodily organs gradually mature. All the organs are present at birth, but many are structurally and functionally immature. Their growth and development depends largely on the action of growth hormone produced by the pituitary gland and given out in pulses, mainly during the night. This hormone has many effects, one of which is to stimulate the production of proteins, the substances out of which much of the body is made. It does this in two ways: firstly by increasing the supply of amino acids, the building blocks for proteins, to the cells; and secondly, by increasing the speed at which DNA (the blueprint for proteins) is checked for details of the correct order in which these amino acids are put together. Growth hormone also increases the rate at which cells divide and thus reproduce. Finally, it acts on the growing zones in the long bones (the epiphyses) causing them to lengthen steadily. Body growth is also greatly influenced by other hormones – namely, thyroid hormone, insulin and the sex hormones. All these, acting together, bring about a progressive increase in the bulk and dimensions of tissues and organs.

BABYHOOD (birth to 1 year)

Except in the case of identical twins, every individual has a unique genetic make-up and experiences a unique set of influences while it is in the womb. The effect of this is that every newborn baby is different from all others, differing in temperament and responsiveness and in the way he or she reacts to the environment. All of them possess a set of built-in protective reflexes that help them to survive. They will, for instance, react to many stimuli in a self-protective way. Babies don't have to be shown how to feed from the breast or from a bottle equipped with a teat. Their hearing is well established and they react in different ways to different sounds. They are startled by sudden loud sounds, but react with alert attention to the sound of the female voice. Within a few weeks of birth babies can distinguish the sound of the mother's voice from those of other women. They find the lower tones of the male voice soothing. They are, however, distressed by high-pitched crying sounds produced by other infants.

The sense of smell is also well developed at birth and babies have strong prejudices in favour of pleasant smells and against unpleasant ones. Within a week or two of birth, they can usually identify their mothers and fathers by smell. They also show definite taste preferences at birth, enjoying sweet flavours and rejecting sour or bitter substances. Vision is somewhat blurred at birth, but the ability to fix the eyes on an object of interest and to follow it is well established by 2 months. Babies have definite visual preferences, favouring images with high contrast, bright colours and curved lines. Their favourite object of gaze is the human face.

Early mental and social development

The first few weeks of life are spent mainly sleeping (initially up to 20 hours per day), crying and feeding. Crying increases to a maximum around 12 weeks because this is the only way the baby can respond to stimuli such as hunger, discomfort, pain, fear or over-stimulation. Later the baby develops other ways of responding and begins to cry less. During the first year of life, the baby's perception of reality is limited to what can be seen, heard, touched or sucked. Objects outside the field of vision no longer exist as far as the infant is concerned. But, around 9 to 12 months, infants begin to develop the idea that objects may have a permanent existence, even when they are not seen. This idea is first related to whoever spends most time with the baby. This person thus acquires great emotional importance for the baby. 'Peek-a-boo' games briefly stimulate the fear of absence (loss) and immediately relieve it: they delight the child because of this.

The parents' response to the baby's attempts at communication are also vital for normal development. If the parents are depressed or emotionally cold and cannot respond to the baby's expressions, future development and the ability to form close human attachments are likely to be seriously damaged.

Early physical development

Many factors determine a baby's size and weigh at birth, but the most important of these are the size, nutritional state and general health of the mother before and during pregnancy. The baby usually loses some weight in the first few days after birth but this is made up again in about 10 days, and thereafter weight is usually gained at a rate of about 30 g (1 oz) per day. If the baby is genetically destined to be large, but is born small as a result of environmental effects (such as, for instance, the illness of its mother during pregnancy), it will generally grow faster than average so as to catch up its deficit. In most cases, such babies will have reached their full, genetically-determined, size for age by about 18 months. Similarly, babies genetically coded for physical smallness, but who are large at birth as a result of such conditions as maternal diabetes, may seem to be failing to grow at an expected rate. In fact, they are reverting to type.

The average rate of growth is such that most babies are 50 per cent longer at the end of their first year and have grown to treble their birth weight. Most babies double their birth weight by about 4 months. This rapid rate of growth soon declines, however, and by about 2 years of age it will have reached a fairly constant rate. This rate will then apply for most of the childhood. On average, infants and young children gain weight at a rate of 2 to 3 kg (4.4 to 6.6 lbs) per year, and increase in height by 5 to 7.5 cm (2 to 3 in) per year. In the early months of life almost half the calories consumed in food are expended on growth. This proportion also declines rapidly, so that by about 2 years of age only 3 per cent is devoted to growth.

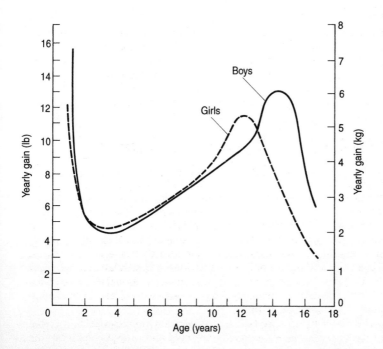

Weight gain from age 0–16

Baby's relationship with mother

Bonding is the close and persistent relationship which develops between individuals, especially those who come into close contact soon after the birth of one of them. Bonding is common to many species of animal and is especially important between a mother and her newborn baby. It is the mechanism that enables an exhausted mother to tolerate a perpetually crying child and to continue to give loving care without resentment. Bonding is essential for the future psychological well-being of the infant. Ninety per cent of parents who batter their children were insufficiently mothered as children.

Bonding is readily disrupted if, for any reason, the mother and baby are separated early. This should never be done unless essential. There is a higher incidence of battering in babies who were so small that they had to be kept for long periods in incubators. The same applies to babies born by caesarian section. Bonding does not occur immediately in all cases. Most women take a little time to fall in love with their babies and should not feel guilty about this.

Ideally, the early physical contact that promotes bonding should occur as soon as possible after birth. This is now widely recognized and mothers will normally be given their babies to hold as soon as they are born. Some babies take this as an invitation to start feeding at once and, if allowed, will attach themselves to a nipple and suck vigorously. This is the exception rather than the rule, however, and most babies will take a little time to recover from the traumas of being born before beginning to think of food.

New babies are very quick to recognize what their mother really thinks of them. In most cases there is no problem; the mother's genuine love and fascination is quickly conveyed to the baby and all is well. But sometimes, perhaps because of postnatal depression, or any other psychological, physical or social disturbance, a baby is resented or rejected. Eye contact is avoided and the baby receives minimal cuddling and close holding. Such behaviour is likely to have serious consequences for the future life and happiness of the baby. All kinds of personality and behavioural problems could result. Unfortunately, many unwilling young mothers do not realise this, and social and behavioural inadequacies can be perpetuated through the generations.

At this early stage, the father's role is less important, but as a recognized member of the group, he has, of course, a future role in the psychological well-being of the child. Later, his role may become even more important.

Newborn babies have been nicely enclosed for 40 weeks or so and need time to get accustomed to the wide open spaces of the alarming new world. For this reason they like to feel that they are still enclosed – whether in the mother's arms or a warm cot blanket, or whatever. Remember, too, that they are frightened of falling, so bear this in mind when picking up and handling a baby. New babies require security of all kinds and especially a secure conviction that they can trust those who are looking after them.

Speech

By about 2 months a baby is capable of producing cooing sounds in response to sounds from adults. By 6 months or so the baby can make spontaneous, repetitive babbling sounds, and by 1 year the child is beginning to understand that there is some relationship between particular sounds and objects. Baby talk is attractive to the child at this stage because it consists largely of sounds that the child can actually make, and there is pleasure and a sense of familiarity in hearing such sounds.

Up to 6 to 10 months nearly all babies spend a good deal of time making arbitrary cooing and babbling noises. Babbling is at a peak at about 1 year and, thereafter sounds begin to become meaningful and the vocabulary of words begins to grow.

Many parents are unaware of the importance of listening attentively to the sounds their baby makes and of responding to them, especially when the child is trying to convey information. If the baby's intentions are clear, the parent should use the appropriate word so as to form the association in the child's mind. This kind of meaningful interaction is most important in promoting the baby's speech abilities. Studies have shown that children deprived of this one-to-one interaction will often end up with poor powers of verbal self-expression. This does not just happen in institutions; it can happen in large busy families in which, although there is plenty of speech going on, there is no one with the time to devote to the patient business of bringing out the new baby's full verbal potential.

Physical ability milestones

Note: Don't worry if your baby does not meet these milestones. It does not mean that he or she is retarded in development.

1 month
- lifts chin
- able to raise head a little
- begins to make crawling movements
- tight grasp of finger
- responds to sounds
- startle reflex present
- looks at faces

2 months
- can raise chest off table when face down
- fists relaxed
- smiles when stroked or addressed
- able to recognize mother or father

3 months
- holds head up
- when face down, can support body on forearms
- follows objects
- hands often open
- vocalizing prolonged vowel sounds
- reaches out for people or objects

5 months
- can sit up when supported
- can roll from back to front and vice versa
- can support body on wrists
- touches objects within range
- moves arms together to grasp objects
- recognizes location of sounds
- looks around with interest

6 months
- sits up unsupported
- can put foot in mouth
- reaches out with either hand
- babbling speech
- recognizes strangers

9 months
- can turn round when sitting
- may be able to crawl
- can pull body up to stand
- holds bottle
- can grasp with fingers and thumb
- may say 'dada' and 'mama' but without discrimination
- interested in exploration

TODDLER (1 TO 3 YEARS)

During the toddler stage of development enormous physical, mental and social changes occur in every department of the child's being. Children, of course, vary widely in the rate of their development, but for many the rate of progress is phenomenal. This is the stage at which everything is new and interesting, often fascinating, and during which the growing child acquires an immense amount of information about the world.

By about 15 months, the child is fully aware that a stranger is not the mother or father or other regular carer. As a result of this awareness, together with the total psychological dependence on the known carers, the child's anxiety in the presence of a strange person may be severe. By about 2 years, however, the development of the nervous system allows the infant to recognize that there are many different people in the world and 'stranger anxiety' largely disappears. By this stage the child's perception of the mother may be so strong that he or she can even recognize her from a photograph.

Walking

Most babies can sit up at 6 months and can get around by crawling, or some other individual method of locomotion, by about 1 year. Some convert upright sitting into a kind of bottom drag and proceed by stretching out and then bending one or both legs. Some find this method of getting around so effective that they seem to have no inclination to get up on their feet and start walking. It is not unheard of for children who have developed a rapid crawling method of moving about to go on using it until they are almost 2 years old. Other babies don't bother with crawling and proceed directly from sitting to walking.

All these are entirely normal as the age at which a child begins to walk varies greatly. This has nothing to do with mental development and can range from 9 months to 17 months. You should not be surprised or concerned by this as different parts of the nervous system may mature at different rates. Walking is, in any case, such a complex accomplishment, calling for the effective action of so many different parts – the brain, the nerves, the balancing mechanism, the muscles, and so on. Some children refuse to walk until long after they have acquired considerable verbal ability.

Walking is a vital stage in development as it allows the child to explore and extend its environment, thus greatly increasing the possibilities of acquiring information. At the same time, the sense of relative independence that the child experiences is an important developmental factor. At this stage you are likely to experience regular conflicts between your concern for the safety of the child and your child's quest for knowledge of the limits of what he or she can observe or control. Exploration and new experiences are important for development, and a balance is therefore necessary between over-restriction and safety. Inevitably, the result will be many stormy scenes. Some mothers may resent the loss of the baby's total dependency on them and special unique intimacy with them.

The toddler's extension of his or her world experience is both pleasurably exciting and alarming. There is a growing awareness that a measure of the former total protection has been removed and that the mother has a life of her own with concerns that are not necessarily wholly related to baby. Because of this, toddler behaviour often seems contradictory. The child will venture away from the mother for a certain distance but will then appear to develop a sudden panic and will hurry back. This behaviour may be extended into the 'I'm running away – you'd better come after me' game. This is partly just fun but is also a way of constantly reassuring the child of mother's continuing concern.

Speech

Once a child realizes that uttering a particular sound can result in acquiring a desired object, this connection is quickly reinforced. The average toddler of 18 months has a vocabulary of between 20 and 50 words, depending largely on how well the child is encouraged, at this stage, to talk. At this age infants understand many more words than they can speak – often well over 100 words. But around the end of the second year there is usually a sudden considerable increase in the power of expression and in the number of words that are understood although not spoken. Vocabulary and the ability to form sentences increase rapidly. These are, of course, rather arbitrary standards, but if the child clearly falls well behind these, help is probably needed.

At this stage parents can help children to enlarge their vocabularies by using simple normal language to refer to objects, rather than by making baby noises. Children brought up in a highly stimulating environment among people with a substantial vocabulary now rapidly develop their powers of expression and are soon prompted to enlarge their environment even more by learning to read.

Security objects

A security object is any particular item that brings comfort and a sense of security to a young child, often for a number of years. Security objects are usually associated in some way with bed and are often made of soft material. A scrap of an old blanket or of a former night garment, a teddy bear, even an old nappy may be chosen as a comforter, and these are often pressed to the face as the child settles down to sleep.

Some children claim that they like the smell of the comforter; most who use security objects are clearly emotionally attached to them and resent attempts to deprive them of the object. Later a kind of ambivalence develops as the child comes to see that the security object is 'rather silly'. Around the age of 6 or 7, the security object is usually repudiated and there may even be a ritual destruction. In some cases the use of the object persists into adolescence or even adult life.

There is no reason to suppose that security objects are in any way undesirable, at any age, and enforced removal may be cruel.

Temper tantrums

These are the expression of frustration in a toddler who has reached the stage of wishing to demonstrate independent action but is prevented from doing so. Tantrums may be very noisy and, especially in public, embarrassing, as they seem to imply lack of parental discipline or effectiveness. The toddler soon learns to exploit the power of screaming, floor-rolling, head-banging and breath-holding and, if injudiciously handled, may come to dominate a household.

Occasional tantrums are normal, but you must not let a pattern develop. Tantrums must be handled calmly, firmly and consistently with minimal necessary restraint, and the child's demands, unless reasonable, should never be met. If necessary, you may have to impose a short period of banishment to a safe cot or playpen in a separate room until the tantrum has passed. Once adequate communication by speech has been achieved, temper tantrums should settle, as the child can express his or her wishes and these can be discussed.

Another important weapon in the toddler's armoury is the breath-holding attack. This is a highly effective form of infantile blackmail, and is usually prompted by annoyance on the part of the child at not being allowed to have his or her own way. Some parents will be convinced that these are manipulative in nature and will feel that the child is making use of the only major weapon at his or her disposal. Others will simply allow themselves to be dominated by the child's use of this effective strategy. Breath-holding attacks are sometimes induced by pain, but the usual causal factors are anger and frustration.

The attack starts with a period of loud crying. At the end of a long wail, during which the lungs are emptied of air, the child simply refrains from taking in a breath and soon turns blue. If his or her resolution allows it, breath-holding continues until consciousness is lost and the child goes quite rigid with arms and legs extended and back arched. Sometimes there are a few muscle twitches or a minor convulsion due to lack of oxygen to the brain, but in a very short time, nature takes over and breathing starts again with rapid recovery. These episodes never involve any danger to life and no treatment is needed. You can, however, often abort an attack by splashing a little cold water on the child's face or blowing on it, or by pulling the tongue forward with a finger hooked round the back of it.

Breath-holding attacks affect only quite young children. They are unusual after the age of about 5 years. They are very common and may be a source of great, but unnecessary, concern to parents. Although they may superficially resemble them, the attacks are of an essentially different nature from EPILEPSY or febrile fits, and observant parents should have no difficulty in making the distinction.

PRE-SCHOOL AGE (3 TO 5 YEARS)

A common preoccupation of parents at this stage is excretory control, and this sometimes provokes anxiety. Most children are clean and dry by 3, but many take longer to reach this stage. Undue concern is inappropriate until about half-way through the third year. By 3, the average child will be anxious to avoid 'accidents' and may become anxious if for any reason access to toilet facilities is delayed. Persistent BEDWETTING after the age of 5 must be considered abnormal and requires attention.

Communication

During this phase of development, parental anxiety may, ironically, switch from concern over failure of progress in speaking to concern over the child's apparent inability to stop talking. To many healthy youngsters, the delightful ability to evoke a response from parents by speech communication, and especially by asking questions, proves irresistible. It is often apparent that questions are not being asked primarily to obtain information. Parents driven crazy by endless questioning might perhaps take comfort in this observation.

Another form of communication important to most children is drawing and painting. Motives for this activity vary but will always include the desire to be admired and the desire to convey to others what the work of art is all about. This is usually quite clear to the child, although often obscure to the observer, and it is important for you to take seriously what will often seem to be no more than a random scribble or a meaningless set of coloured blobs. Children are usually very proud of their artwork and will often elaborate a story which they are purporting to illustrate. They should be encouraged to explain what their paintings are all about and should, at this stage, always be praised for the quality of their productions. At this age, the child has few opportunities of demonstrating what he or she can do and needs reassurance.

Proprietary rights

This is also the stage at which personal property and individual rights assume great importance for the growing child. Jealousy in childhood or sibling rivalry is a common result of competition, often between brother and sister. Much parental patience and diplomacy is often needed to resolve, or at least limit, the resulting conflicts. Ensure that children's proprietary rights are respected by their siblings and that attempts to infringe these by siblings – a common manifestation of jealousy – are firmly repressed.

Alternatively, jealousy may be prompted by the arrival of a new baby. The usual signs are BEDWETTING, a regression to a simpler and more childish mode of behaviour, TEMPER TANTRUMS, or sometimes evident anxiety. Children should be warned, well in advance, of an expected addition to the family and should be clearly told that time and attention will have to be given to the new baby. You must understand and tolerate the signs of jealousy and should give as much attention as possible to the older child(ren). So far as is possible, the baby should not be allowed to intrude into the older child's possessions and living area, as this will make the jealousy worse.

Nutrition

It is during this period that faulty appetites are commonly established and these can have a most important effect on the later health of the individual. So it's a good idea to be as well informed as possible on the subject of diet in childhood.

There is increasing evidence that ATHEROSCLEROSIS, which affects the linings of arteries, narrowing them and making them prone to obstruction, begins in childhood. atherosclerosis is one of the two or three most serious of all diseases and is the underlying cause of heart attacks, strokes, limb gangrene and many other devastating disorders.

Quite young children have obvious fatty streaks in their arteries and these are where atherosclerosis later develops. The fully established condition is now regularly found in adults as young as 30, examined at autopsy after accidental death.

Atherosclerosis is proportional to the levels of cholesterol carriers – low density lipoproteins (LDLs) – in the blood, and these relate to the amount of *saturated* fat consumed. Saturated fats come from animal and dairy products. Fish and vegetable fats are unsaturated. Most children get about 40 per cent of their calories from fat, and those with a regular junk food intake, get over 50 per cent from fats. The average fast-food hamburger provides half its calories in fat.

Experts do not, at present, think that there is any justification for amending the diets of infants under 1 year. During the first year of life, fats from milk are an essential source of calories and fat-soluble vitamins. Any reduction in fat intake – as, for instance, by feeding skimmed milk – might lead to a failure to thrive or even vitamin deficiency. Infants and young children need plenty of calories for energy and growth and a low-fat diet might be so unattractive to children that they won't want to eat it.

> The diets of children over 1 year should be modified to reduce the levels of total fats and LDLs. Post-toddlers who have begun to have a regular daily intake of hamburgers, crisps, French fries and other junk foods need to be protected from their natural appetites for high-fat food. Dairy products such as butter, high-fat cheeses, whole-cream milk, and animal fats should be avoided. Children's food should be grilled rather than fried, replace animal cooking fats by vegetable fats; meat and dairy products replace by fish and foods of vegetable origin; creamy milk by skimmed milk; and butter by polyunsaturated margarines.

A satisfactory diet at home will achieve little if you allow children to spend money on junk food or fat-containing sweets, or if they are having high-fat food in school lunches.

There is a small group of children at particular risk and these should be identified as early as possible. One person in about 500 suffers from a condition called familial hypercholesterolaemia. This is a hereditary condition in which the levels of LDL cholesterol in the blood are particularly high. The condition invariably leads to early and severe atherosclerosis and may be suspected if there is a family history of heart attacks or strokes at an unusually early age.

It has been recommended that all children and other immediate relatives of people who have had a heart attack or a stroke, under age 55, should have laboratory checks of their blood cholesterol levels done, under properly controlled dietary conditions. The blood pressure should also be checked. Children found to have raised cholesterol levels should be referred to a specialist for management. Many will be able to be controlled on diet alone, but some will need treatment with cholesterol-lowering drugs.

Underdevelopment

There are many reasons why a child does not achieve abilities and behaviour patterns appropriate to his or her age.

> **Causes of underdevelopment**
> - serious and prolonged general diseases especially of the heart and lungs
> - poor nutrition
> - brain damage before, during or after birth
> - severe deafness
> - very poor vision
> - lack of parental affection or attention
> - lack of adequate guidance in acceptable conduct
> - lack of mental or physical stimulation

Routine checks on development are most important and follow a fairly standard pattern. For newborn babies, attention will be paid to:

- weight
- length
- head circumference
- presence of any congenital abnormalities
- reaction to noise
- reaction to light
- clarity of lenses of the eyes
- state of the FONTANELLES
- possible hip dislocation
- possible jaundice
- pulses
- whether testes present in scrotum
- possible floppiness

At 6 months, the doctor will be interested in:

- interaction with environment
- interaction with parents
- physical parameters
- vision
- hearing
- sounds produced
- possible SQUINT
- ability to roll over
- ability to sit up without support
- laughter

At 2 years, all these points will be reviewed and the doctor will check:

- walking
- ability to climb stairs
- speech
- vocabulary
- response to commands
- tightness of sphincters

Developmental delay does not necessarily imply permanent damage to the future quality of life. Human beings are remarkable for their adaptability and for their powers of recovery even from the seemingly most disastrous early experiences. See also FLOPPY INFANT SYNDROME.

JUNIOR SCHOOL AGE (5 TO 11 YEARS)

By the time they reach school age children have acquired a considerable range of personal skills – feeding and often clothing themselves, using the the toilet, washing, and effectively communicating needs and wishes to others. These skills confer a degree of independence that is usually greatly valued by the child, especially if they are clearly appreciated by the parents. This stage, however, brings with it new challenges and anxieties, the most significant of these being the move from an exclusively home and family environment to one that includes the school.

For most, the early experience of school involves at least a degree of separation anxiety and, at first, tears and refusal to attend are to be expected. At its worst, separation anxiety is a significant childhood disorder in which excessive and inappropriate alarm is shown whenever there is separation, or the threat of separation, from one or both parents. The child suffers unrealistic fear of abandonment and of danger to the parent. In addition to dramatically demonstrating concern at the time of separation, by a show of terror or panic, the child may complain of headache, tummy pain and nausea, and may often vomit. Such children make abnormal demands to be held and cuddled and can obtrude unduly into adult affairs. In addition to persistent refusal to go to school, they may refuse to sleep away from

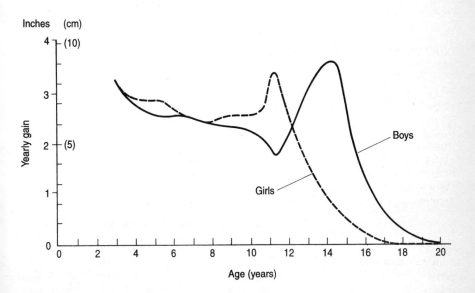

Growth rate from age 3–20

home or even to go to bed unless accompanied by a parent. Separation anxiety is managed by constant reassurance of love and support, fair treatment, explanation, firmness and natural responses. Occasionally, a doctor may prescribe tranquilliser drugs and night sedatives.

Such extreme cases are rare, but it is not at all uncommon for children at the stage of starting school to show signs of real anxiety such as night terrors or complaints of various symptoms. The most popular is abdominal pain. No one need be surprised at these reactions. For the whole of the child's life, he or she has had constant access to a parent; suddenly, for periods of hours at a time, this individual support is withdrawn. In the face of these child anxieties, it can be hard for parents to insist on taking children to school. But it is rare for the anxiety to persist for more than a few days. Sometimes, asking the child to look after some small object until the parents return provides vital reassurance.

Primary school teachers are thoroughly familiar with these problems and will almost always deal with them sympathetically and understandingly. Children are so accustomed to having, and needing, a parental figure that successful primary school teachers are often unconsciously treated by children as temporary surrogate mothers. It is commonplace for a child to address a popular teacher as 'Mummy' and then to look embarrassed or to laugh.

At first, children new to school may find it difficult adapt to the new, and possibly more disciplined and structured, routines of school. There may also, especially in the case of first or only children, be problems in relating to larger groups of other children. For some, there may have been little or no experience of taking account of the needs of other children so that work and play can be cooperative. A child who appears unduly selfish may simply be a child who has never learned this elementary lesson. The school environment provides plenty of opportunities for acquiring essential social skills of this kind.

Because of their inherent fascination with all things new, school imposes great assimilative demands on new junior pupils. For many this huge new spectrum of experience can be exhausting, and parents may find that, at first, children are apt to fall asleep as soon as they get home, or even when being driven home from school. There is no harm in this and it can be regarded with satisfaction as indicating the intensity of the child's educational experience. Regrettably, few children maintain the same depth of concentrated interest throughout the whole of their schooling.

The period of junior school is also notable for a new and growing awareness by the child of the need for rules and regulations. Rules are important to the young child in two senses. They provide a stable framework for behaviour which allows the child to recognize the limits in which he or she may operate. Anarchy is no more comfortable in childhood than it is in adult society. Rules also give the child an opportunity to become accustomed to conforming to the kind of discipline which forms an inevitable part of the child's future life.

Many vitally important things happen to the child during the period of primary schooling. From the point of view of social and mental health, these early years are by far the most important formative period of the child's whole life. This fact has been recognized by sages throughout the centuries and there is now a mass of neuro-physiological and psychological evidence to back it up. The primary responsibility for the quality of the child's conditioning during this period of remarkable neurological plasticity rests, of course, with the parents, but a great deal of the responsibility devolves on the teachers who may often be perceived by the children as figures of greater authority than the parents.

TEENAGE (11 TO 19)

The principal developmental feature of the teenage is, of course, puberty. This is the period of physical development during which the young person becomes sexually mature and capable of sexual intercourse and reproduction. Puberty is not the same as adolescence, which is a social concept referring to the period of transition from childhood to adulthood. Puberty occurs during adolescence, but puberty is a purely physical and physiological process.

Adolescence, on the other hand, involves, in addition, mental and emotional changes. Before puberty, children grow in body and mind but undergo no fundamental change. At puberty, basic changes begin that fully differentiate children into sexually oriented women and men.

Puberty occurs, on average, at age 10 in girls and 12 in boys. Just before it there is a striking acceleration in the rate of growth. This jumps to about 9 cm (3½ in) per year in girls and over 10 cm (4 in) per year in boys. The prepubertal growth spurt often affects different parts of the body at different times so that, while it is in progress, the body may appear temporarily out of proportion. This growth spurt usually affects first the feet, then the legs, followed by the trunk, and finally the face, especially the lower jaw. In boys the prepubertal growth spurt lasts longer than in girls and leads to a significant advantage in height over girls.

Puberty in girls

Since the middle of the 19th century, puberty in Western European and North American girls has been getting progressively earlier. The average age of the onset has dropped at a rate of four to six months every decade. This phenomenon, which is thought to be due to improvements in nutrition, has now stabilized. Puberty in girls now occurs at any age between 10 and 13, and takes three or four years in all. Because of this variability, some girls reach physical sexual maturity while others of the same age may still have a childlike physique. A similar phenomenon occurs with boys and, in both sexes, can be a cause of distress. But by the age of 16 or 17, almost all the late starters will have caught up. Late onset of puberty has no bearing on the adequacy of future sexuality.

The period of puberty features considerable body growth, changes in body proportions and major changes in the sexual organs. The first sign is usually breast budding, although pubic and underarm hair may sometimes appear first. Breast buds may appear as early as the age of 8, but, on average, they appear at the age of 11. Menstruation usually starts a year after this. By this point, the other changes associated with puberty are well established.

Breast growth is often rapid, and for a time, one side may grow more rapidly than the other. It is rare, however, for the breasts to remain significantly different in size. Bony deposits in the pelvis cause it to widen relative to the rest of the skeleton, and the visual effect of this is emphasized by new deposits of fat laid down around the hips. The general contours of the female body are considerably influenced by these specific fat deposits, which also occur under the skin of the breasts and buttocks.

In girls, puberty is deemed complete when menstruation is occurring regularly. This means that eggs are being released from the ovaries (ovulation) and that conception and childbirth are possible. To begin with, however, menstruation may often be irregular, in both flow and rhythm, and this can last for up to two years. In some cases, scanty periods occur during the summer months throughout adolescence. This is quite normal and is caused by the fact than many cycles do not feature ovulation, and it is because of this that the irregularity occurs. The onset of regular menstruation, however, can be affected by various factors such as obesity, which tends to bring on periods earlier, and malnutrition (from dieting) and excessive athletic activity, which tend to delay onset.

Puberty in boys

All the physical changes that occur during male puberty are caused by the male sex hormone testosterone. This is an anabolic steroid (growth-promoting hormone) produced in the testicles by cells lying between the sperm-producing tubules. Until shortly before puberty the testicles contain only numerous solid cords of cells, and there is no sign of sperm production. At puberty, however, the cells at the centre of these cords atrophy so that the cords become tubes. These are the seminiferous tubules in which the sperm develop. This process is completed early in puberty, and thereafter sperm production is active and rapid. Very large numbers of sperm are produced – about 300–600 per gram (10,000 to 20,000 per oz) of testicle every second.

Testosterone is a powerful hormone and has many effects. It causes the testicles, scrotum and penis to enlarge, and enables the penis to erect fully. It also causes the seminiferous tubules to begin to produce sperm, and causes the sperm-carrying ducts and the semen-storage sacs (the seminal vesicles) to increase in size and mature. It enlarges the prostate gland and causes it to begin to secrete fluid that makes up part of the seminal fluid. It makes the voice box (larynx) bigger and causes the voice to drop in pitch as a result. It promotes the growth of pubic and underarm hair and of the beard, and may cause hair to grow on the chest and abdomen. Finally, it accelerates general body growth and muscular development.

These changes usually occur roughly in the order given above. Puberty may start at any age from about 10 to 15 and usually takes about two and a half years, so it may not be complete until after the age of 17. Most boys have reached about 80 per cent of their adult height before puberty, but there is nearly always a large growth spurt during puberty too.

PSYCHOLOGICAL ASPECTS OF PUBERTY
The main psychological consequence of puberty is the initiation and growth of sexual interest and sexual drive. Both boys and girls quickly become aware of the physical differences between the sexes and this awareness often arouses their intense interest in the opposite sex. In many cases, this becomes the chief preoccupation. There is often a new and uncharacteristic concern over personal appearance and clothes, and adolescents may become increasingly anxious to conform to current fashions in dress.

Adolescence is a difficult time for many. Growing knowledge and intellectual powers often bring with them a kind of arrogance and a contempt for the opinions of older and more experienced people. Adult ways and views are often rejected by adolescents and they may be extremely impatient with imposed rules and regulations. There is a growing recognition of the importance of success, and if they fail to achieve this, as it is defined by adults (good school reports, for instance) adolescents may then make attempts to succeed in the eyes of their peer group. This may lead to delinquency, but this is usually only a temporary phase. To some extent, a degree of rebellion is natural, and part of the need to define an identity that differs from that of the parents.

Few young people pass through adolescence without some psychological and emotional upset, for there are many conflicts between the innate desires and the still inadequate capacity to fulfil them. Suicide is common in adolescents, particularly among boys. During this period most young people begin to acquire self-assurance and self-reliance and become aware of the possibilities of deep relationships with people outside the immediate family. (See also SUICIDE of a young person).

Many adolescents never reach the stage of mental development characteristic of the fully adult formal way of thinking in which abstract reasoning predominates. In many, thinking continues to be concerned with the particular rather than with the general, the concrete rather than the conceptual. Thinking often remains egocentric (unable to see things from another person's point of view) and some adolescents have difficulty in appreciating the relationship between present action and future consequences.

ABNORMAL PUBERTY
The whole process of puberty is initiated by the production of gonadotrophin-releasing hormone by the hypothalamus of the brain. Why this occurs is not clear. This hormone acts on the pituitary gland, causing it to begin to secrete a new group of hormones, the gonadotrophins, around 10–14 years. The term 'gonadotrophin' simply means 'sex gland stimulator'. Gonadotrophins cause the ovaries to secrete oestrogens, and the testicles to produce testosterone.

Very rarely, abnormal changes in the hypothalamus, such as a brain tumour, may start this sequence going at a much earlier age than normal. As a result, puberty may occur at almost any earlier age, even in infancy. Because the adrenal glands also secrete male sex hormones, a tumour of an adrenal can have a similar effect in a small boy. There have been cases of extreme precocious sexual development, in which full sexual maturity and reproductive capacity have been reached at the age of 5 years in both boys and girls. The youngest known mother gave birth to a healthy baby four months before her 6th birthday.

Homosexuality may be a serious preoccupation with young people who are in doubt as to their sexual orientation. Homosexuality is a sexual preference for a person of the same anatomical sex. The term comes from the Greek root *homos*, meaning 'same', not from the Latin *homo*, meaning 'man'. Human beings are never completely hetero- or homosexual: sexual preference lies somewhere on a spectrum between exclusively heterosexual and exclusively homosexual. It is entirely normal for young people to experience some homosexual interest or engage in homosexual activity at some point in their lives. The stereotypes of the homosexual person are misleading; most homosexual people merely want to express, in private, the emotions and inclinations that seem normal to them.

The prevalence of homosexuality is unknown, but many researchers believe that the frequency of exclusive homosexual preference is about 1 per cent for both sexes, and that the same figure applies to bisexual preference.

A distinction needs to be made between homosexual preference and homosexual behaviour. The latter is common in conditions where heterosexual contacts are limited or absent, such as boarding schools, convents and so on, but such behaviour is often merely a substitute for heterosexual activity and is usually accompanied by heterosexual fantasies. There is no particular reason to believe that homosexuality is caused in this way. The experts do not believe that homosexual preferences are caused by experience, but it is clear that a pre-existing homosexual identity can be, and often is, reinforced and established by homosexual experience.

The causation of homosexuality remains obscure. The suggestion that there is a genetic basis for homosexuality was strongly supported in mid 1993 when an American team of researchers at the National Cancer Institute, Washington, DC, published the results of their studies of the families of 114 homosexual men and found that their close relatives were far more likely to be homosexual than expected from population statistics. There were also far more homosexual people on the maternal than on the paternal side. This prompted the view that homosexuality might be connected with the X chromosome. (Women are XX; men XY.) DNA was then taken from 40 pairs of homosexual brothers and the X chromosome studied. Thirty three of these 40 pairs had genetic markers in the same region of the chromosome. This region is called Xq28 and it is long enough to contain several hundred genes.

These findings are unlikely to have arisen by chance or coincidence, and suggest that 65 per cent of the families studied were transmitting a gene that predisposes to homosexuality. The researchers believe that within a few years it will be possible to isolate the gene.

BABY CARE
Feeding

The first feed in life usually occurs at the age of 2 to 6 hours and, as we have seen, may even occur in the delivery room. Healthy newborn babies are best fed on demand and this may involve feeds at intervals of two to five hours. You can judge whether a new baby is ready to feed by checking that he or she has a good strong and rhythmical suck, has a soft, non-distended stomach and has good bowel sounds. Breast-feeding is always preferable to bottle-feeding (see below), but in some cases bottle feeding may be unavoidable. The amount taken by a newborn baby usually starts at about ½ to 1 oz and increases up to 2 oz on the third day of life. By then, the average baby has a daily intake of about 100 ml for each kilogram of body weight.

Demand feeding is all very well in the first month or so when the needs of the baby are paramount, but can cause serious domestic upheaval if continued much longer than this. At the same time, the enforcement of a rigid, unalterable routine can cause its own difficulties, especially in the context of the baby's reaction to such an unnatural regimen. So the ideal probably rests somewhere between the two – the gradual establishment of a pattern of feeding, not strictly and invariably by the clock, but based on one with flexibility.

Normal breast milk is deficient in vitamins K and D. All new babies should have vitamin K at birth to prevent the bleeding tendency known as haemorrhagic disease of the newborn. Supplements of vitamin D (7 micrograms daily) are also required and breast-fed babies should also have small daily doses of vitamin A (200 micrograms) and vitamin C (200 mg). If the mother is a strict vegetarian, her breast-fed baby may not have a sufficient supply of iron, folate and vitamin B_{12}. The baby may need supplements of these. Note that most formula milks contain all the necessary vitamin and mineral supplements, apart from vitamin K, which is usually given by injection in hospital but which may be given by mouth. See also VITAMIN K CONTROVERSY.

With these provisos, breast milk provides *all the nutritional requirements* of the baby and infant for the first four months of life. There is no nutritional advantage in early weaning; there is the possible disadvantage that it may encourage obesity. British mothers prefer cereals and rusks as the first solid foods, but there is a wide range of semi-solid proprietary baby foods such as various purées of meat, fish, fruit or cereals, and these can be offered from 4 to 6 months of age. During weaning, these foods should be offered on a spoon prior to breast feeding.

From 6 to 9 months, babies need foods rich in iron for growth; by 9 to 12 months, they are usually ready to follow the three meal a day pattern. Many foods can simply be chopped or minched, but avoid giving them sugary things, fatty meats, salt and tea and coffee.

Babies quickly form preferences and dislike change of diet. For this reason it is helpful to introduce new flavours early on, although only one should be tried at a time. Rejected foods should be deferred for two or three weeks and then tried again. Babies should be encouraged to use suitable spoons and feeding cups as early as possible after weaning; there is always a risk that a baby might be very reluctant to give up breast- or bottle-feeding. By about the age of 9 months most babies should be able to join the rest of the family at table for at least one meal a day – however messy they may be.

Milk

Cow's milk differs from human milk (see below) but, because of its similarity in composition, it is a good food for older children, providing an excellent balance of carbohydrate, fat, protein, minerals and vitamins. It has therefore been commercially exploited on an enormous scale.

The chief difference between cow's milk and human milk is with the composition of the milk fats. Human milk fats contain a higher proportion of long chain and unsaturated fatty acids, and these provide greater resistance to germs commonly affecting the bowel, such as those causing dysentery, than do fatty acids from cow's milk. Even more important, human milk contains protective antibodies produced by the mother's immune system, which provide the baby with protection against many organisms, until such time as the baby can produce its own.

The main carbohydrate in milk is lactose. Some people do not have the enzyme which breaks this down to simpler sugars and, as the unaltered lactose cannot be absorbed, it remains in the bowel and ferments, causing bloating, distention, pain and diarrhoea. This is called LACTOSE INTOLERANCE.

Milk protein allergy occurs rarely in some infants and can cause eczema or vomiting and diarrhoea. See ALLERGY IN CHILDREN.

COMPOSITION OF MILK			
Per 100 Calories	**Human milk**	**Cow's milk**	**Formula**
Protein (g)	1.3–1.6	5.1	2.3
Fat (g)	5	5.7	5.3
Carbohydrate (g)	10.3	7.3	10.8
Vitamin A (IU)	250	216	300
Vitamin D (IU)	3	0.3	63
Vitamin E (IU)	0.3	0.1	2
Vitamin C (mg)	7.8	2.3	8.1
Thiamine (μg)	25	59	80
Riboflavine (μg)	60	252	100
Niacin (μg)	250	131	1200
Folic acid	4	8	10
Vitamin B_{12} (μg)	0.15	0.56	0.25
Calcium (mg)	50	186	75
Phosphorus (mg)	25	145	65
Magnesium (mg)	6	20	8
Iron (mg)	0.1	0.08	1.5
Iodine (μg)	4–9	7	10
Zinc (mg)	0.1–0.5	0.6	0.65
Copper (μg)	25–60	20	80

BREAST-OR BOTTLE-FEEDING

There can be no question that, from the point of view of the baby, breast-feeding is preferable to bottle-feeding. Breast-feeding promotes better bonding between baby and mother and this may have some bearing on the future personality of the child. In calorific terms, breast milk contains 55 per cent fat, 38 per cent carbohydrate (lactose) and 7 per cent protein. This is an ideal ratio. The proportion of the watery liquid protein (whey) to the casein protein (curds) is 60:40 and this facilitates ready digestion of the protein. Cow's milk contains 80 per cent casein. Formula milk cannot be made identical to human milk.

The bottle-fed baby is deprived of many valuable antibodies present in the mother's milk. There is evidence that breast-fed babies may be less likely to develop atopic conditions such as ECZEMA and ASTHMA. The risks of contamination of the feed are also greater with bottle- than with breast-feeding and care must be taken with sterilization. Gastroenteritis is a special and this is encouraged by the absence of antibodies, the ease with which a bottle, the teat, or the milk itself can be contaminated, and the fact that milk at feeding temperature is an excellent culture medium for bacteria. This risk is, of course, greater if the milk is not used immediately but is kept warm artificially.

The advantages of bottle-feeding are too obvious to require enumeration, especially to a working mother, and these are often socially overwhelming. Breast milk, however, can be expressed into a wide-necked feeding bottle or sucked out with a breast pump and poured into a feeding bottle.

Weaning

Solid food should be started between 4 and 6 months, depending on weight and rate of growth. Large babies take to solid food earlier and are often dissatisfied with milk. A small supplement of fruit or vegetable purée or cereal can be given by teaspoon before or after a breast- or bottle-feed at about 4 months, and the proportion of purée to milk can then be gradually increased. By 6 months babies should be happily consuming finely chopped meat and vegetables, and by 7 or 8 months baby foods will usually have taken precedence over milk as items of diet. Cow's milk is best avoided during the first year of life; some experts recommend it should be avoided for the first two years. See also ALLERGY IN CHILDREN.

Weaning from milk can cause problems as some babies are sensitive to certain foods and may develop DIARRHOEA, VOMITING or skin rashes. So it is best to start new foods one at a time, to be sure that any which might be causing trouble can be identified. Most babies are fully weaned from the breast by 9 months.

Crying

Crying can be a real problem. Fortunately, most crying results from minor discomforts such as wet nappies or infantile colic. It can also be part of manipulative behaviour (see BEHAVIOUR PROBLEMS and SLEEPING PROBLEMS). A very few cases result from organic disease or from constitutional problems such as AUTISM, the CRI DU CHAT SYNDROME or PHENYLKETONURIA. A few disorders that may cause crying in a previously quiet child include:

- bowel obstruction
- strangulated hernia
- INTUSSUSCEPTION
- COLIC
- OTITIS MEDIA
- fever from any cause
- MENINGITIS
- urinary tract infection
- raised pressure within the skull from any cause

Most of these conditions will have other signs and the quality of the child's crying and general response will be obviously different from its usual crying and behaviour. If in doubt, call the doctor.

The term 'infantile colic' is often applied to a distressing baby problem that has nothing to do with real COLIC. The affected infant is healthy, feeds well and gains weight, but seems exceptionally hungry and will suck vigorously on anything offered. The feature which can drive you crazy is the apparently endless frantic crying, often at around the same times of the day or night. This crying regularly occurs after the evening feed, when you are most likely to be exhausted and when your anxiety and tension are most likely to be transmitted to the baby. In addition, vigorous crying often causes the baby to swallow air and this may lead to distention of the abdomen and the passage of wind from either end.

There is no reason to believe that the original cause of the crying is colic, or anything else connected with the bowels. If crying is due to insufficient feeding, the baby will not gain weight; if due to bowel upset there will be other signs, such as diarrhoea, fever and dehydration. In bottle-fed babies, milk intolerance may sometimes be the cause, and a change of brand may be worth trying. Sometimes the problem can be solved by deferring the evening feed.

Some babies are naturally hyperactive and these can often be calmed down by being firmly wrapped up in a small sheet. Powerful crying is never harmful to the baby, however severely it may affect the unfortunate parents, and the problem nearly always disappears by the age of 3 or 4 months.

Potty training

Feeding a baby sets off a reflex that starts things moving down the intestine. So the older material at the bottom end is liable to be ejected during or shortly after a feed. Trying to anticipate this event and getting a potty in place beforehand is not really a good idea. The baby doesn't like it and it could interfere with the bonding process.

Towards the end of the first year of life most babies can sit up quite stably. Many mothers feel that this is the time to start potty training. This is also a mistake. Babies of this age simply don't have the awareness to cooperate. Defecating without thought is natural to them and, up to the age of about 15 months, they will do it almost unconsciously, whatever else is going on. Sitting on a pot is uncomfortable and very boring and your baby will want to be doing something else. Whether or not you catch anything in the pot is a matter of pure chance. You are just wasting time and effort in taking off the nappy. And you are running the risk of setting up a revulsion for the potty in the baby's mind.

Around 18 months, most babies begin to become conscious of bowel and bladder function and it is time to let the infant know that there is a receptacle dedicated to the purpose. This introductory stage should precede the actual use of the pot. Tell your baby that a time will come when he or she will no longer need nappies, and everything that usually goes into the nappy will have to go into the pot.

It is a mistake actually to put the infant on the pot until he or she is able to indicate that a defaecation or urination are imminent. This indication is usually obvious. The child suddenly stands still, the face may redden and there may be self-clutching. In some cases there may even be a verbal indication. This is the time to suggest that the potty might be used. Never force the child to sit on the pot, but if the suggestion is accepted and the result satisfactory, say so, but try to avoid being too lavish in your praise. Your reaction will probably be heartfelt and genuine but it is best not to make a big deal out of this. Equally important is not to pass on any abhorrence you may have of faeces to your child. The faeces are the child's own possessions and, at this stage, he or she is not too well endowed with worldly goods. So don't spoil it.

Potty training can be heart-breaking and requires a good deal of patience. Just remember that nearly all infants are reliably clean and dry by the age of 3½.

So far as fear of CONSTIPATION is concerned, the first thing to appreciate is that it is not unusual for a baby's bowels to remain unopened for as long as a week. So long as the baby is otherwise well, there need be no cause for panic. Bottle-fed babies usually have firmer stools than breast-fed ones. Small children will sometimes deliberately prevent themselves from defaecating as a response to undue parental concern over potty training.

Such deliberate stool-holding by children really has nothing to do with constipation. The practice is very common in children aged between about 3 and 5. This is by no means always due to perversity. Very often the child is so interested in what he or she is doing that there is no question of taking time off to go to the toilet. In other cases, the child actually comes to enjoy holding back. This, unfortunately, usually causes parental distress and anxiety and the child may soon become aware that it has acquired another effective weapon in the power struggle. Another effective ploy is to stool-hold for long periods while sitting on the potty and then to defaecate in the clothes.

Determined stool-holding will, of course, lead to constipation. Water is absorbed from the faeces in the rectum and these become harder. Eventually this may lead to painful defaecation and the recollection of this will increase the child's tendency to stool-hold. In this way a vicious cycle can be set up. In such cases, a safe bulking laxative, such as Lactulose, may be needed. Try to avoid enemas in children.

Bathing

New babies have no sense of hygiene and will simply let everything go whenever this is necessary to their comfort. So every baby needs a great deal of cleaning up – at both ends – and should also have a bath or a complete overall wash every day. As an absolute minimum, you must keep baby's bottom, face and hands clean.

Many new mothers are very nervous at the thought of bathing their babies, but remember that a watery environment is more familiar to a new baby than a land-based one, so although you may be worried, baby is not. It is best to use a baby bath rather than a normal sized bath, but the latter is acceptable if the environment is warm and you are, as always, particularly careful about water temperature. It may be more convenient to use a suitable sink rather than a bath. If you do, however, remember the danger of baby kicking the taps and turning on the water. This could result in scalding.

When filling a bath always put cold water in first so as to avoid making the bottom of the bath too hot. Add hot water until the temperature is no more than 30°C (86°F). A depth of two inches is adequate. Test the temperature by the time-worn method of dipping in your elbow. It should feel neither obviously hot nor obviously cold. Some mothers use a thermometer. Always clean up the baby's bottom thoroughly with a corner of the nappy, followed by a baby lotion on cotton swabs, before putting the baby into the bath.

Support the baby's head and shoulders with one hand and forearm. Curl your fingers around the far shoulder and under the armpit. Put the other hand under the buttocks. You can now lower the baby into the bath while still controlling the position of the head and shoulders and keeping the face well above water level. You can now release the hand under the buttocks and allow the lower half of the body to be immersed in water. Use your free hand to wash the baby.

SAFETY AND FIRST AID
Safety measures

Accidents are a very important cause of death and long-term disability in children. Indeed, accidental and other injury is the leading cause of death in children aged between 1 and 14. Three children die every day in accidents in Britain, and each year some 1,250,000 children are seen in accident and emergency departments of British hospitals. That is one child in five.

You can avoid most accidents by exercising vigilance and imagination. You should constantly be aware of the risks, both in your home and in play areas. The home can be a dangerous place for the young; asphyxiation; poisoning; burns; electric shocks; wounds from broken glass panels; falls and even drowning can all occur.

CHOKING

During the first year of life, the commonest cause of accidental death is choking on an object accidentally inhaled into the larynx, the upper part of the wind pipe. This may be a lump of food, a small toy, or any other object small enough to pass over the tongue. Children automatically put things in their mouths, so dangerous objects should be kept out of reach. A sudden inhalation, perhaps during laughter, while something is in the mouth can lead to laryngeal obstruction and death. Every parent should be alive to this danger and do everything reasonable to avoid it. Parents should also be aware of the first aid treatment for choking (see **First Aid**). Tragically, death from smothering, by plastic bags, bedclothes or other material still occasionally occurs. The former practice of placing babies face down in their cots has now been abandoned. This is known to have been a cause of sudden death ('Cot Death') in many babies.

BURNS

Very small children should never be allowed access to electric outlets or equipment. Little fingers can penetrate non-shuttered electric sockets. Larger children must be made to understand the dangers. Most electric mains outlets are fitted with automatic internal shutters nowadays. If yours are still exposed, it is time you had them changed.

Babies and young children are very vulnerable in house fires, and often succumb to smoke asphyxiation or burns. In the USA, burns are the second most common cause of accidental death in children under 5 years. The first priority, in a fire, must always be to get the children outside. In anticipation of fires, smoke detector alarms are mandatory and have saved many lives. It is not enough to fit these, however; they should be regularly tested. Familiarity with possible escape routes is also important. Possible escape windows should not be painted tight shut so that they can readily be opened.

Burns in the home are common and can be very serious. Never leave a hot bath running in the presence of a toddler. Never leave a toddler unattended in a kitchen where food is cooking on open rings. Numerous severe burns have been caused by children pulling pans of boiling water or hot fat down on top of themselves.

Another often forgotten source of first degree burns is sunlight. Even in Britain, undue exposure of unprotected and untanned skin to the sun can produce quite severe burns. In sunnier countries the danger can be be even greater. Sunburn is more likely in children unaccustomed to exposure to bright sunlight and in those with fair skins. You should never allow a child's skin to turn red. Remember that this can occur after only 20 minutes' exposure. Unfortunately, the redness does not appear at once, so you have no direct way of knowing when the child has had enough. Reddening occurs after anything up to six hours. Carefully graduated exposure, for periods starting with no longer than 15 minutes a day and increasing progressively, but very gradually as the skin pigmentation builds up, can prevent sunburn.

There is evidence to suggest that sunburn sustained in early childhood can increase the risk of developing malignant MELANOMA later in life.

> **Preventing burns in children**
> - always turn pan handles away from the reach of children
> - avoid dangling electric kettle cables
> - keep cables short
> - never drink anything hot while you have a baby on your lap
> - use heavy, wide-bottomed mugs rather than cups
> - avoid tablecloths that a toddler can pull; use mats
> - fit effective guards round all electric and other heaters
> - when running baths, put in cold water first
> - keep matches out of reach of children
> - keep inflammable material away from children out of reach
>
> Burns are not only immediately dangerous; they can also lead to permanent disfigurement.

FALLS

Falls are a very important and common cause of injury to children. They lead to more than one child death every week, and 300,000 hospital visits. As children grow and acquire new abilities, it is in their nature to explore and to be adventurous. As soon as they are able, children, unless prevented, will climb. Recognize potential climbing sites, and try to anticipate and prevent dangerous climbing. Other factors to be borne in mind in trying to avoid falls include:

- quality of lighting over stairs and in hallways
- provision of stair gates and barriers, not only at the top of stairs but also at the bottom
- importance of safety catches on windows to prevent easy opening
- avoidance of unnecessary floor obstacles
- avoidance of polished floors and mats that can slip
- remembering that even small babies can roll off tables and other raised surfaces

DROWNING

Drowning is also a very common cause of death in the young. A high proportion of all deaths from fires and drowning occur in young children under 5. Drowning in the home is largely confined to small babies immersed in the bathtub. Babies can drown in just a few inches of water. In homes with swimming pools and even ornamental garden ponds, however, the risk to small children is, of course, much greater. Domestic swimming pools claim many victims. Most cases of drowning out of doors occur during swimming or play paddling, but may follow accidental falls into water, during boating, or when crossing bridges. Never be complacent about children who have not learned to swim; ensure that they have swimming lessons as soon as possible.

Remember that recovery from apparent drowning is possible after long periods of total immersion in very cold water, even under ice. This is because the vital metabolic processes of the body are greatly slowed by low temperatures. So every attempt should be made to resuscitate such children even if it seems impossible that they could have survived.

POISONING

Death from poisoning is less common in children than it is in adults and is almost always preventable. All poisons, especially corrosive poisons and medical products, must be kept out of reach of children. The pharmaceutical industry has cooperated in producing 'childproof' caps to tablet containers, but new EEC legislation will mean that most drugs prescribed as tablets will be dispensed as calendar packs in non-childproof containers. This means that extra care will have to be taken to lock away medicines.

Often, children show no immediate ill-effects from poisons they have taken. So, if this seems to be a possibility, the child concerned must be taken to a casualty department right away. If a child is strongly suspected of having taken a potentially dangerous substance within the previous four hours, it is usual for doctors to promote vomiting with the drug ipecacuanha. In the case of aspirin, opiates and tricyclic drugs, which slow the action of the stomach, ipecacuanha may usefully be given up to 12 hours after ingestion of the drug. You will find more about poisoning and poisons in the section on **First Aid** below.

TRAFFIC ACCIDENTS

Car accidents are still a very common cause of accidental death and severe injury in the young, but seat-belt legislation has gone a long way to reducing the carnage. Even more important is your responsibility, imagination and foresight when you are driving. Speeding and aggressive driving are dangerous at any time. Ensure that the children's car seats are safe, and properly fitted and secured, and that children are properly strapped in. Children are usually safer in the back seat, as long as they are properly secured. Adult seat-belts are useless for small children and may simply give you a false sense of their security.

Many children are killed or seriously injured while out of cars. Indeed, the majority of accidental deaths of children occur in pedestrians. In 1991 in England and Wales, 185 child pedestrians were killed and 3,965 were seriously injured in road accidents. The major risks are to children who live in environments with heavy traffic and high traffic speeds. Never assume that your young children are able to cross roads safely. Even children as old as 10 are unable reliably to judge the speed of oncoming traffic. If they have a strong motive to cross, they may do so at great risk to themselves. Remember that toddlers may suddenly pull away from you and step onto a busy road. This is especially dangerous if you are on crowded pavements in shopping areas and are forced to the outside. It is better to use child reins than to rely on hand-holding.

Child cyclists are also at great risk. Many motorists resent cyclists on the roads and some behave aggressively towards them. Children who have recently learned to cycle are particularly vulnerable and should never be allowed on roads. Most deaths in child cyclists involve head injuries. Properly fitted and effectively protective helmets should be worn by all cyclists.

Remember the dangers of your own immediate environment. Never reverse your car unless you are quite certain that your toddler is not in the vicinity.

First Aid

The general principles of first aid are much the same for children as for adults, but some methods have to be modified because of the size of the patient. The immediate assistance you can give to an injured child is often more important than expert medical care given later. In some cases it is only the person on the spot who can save a life or prevent serious long-term disability. If you have a few basic facts and a little vital knowledge on procedure, you can save a life rather than just stand around watching a child die.

You need to understand the priorities and how to act accordingly. There are only a few really essential points everyone should know. Apart from these, most of the detail contained in first aid manuals is unimportant and may even direct your attention away from what really matters. Most accidents occur in the home, and far more deaths and serious disability occur from home accidents than from car or other accidents away from home. So it is up to you to know what to do.

In all cases, get medical help as soon as possible, but if action is urgently needed to ensure breathing, this has priority. If necessary, send someone else to phone for an ambulance. Don't delay arranging to call an ambulance, however. Ambulance paramedics are highly trained and experienced in all measures necessary to save life in emergency, and they carry all the necessary equipment. They can:

- pass tracheal tubes to maintain an airway
- carry out cardiac compression
- perform defibrillation in cases of cardiac arrest
- start a transfusion when required

And they have the equipment and skills to control serious bleeding.

But until expert help arrives your own action may be critical. The priorities are: **airway**, **breathing** and **circulation**. Remember, ABC.

BREATHING STOPPED

The most immediate life-threatening situation is loss of the air supply. This is the first and most urgent requirement, so that the brain can get its oxygen supply. A child who cannot breathe for whatever reason, or whose airway is obstructed, is dying, and *everything else* is secondary to the critical requirement of restoring the supply of air. Brain damage from partial deprivation of air is usually more serious than any other kind of injury.

Obstruction to the airway can occur in many ways. In an unconscious child the tongue may fall back and block the air passage. Blood, vomited food, even collected saliva can block the airway. The child may have choked on a small toy or a large piece of food accidentally inhaled into the voice box in the neck (larynx). (see section on CHOKING). Whatever the cause, the situation is critical and the obstruction must be relieved at once.

Clear the mouth with your finger. Remove loose dentures and all foreign material. Mop out the mouth with a handkerchief. Bend the head as far back as possible and push the lower jaw upwards until the teeth are clenched. Check for breathing. If this is occurring, and the child is unconscious, maintain the position of the head. If there is no breathing, start mouth-to-mouth respiration.

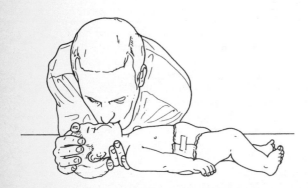

Mouth-to-mouth artificial respiration

You can perform the 'kiss of life' (mouth-to-mouth respiration) on your own, but it is easier if there are two or more people present. Turn the child on to his or her back on the floor or ground and ensure that the airway is cleared (see above). In an unconscious child the tongue will often have fallen back to obstruct the airway and this must be overcome by tilting the head backwards and pulling the chin forward and up. If there is any possibility of a broken neck, don't do this. With the head kept in the extended position by one hand under the chin, use your other hand to pinch the nose. In a very small child this is unnecessary, as you can easily get your mouth over both the nose and mouth of the child. With a larger child, apply your wide open lips to the mouth of the child, making a good seal around the mouth. Now blow in hard and regularly, at first as quickly as possible, then at a rate of 16 to 20 blows a minute.

If you do this properly, the child's chest will rise well with each blow, and between blows the air will come out. It is essential to check that this is happening. You will do no good at all unless you are actually blowing up the lungs like a balloon; you will be able to see that this is happening. Forget what you may have seen on TV. They never get it right. If there are no chest movements there may be obstruction in the larynx. See section on CHOKING below. Keep this up for at least an hour, or until the child breathes spontaneously.

HEART STOPPED (CARDIAC ARREST)

Oxygen to the brain is literally vital and this implies that the blood, which carries the oxygen, is circulating. If the heart has stopped beating (cardiac arrest), the blood has stopped circulating, so the heart must be started again, or must be squeezed repeatedly so that the blood is circulated. If nothing is done the child will die. A knowledge of cardio-pulmonary resuscitation will save life in such a case and may restore a child to normal. Out of hospital, there is *never* time to summon medical assistance.

Cardiac arrest does not necessarily mean that the heart has stopped contracting completely. The heart may be stopped or it may be in a state of rapid, ineffectual twitching, called ventricular fibrillation. In either case, no pumping action is occurring and, unless something is done within three or four minutes, death is inevitable from failure of the oxygen and sugar supply to reach the child's brain.

> Within seconds of a cardiac arrest, consciousness is lost, the breathing becomes rapid and shallow and soon stops. No pulse can be felt and no heart sounds heard. Within minutes, the pupils of the eyes become very wide (dilated), and the skin turns bluish (cyanosis). To save the child's life, immediate artificial respiration and cardiac massage are needed (cardio-pulmonary resuscitation).

This is what you should do:

1 If there is someone else around, send them to call an ambulance or get medical help.
2 Check if the child is conscious. If so, the heart has not stopped.
3 Check for breathing. Tilt the head back by pushing the chin upwards and lift the jaw forward. Put your ear close to the child's mouth and watch the chest for breathing movement. If you hear or feel the breath or see the chest moving, the heart has not stopped.
4 Get the child flat on his or her back on the floor.
5 Clear the mouth and throat with your finger. Make sure there is no obstruction and that the tongue is well forward.
6 If there is no breathing, pinch the child's nostrils closed with your fingers, seal your mouth tightly around the mouth, and blow until the child's chest rises well. With a small child, seal your mouth around both mouth and nose and blow into both. Remove

your mouth and listen for the air coming out again. Repeat this steadily, using full breaths and allowing the child's lungs to deflate completely between each breath.

7 Do this five times and feel for a pulse in the child's neck, along the side of the Adam's apple. If there is a pulse, carry on with mouth-to-mouth respiration, at a rate of 16 to 20 blows a minute, until the child breathes spontaneously.

8 If there is no pulse, place the heel of one hand over the lower part of the breast-bone two finger-breadths above the angle of the ribs. Use one hand only. Keep your arm straight and use the weight of your body to press down firmly so that the child's heart is compressed about 3 cm (1 in) between the breast bone and the backbone. Little force is needed. In a very small child or infant, do the compression with two fingers only. Do this, evenly and smoothly, five times in 10 seconds, and then give two full mouth-to-mouth ventilations. Continue alternating cardiac compression with respiration in this way until the child's heart starts, or help arrives. If you have someone to help you, one of you should perform the cardiac compression and the other the mouth-to-mouth respiration.

CHOKING

Anyone present at the time choking occurs is hardly likely to be unaware of what has happened. The affected child is obviously distressed, turns blue and often clutches his or her throat. A choking child cannot speak.

Very small children are best turned upside down and patted firmly on the back. Give this a short trial but do not waste too much time. If this fails or if the child is too big to be easily inverted, the recommended first aid in choking is the abdominal thrust. This is also called the Heimlich manoeuvre. It aims to dislodge the obstruction from the larynx by a sudden increase in the pressure of the air in the upper air tubes below the obstruction, so that it is forced up and out. Conscious children can sometimes do this for themselves by forceful coughing or by sudden inward and upward compression of the upper abdomen in the 'V' below the ribs.

Stand behind the child and put your arms around him or her, just above the waist. Make a fist with one hand and grasp it with the other. Position the hands, with the thumb pressing inward, just below the point of the 'V' of the ribs. Give a powerful, sudden, upward thrust or hug. Repeat, as necessary. If the child is unconscious and lying on the ground, turn him on his back and give double-handed thrusts from the front. If breathing stops, begin mouth-to-mouth artificial respiration (see above).

Remember that a child in this situation is dying. Details like bruised or torn muscles are of no concern by comparison with the over-riding necessity to restore an open airway.

UNCONSCIOUSNESS AND THE RECOVERY POSITION

An unconscious but breathing child may vomit and obstruct his or her airway. The tongue may fall back and do the same. To prevent obstruction, the child should be placed in the recovery position while you wait for help to arrive. The recovery position keeps the child still, makes the jaw and tongue fall forward so that breathing is free, and allows vomit or secretions to drain easily from the mouth.

The unconscious child should be turned face down, head turned to one side, and one leg bent to prevent rolling. Check at frequent intervals that breathing is continuing. If breathing stops, turn the child over and start mouth-to-mouth respiration (see above).

NOTE: If the injury was such that a fracture of the spine is probable, in turning the child, you risk further damaging the spinal cord, causing permanent paralysis or even death. In such a case, any movement, except under the supervision of a skilled and knowledgeable person, is dangerous.

BLEEDING

After ensuring an air supply and a circulation, the next priority is the control of severe bleeding. This, too, is largely in the interests of a continued supply of oxygen to the child's

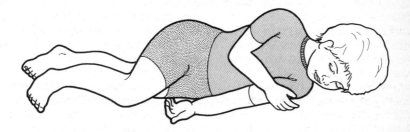

The recovery position.

brain. If there is not enough blood, insufficient oxygen will be carried to the brain. External bleeding is easily controlled. Internal bleeding requires surgical intervention, so it is imperative to get the injured child to hospital immediately.

The first aid management of obvious external bleeding is easy. Apply direct pressure to the bleeding area and maintain it. Use your hand until you have time to think. Look for something with which to make a pad. Apply it firmly and fix it in place, using an encircling tie. Try to elevate the bleeding part and to keep it at rest, so that a clot can form. Make sure you can see what is happening and that continued bleeding is not just seeping into the child's clothes. Direct pressure, properly maintained, will stop almost any bleeding. Forget about pressure points and *never* use tourniquets. These can lead to gangrene.

SHOCK

Severe injury often leads to a dangerous condition in which the blood, instead of circulating normally through tight arteries and veins, forms useless pools or depots in widely dilated vessels in the skin, digestive system and legs. This is called surgical shock and it has nothing to do with fright. Shock is another way in which the brain can be deprived of oxygen, and the prevention of shock is the third priority.

Prevention of shock is simple. It is essential for the child to make the fullest use of the blood available and this must not be wasted by flushing the skin or filling the legs. So, do not pile up the injured child with blankets. Shivering and complaints of cold do not matter. Use one blanket only. Elevate the legs, if possible, to improve the blood return to the child's heart and brain. A child in surgical shock desperately needs more fluid in the circulation and a drip, even of saline solution, can be life-saving. Ambulance paramedics can give this.

Do not give the child anything by mouth, unless the injury is limited to minor burns.

NEAR-DROWNING

Near-drowning is another important cause of oxygen deprivation and, again, urgency is of the essence. Mouth-to-mouth artificial respiration must be started at once (see above) even before the child is out of the water, if this is possible. If the abdomen is distended with water, the child should be placed face down and then lifted with the hands under the midriff. Clear the airway, check for breathing and pulse. If no pulse is felt, begin cardiopulmonary resuscitation (see HEART STOPPED, above). Survival is possible after long periods of immersion in cold water because the lowered temperature reduces the body's requirements for oxygen and brain fuel.

POISONING

There is no first aid for poisoning, unless the child is unconscious. In this case put him or her in the recovery position (see above) and get to hospital, together with all available evidence of the type of poisoning – empty bottles, samples of vomit, tablets, plants or berries – as soon as possible. Do not make the child vomit. Do not give anything by mouth. Just get him or her to hospital by any means, with the minimum delay. Inform the ambulance people that it is a poisoning case and state whether or not the child is conscious. If going by car, get someone to telephone the hospital casualty department and warn them.

About poisons

Children are particularly susceptible to poisons and in some cases can be killed by a dose that would not seriously harm an adult. The matter of dosage is important because most substances, even some of those taken as nutrients, are poisons if taken in sufficient amount. Almost all drugs are poisonous if taken in excess, but are safe if taken in correct dosage under medical supervision. Normal adult doses may be poisonous to children.

It is impossible to list all the poisonous substances with which one might come in contact. Some substances, however, are commonly accessible to children and are particularly toxic and dangerous.

Poisons in the home:

- ammonia
- liquid bleach
- toilet bowl cleaning powder or liquid
- fungus-killing liquids
- oven-cleaning liquids and sprays
- corrosive agents, such as acids, alkalis, bleaches and disinfectants.
- rust removers
- paint-strippers
- spot removers, especially if inhaled
- sterilizing fluids such as phenols or Cresol
- various liquid glues, if inhaled
- coumarin and warfarin rat and mouse poisons
- methylated spirits
- rubbing alcohol
- antifreeze
- drugs (see below)

Poisons in the garden and countryside:
- organophosphate weedkillers, such as Paraquat
- insecticides, such as Parathion and Malathion
- laburnum berries
- yew leaves and bark
- deadly nightshade
- common inkcap mushroom
- deathcap mushroom
- 'magic' mushrooms, such as *Psilocybe* and *Amanita* species
- fly agaric mushroom

DRUG OVERDOSE

Prescription drugs are often dangerous to children. If a child is suspected of having taken a drug, whether normally used for medication or otherwise, there are often some characteristic indications of what they may have taken.

Features of poisoning with drugs

Drowsiness – narcotics, sedatives, sleeping pills, aspirin, tricyclic depression tablets, atropine, diphenoxylate, alcohol

Excitement or confusion – asthma drugs especially salbutamol, antihistamines, amphetamines, cocaine, alcohol, solvent inhalation

Convulsions – amphetamines, tricyclic drugs, asthma drugs especially theophylline, lithium, alcohol

Irregular pulse – amphetamines, tricyclic drugs, theophylline, salbutamol, potassium, digoxin, beta-blocker drugs

Vomiting blood – iron tablets, aspirin and other salicylates

Wide pupils – atropine, diphenoxylate, tricyclic drugs

Pinpoint pupils – opiate narcotics

Here are some details of the drugs that commonly poison children. Check the labels to identify the drug:

Tricyclic antidepressants (Tofranil, Tryptizol, etc). These are very poisonous to children and are the commonest cause of death in childhood poisoning. Symptoms start within four hours, and include dry mouth, wide pupils, inability to urinate, hallucinations, twitching and loss of consciousness.

Paracetamol (Panaleve, Calpol, etc., etc). Overdose is very dangerous especially in adolescents. Those who take more than 20 tablets are in danger of developing fatal liver damage unless treated quickly. Younger children are more resistant but always need treatment. The early symptoms are fairly mild – no more than nausea and vomiting. The danger is in what happens to the liver after 36 hours.

Benzodiazepines (Valium, Librium, etc). These are safer than many other drugs but can seriously depress the nervous system in a child. Symptoms are staggering, dizziness, drowsiness and shallow breathing.

Beta blockers (Sectral, Visken, Angilol, etc). These produce a very slow pulse, collapse, drowsiness, delirium, seizures and cardiac arrest.

Digoxin (Lanoxin). This heart drug causes nausea, vomiting, diarrhoea, complaint of yellow vision and a slow, irregular pulse.

Iron (Ferrocap, Ferromyn). Iron salts are very poisonous to children and may cause severe bleeding from the stomach and shock. Early symptoms are stomach pain, nausea, vomiting, diarrhoea and rapid pulse. The stools soon become blackened.

Lithium (Camcolit, Priadel). This antipsychotic drug causes nausea, vomiting, apathy, tremor, muscle twitching and convulsions in children.

Non-steroidal anti-inflammatory drugs (NSAIDs) (Brufen, Ebufac). In overdosage, these painkilling and anti-inflammatory drugs can cause nausea, vomiting, abdominal pain, headache, rapid breathing, disorientation, jerking eyes, seizures, drowsiness, coma and cardiac arrest.

Salicylates (Aspirin). Poisoning with salicylates has become less common since aspirin was banned from child medicine. Children, however, are very susceptible to salicylates and can be poisoned by a dose only moderately higher than the normal dose. Symptoms include deafness, complaint of ringing in the ears and of blurring of vision, profuse sweating, convulsions, coma and cardiac arrest.

Children should, of course, never have access to 'recreational' drugs. They are extremely sensitive to any of these and a small dose may have a marked effect. Some of these effects are as follows:

- heroin and morphine – vomiting, depressed breathing, pinpoint pupils
- cocaine (Crack) – excitement, euphoria, restlessness, trembling, wide pupils, fast pulse, overbreathing, cardiac arrest
- amphetamines (Benzedrine, Dexedrine) – jumpiness, excitement, confusion, aggression, indications of hallucinations
- barbiturates (Amytal, Luminal, Seconal) – drowsiness, coma, a drop in body temperature, slow and shallow breathing

See also SOLVENT ABUSE.

POISONOUS ANIMALS
A few animals, insects and marine creatures produce toxins harmful to humans and especially to children in the doses normally acquired. These include:

- venomous snakes
- sea snakes
- ciguatera (an alga eaten by fish in the Pacific and Caribbean)
- certain shellfish contaminated by toxic protozoa
- puffer fish
- sting rays
- scorpion fish
- cone shell molluscs
- jelly-fish
- land scorpions
- centipedes
- a few tropical spiders

Children who have been affected by any of these should always be seen by a doctor without delay.

BURNS
Put the fire out and cool the burned area as quickly as possible. Heat destroys tissue and immediate cooling is the only measure that can help. So get the affected part under the cold tap and keep it there. Chemical burns need prolonged washing. You cannot overdo this.
Don't burst blisters. Don't apply any medication, grease, oil or anything else to a severe

burn. Burns rapidly lead to loss of fluid from the blood, especially in children and this has to be replaced. A moderately burned *conscious* child is the only kind of casualty who should be given plenty of fluids by mouth.

HEAT CRAMPS
These are due to abnormal loss of salt from excessive sweating and inadequate replacement. They usually occur after strenuous exercise in conditions of high ambient temperature. The onset is often sudden and incapacitating with hard spasm of the leg, arm or abdominal muscles. Heat cramps are usually rapidly relieved by drinking plenty of fluid containing a little salt. Prevention is easy, if the danger is understood and a good fluid and salt intake ensured.

HEAT EXHAUSTION
This is not particularly common in children, but is more serious if it does occur. It is simply due to excessive loss of water from the body, so that there is insufficient fluid to maintain the circulation. It is a form of shock and the signs are similar to those of severe blood loss. There is:

- weakness
- fatigue
- collapse
- pale clammy skin
- very weak but rapid pulse
- abnormally low blood pressure
- sometimes unconsciousness

The temperature is usually below normal.

Heat exhaustion occurs when fluid loss from sweating substantially exceeds the intake. The treatment of heat exhaustion is urgent replacement of fluid, by mouth, if possible, or by intravenous infusion if the child is in coma.

HEAT STROKE
Heat hyperpyrexia, or heat stroke, is the most dangerous of all the heat disorders. Fortunately, it is rare in children. It occurs when the temperature-regulating centres are unable to cope with excessive heat production, as may occur from excessive exertion in very hot conditions, or when, as a result of disease or other causes, they fail altogether to control the temperature of the body. The temperature rises rapidly and the situation quickly becomes critical. Initially, there may be warning indications in the form of faintness, dizziness, headache, dry skin, absence of sweating, thirst and nausea. Later there may be lethargy and confusion, or agitation progressing to epileptic-like fits, coma and death.

This is a medical emergency. The rising temperature causes brain damage which worsens with duration and level and, if the child survives, this damage is often irreversible. A rectal temperature of 41° C (106° F) is a sign of grave danger.

The treatment is to get the temperature down by any available means. The whole body should be immersed in cold water, and ice-packs and fans used to supplement the cooling. The temperature must be monitored continuously and not allowed to drop below 38° C (101° F) as excess cooling may convert hyperthermia to hypothermia.

ELECTRIC SHOCK
Electric shock injuries are made worse by continuing flow of current. Switch off, if possible. Do not touch the child until current is off or contact broken. Move the child from the current source with a wooden chair, a dry cloth or a plastic garment. Start mouth-to-mouth artificial respiration if breathing has stopped. If the child is breathing place in the recovery position (see above).

CORROSIVES IN THE EYES

Although there is no danger to life, this does call for urgent action if damage to the child's vision is to be avoided. The accidental contamination of the eyes with corrosive chemicals, such as lime or other alkalis, strong acids or even dishwasher machine detergent, calls for *immediate*, vigorous, and prolonged washing with a large quantity of water, so that the chemical can be diluted and washed off before it has time to cause permanent damage to the transparency of the corneas (front lens).

You may have to be a little rough with the child to do real good. Ideally, tap-water should be run on to the open eye or eyes, or a hand-shower directed on to them, for a minimum of 10 minutes, preferably longer. The longer the interval between the accident and the start of the wash, the longer you should continue the washing. Hold the child bodily under a tap and ensure that the lids are kept wide open. You will have to hold them open. Turn the head so that the water does not run from the contaminated eye into the other eye. You cannot damage the eye by pouring water on it; if there has been contact with a corrosive, especially alkaline, substance, you can do much harm by not doing so. If water is not available, any bland fluid, including urine, should be used.

FOREIGN BODY IN EYE

This is a common hazard, especially if the child is watching you working with a high-speed tool or grindstone. You should never allow this without eye protection. The danger depends largely on the velocity with which the foreign body strikes the eye. A penetrating foreign body must always be suspected if the eye was struck while the child was watching any activity which could produce high-speed missiles. Especially dangerous are grinding, turning, milling and hammering metal. The cold chisel with the mushroomed head is a prolific cause of serious eye injury. X-ray examination is mandatory in all such cases, for a retained metallic intra-ocular foreign body will usually do serious harm to the eye – often after many months.

Most foreign bodies do not penetrate the eye, but lodge on the membrane covering the white of the eye (the conjunctiva), or behind the lids. Foreign bodies on the transparent front lens (the cornea) cause exquisite pain and intense awareness and induce an uncontrollable tendency to squeeze the lids – an activity that increases the pain. Unless sharp and on the centre of the cornea, however, superficial foreign bodies are unlikely to do much harm. A child who has suffered this misfortune is likely to be almost unmanageable and you should get him or her to a hospital as soon as possible where local anaesthetic drops can be used to abolish the pain and allow examination.

A foreign body behind the upper lid may sometimes be dislodged by grasping the lashes and pulling the upper lid down over the lower lid so that the lower lashes can brush it off. Eversion of the upper lid, to examine its underside, may be very easy or very difficult, depending on whether or not the affected child trusts you. A cotton bud, or even a match stick, will help. Get the child to look *down*, pull the upper lid lashes downward, press the tip of the bud against the skin, 1 cm above the lid margin, and pull on the lashes, outwards and then upwards. The whole thing can be done quite gently and painlessly so long as the child refrains from squeezing the lids and continues to look down.

Superficial foreign bodies may safely be removed from the conjunctiva using a piece of paper folded to a point. Attempts to remove foreign bodies on the cornea may cause further damage and if the foreign body is central, permanent visual loss may result. A wash with an eyebath may occasionally be successful, but attention by an ophthalmologist (eye specialist) will usually be necessary.

FRACTURES

Broken bones call for immobilisation. Unnecessary movement may cause increased loss of blood and may precipitate surgical shock. Effective emergency splints always need to be longer than might be expected. The principle is that to immobilise a fracture, the joint above and below the fracture must be prevented from moving. Almost any firm, elongated object may be used as a splint. Plenty of padding, of any kind, is needed and splints must be securely tied in place. It is often helpful, in leg fractures, to tie the legs together. Arms may be tied to the side for upper arm fractures. A sling is usually sufficient support for a lower arm fracture. Children need great reassurance and very gentle handling. In many cases it may be better to wait for the ambulance crew than to attempt any emergency splinting.

NOSE BLEEDS

These are very common in children and usually result from minor injury, such as nose-picking, or a blow to the nose. Very occasionally a nose bleed may be serious. This is rare in children. A nose bleed can almost always be controlled by pinching the nostrils firmly together for five minutes and persuading the child to breathe through his or her mouth. Pressure maintained for this length of time will allow the blood to clot, and the bleeding is unlikely to recur unless the site is disturbed. Failure to control bleeding by this method may call for medical attention – the doctor may cauterize the bleeding area by touching it with a tiny wool swab moistened with a corrosive chemical, or the nose may be firmly packed with ribbon gauze.

Bleeding in children, arising from persistent crusting of the insides of the nostrils, is best treated by the use of a softening ointment, such as petroleum jelly.

See also BITES AND STINGS.

HOW TO RECOGNIZE SERIOUS ILLNESS

This is one of the commonest worries for parents, anxious not to trouble doctors unnecessarily. Unfortunately, it can often be difficult, even for the expert, to distinguish the early stages of a serious illness from one of the common minor disorders of childhood. The situation is further complicated by the fact that particularly severe forms of normally harmless common diseases may sometimes be dangerous.

There are, however, some useful indications. Seriously ill children remain quiet. Loud crying or screaming is seldom, if ever, a feature of serious illness. When seriously ill, the child must harness all his or her resources to combat the problem and this means lying still, and not wasting energy in crying.

Certain symptoms, although not necessarily indicating serious illness, must always be taken seriously. These include:

- breathing difficulty
- the onset of blueness of the skin
- very high fever
- unrousable coma
- uncharacteristic and inappropriate drowsiness
- any alteration in the state of consciousness
- any interference with easy breathing
- weak or inadequate breathing efforts
- any obstruction to breathing
- convulsions
- irregularity of the pulse
- weak, thready and rapid pulse after bleeding, severe vomiting or diarrhoea
- sudden projectile vomiting for no apparent reason, especially if associated with headache
- persistent vomiting
- persistent diarrhoea in small children
- a visible writhing movement in the abdomen

As always, the most urgent and critical signs are those of airway obstruction or difficulty in breathing. Parents of children with asthma will know what to do about this, but any

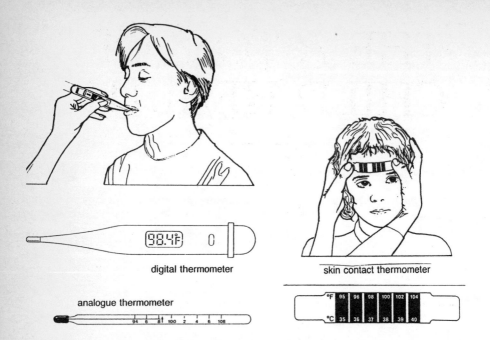

digital thermometer   skin contact thermometer

analogue thermometer

Various types of thermometer are used to measure temperature, involving colour changes, digital readouts or simple analogue mercury expansion.

indication of oxygen lack from any cause – especially blueness around the mouth – is an indication of an acute emergency, calling for immediate hospital attention.

Ill children often seem to take longer than usual to wake up and readily become drowsy. They do not show the usual degree of alertness and are often irritable and uninterested in toys and in socializing. They will often fail to maintain eye contact or smile in circumstances in which they would normally do so.

Many parents worry that symptoms, such as fastidiousness in diet, loss of appetite, INFANTILE COLIC and SKIN PALLOR imply serious illness. Such concern is nearly always unjustified. The golden rule, however, is always – if in doubt, call the doctor.

THE A TO Z OF CHILD HEALTH

—

A

Absence attacks

These are short periods of loss of consciousness or awareness that occur in the mild form of EPILEPSY known as 'petit mal'. Absence attacks are fairly common in children and adolescents, but rare in adults. The attacks last for two to 10 seconds and are often unobserved by the sufferer. They may be mistaken, by an observer, for moments of inattention or absentmindedness, but there is, for the child concerned, a complete interruption of consciousness. The child remains motionless, stares, stops talking, ceases to respond, and is, for the duration of the attack, inaccessible.

Sometimes absence attacks feature small, jerky contractions of the muscles of the eyelids, face or fingers at a rate of about three per second. If the brain waves are being recorded on an electroencephalograph (ECG) when an attack occurs, the associated abnormality of brain electrical activity shows up prominently on the tracings. There may be lip-smacking or chewing movements, especially if the attack is brought on by voluntary over-breathing (hyperventilation). In an absence attack, the affected child does not usually fall and may even continue to walk or ride a bicycle.

As many as 100 attacks may occur in a day and the total loss of time and educational input may be serious. By causing gaps in consciousness, these attacks also derange thinking and this, too, can affect educational performance, especially if you do not suspect epilepsy. It is particularly hard on a child to be blamed for daydreaming or lack of concentration when, in fact, he or she has actually been repeatedly shut off from everything that is going on. Attacks tend to diminish in frequency towards adolescence and may disappear. Unfortunately, petit mal can progress to major epilepsy (grand mal).

Try to manage absence attacks by:

- attempting to eliminate anything you notice brings on an attack.
- ensuring regular sleep, a good balanced diet and a physically active life.
- promoting healthy family attitudes and avoiding over-solicitude and over-protection.

The drugs ethosuximide (Zarontin) and acetazolamide (Diamox) can greatly reduce the tendency to attacks. In many cases, absence attacks are of no significance but they should always be reported as they may lead to more serious forms of epilepsy, and treatment may be necessary.

Absent testicle see
CRYPTORCHIDISM

Accidents see introductory section (Safety and First Aid).

Achondroplasia

This is a form of dwarfism, present from birth and caused by a rare, dominant genetic disorder of bone growth (see GENETICS – AN OUTLINE). Achondroplasia affects about one child in 30,000. The shortness of stature is mainly due to a failure of full development of the long bones of the arms and legs. Normally, the long bones grow at special cartilage zones near each end of the bone. In achondroplasia, these growing areas are converted to bone too early, so further limb growth ceases. The other bones grow normally.

Affected children have well-developed bodies and heads of normal size except for protruding foreheads, but short, strong limbs. They also have:

- bowing of the arms and legs
- shorter upper arms and thighs than forearms and lower legs
- a waddling gait
- short, stubby fingers of nearly equal length
- a small face
- a depressed bridge of the nose
- marked forward curvature of the lower spine (lumbar lordosis)
- limitation of movement in the major joints

Intelligence and sexual development are unaffected, and the expectation of life is normal. The gene for achondroplasia is dominant, so the children of achondroplastics have a 50–50 chance of inheriting the defective gene and developing the disorder. Surprisingly, the parents of most achondroplastics are normal, so the condition must often arise as a mutation of a normal gene. Unfortunately, there is no treatment. Achondroplasia cannot yet be diagnosed before birth. It is usually apparent within the first year of life from the disproportion between the length of the limbs and the size of the head.

Surgical advances have made it possible for legs to be lengthened, thereby making life easier for those with achondroplasia to live in a world designed for taller people.

Acne

Acne is, of course, most common in adolescence and early adult life, but it can also occur in infancy. Most of the very young children who develop infantile acne are boys; such cases are often mild and soon pass. In other cases, however, the child is less fortunate: a severe and very persistent form, with nodules and cysts, develops. The features are similar to those of adolescent acne (see below). One of the principal drugs used to treat acne in older people is the antibiotic tetracycline. This must *never* be given to children under 12 as it becomes incorporated into the growing permanent teeth and produces life-long staining.

Adolescent acne causes great distress and unhappiness to young people and, indeed is often severe and disfiguring enough to justify this distress. It is a disorder of the oil-secreting (sebaceous) glands of the skin in which there is excess production of their secretion (sebum) and obstruction of the outlets of the glands, resulting in accumulation of sebum under the skin surface. Blackheads are not the cause of the obstruction; blackhead formation is believed to be a consequence of the sluggish flow of thickened sebum.

Technically known as comedones, blackheads are bodies composed of compressed sebum, produced excessively in acne. They occur when excess sebum cannot escape on to the surface of the skin and accumulates in the ducts of the sebaceous glands. The darkened outer part of the blackhead is caused by chemical changes in the exposed sebum, and has nothing to do with any lack of cleanliness.

Other chemical changes, caused by certain resident bacteria, break down the neutral fat in the blackheads, releasing fatty acids which are very irritant to the surrounding tissue. This is the main cause of the inflammation which so commonly surrounds blackheads, especially when the sebaceous gland is ruptured by squeezing. The rupture of blackhead contents into the surrounding skin causes spots and sometimes even small abscesses called pustules. Most acne spots are not infected, but some may become so, and pustules form. Pustular acne can lead to severe permanent scarring, but, given expert medical care, this need never happen.

The cause of the excess production of sebaceous material is still a matter of debate. The sebaceous glands are under the control of the sex hormones: the male hormone, testosterone, stimulates the glands and the female hormone, oestrogen, damps them down. Most acne sufferers do not have raised male sex hormone levels, but this is sometimes the case in girls with severe acne. Acne is most common at and after puberty with the flare-up of hormone activity, and reaches its peak in the late teens. It does, however, often persist into the 20s or even, occasionally, 30s. It mainly affects the face, shoulders, back of the neck and upper trunk. Acne is not caused by eating sweets and rich, fatty foods, but these are best avoided for other reasons.

Affected areas should be washed with ordinary soap and water, but not more than twice a day. On the whole it is better not to squeeze blackheads, but many young people are so self-conscious about them that they will do this whatever advice is given them. Unless they are very large indeed, they will not produce permanently enlarged pores. But if cosmetic considerations demand the removal of blackheads, this should be done with great care, using a proper clean instrument that applies even pressure all round the darkened head.

Courses of ultraviolet light under medical supervision, or controlled and graduated sunbathing, are helpful. Antibiotic ointments are often prescribed and are useful in infected cases, or to prevent infection. Many other preparations, such as ointments containing benzoyl peroxide or sulphur, are recommended by dermatologists. In severe cases, a doctor may prescribe tetracycline, to be taken by mouth, over a period of several months. This can work very well, but the drug should never be taken during pregnancy, as it will affect the baby. If these measures fail, the doctor will consider giving a female sex hormcne combined with an anti-male sex hormone known as cyproterone acetate. This preparation, marketed as Dianette, is effective in controlling severe acne in girls who also require contraception.

Probably the most effective remedy of all for adolescent acne is the drug tretinoin (Retin-A), a vitamin A derivative used externally as a cream or gel or, under specialist supervision, taken internally in the form of isotretinoin (Roaccutane). This drug can cause fetal abnormalities if taken during pregnancy. Girls using it must be on a reliable contraceptive. Most acne is treated by GPs who can prescribe the whole range of therapies except isotretinoin. It is the exception rather than the rule for cases to have to be referred to a hospital specialist.

Adenoids

Adenoids are swellings on the wall of the back of the nose above the tonsils. They contain masses of immune system white cells (lymphocytes) that help to combat infections. In doing so, they enlarge and this may cause complications. Most children's adenoids shrivel away after the age of about 5/6 yrs, and it is uncommon for them still to be present at puberty.

Trouble starts if adenoids get so big that they obstruct the movement of air from the nose to the throat. This causes, or can cause:

- mouth breathing
- an open, dry mouth
- a nasal quality to the voice
- snoring
- recurrent sore throat
- chest infections
- sinusitis

Enlarged adenoids can block the openings of the eustachian tubes which connect the nose to the middle ear. This can cause deafness and, by preventing drainage of secretions from the middle ear, encourage middle ear infection – OTITIS MEDIA. The child may require ANTIBIOTICS or even a minor surgical operation to drain pus from the middle ear.

Adenoids can be diagnosed from the patient's medical history and by direct examination. The operation to remove adenoids is called ADENOIDECTOMY.

Adenoidectomy

This is the operation to remove ADENOIDS which are large enough to cause troublesome effects. Adenoidectomy is often done at the same time as removal of the tonsils (TONSILLECTOMY).

The operation is performed under general anaesthesia. An instrument with a sharp edge, called a curette, is passed in through the open mouth and up behind the soft palate into the space at the back of the nose. The sharp edge is then pressed against the back wall of the nose to cut off the adenoids with a scraping action. Bleeding is usually slight and soon stops on pressure with a gauze swab. Brisk bleeding is controlled by packing the nose. Adenoidectomy takes only a few minutes and can save a child considerable risk to health. There is little or no postoperative pain and, if the operation has been done along with tonsillectomy, any discomfort will be submerged in the temporary throat pain experienced as the tonsillectomy sites heal.

Adolescence see introductory section (Puberty and Adolescence)

AIDS

HIV, the virus that causes AIDS can be transmitted to babies before they are born, by passage through the placenta. The infection can also be acquired from the vagina during birth. This is not inevitable, however. The reported figures for the proportion of children born to HIV positive mothers who become infected by the virus vary widely. In Europe as a whole, the figure is said to be about 14 per cent; in New York 29 per cent; in Kenya, the infection rate is said to be about 45 per cent. These figures must be accepted with caution, but it is clear that a substantial proportion of children born to HIV positive mothers do not become infected with the human immunodeficiency virus (HIV) or develop AIDS.

The question of whether HIV is readily transmitted by breast feeding remains open and has caused a good deal of argument among the experts. Research has shown that HIV-infected cells are present in the milk of over 95 per cent of HIV positive mothers. At the same time, antibodies against HIV are also present in breast milk, and breast milk is well known to afford protection against a wide range of infections. In the case of women who were HIV positive during their pregnancy, and whose babies become HIV positive, those who are breast-fed take longer to develop AIDS than those who are bottle-fed. It seems, also, that women whose milk contains large quantities of the antibody IgM are less likely to transmit the virus to their babies. IgM is concerned mainly with the breakdown of foreign cells and with the preparation of foreign material for destruction by the immune system cells. It is particularly effective in dealing with viruses.

There have been cases in which it is known that the mother was infected (mainly by a blood transfusion) *after* the child was born. The limited data available suggest that in these cases the risk of infection of the baby from the breast milk is about 30 per cent. The advice of the World Health Organization is that HIV-infected women should not breast-feed if a safe alternative exists. In the Western world, there is always a safe alternative.

A report in the *Lancet* in 1994 showed that of 624 children infected with HIV-1 at the time of birth, 60 per cent reached their 10th birthday. One hundred and thirty (19 per cent) died of AIDS before they were 5. One hundred and eighty-two children who lived longer than five years were studied. Of these, 28 (15 per cent) were entirely free of symptoms and 154 had symptoms. A third of those with symptoms were very mildly affected. Only about 30 per cent of these long-term survivors had symptoms severe enough to warrant a diagnosis of AIDS.

In all the cases, bad signs, which tended to predict a poorer chance of survival were:

- failure of normal growth
- ANAEMIA
- FEVER
- DIARRHOEA
- frequent infections
- heart problems
- HEPATITIS
- neurological problems

Even these indications, however, did not necessarily prevent survival after five years. Interestingly, children who developed enlarged lymph nodes and a mumps-like enlargement of the salivary glands (parotitis) were more likely to be in the long-term survival group. This suggested that they suffering from a less severe form of the infection.

Fully-developed AIDS in young babies may be more rapid and aggressive than in adults. If this occurs within the first six months, the outlook is very poor and the chances of surviving for two years are small. Treatment with immunoglobulin can help to prolong life. The first indications are usually failure to thrive, followed by the development of many infections, especially severe thrush of the mouth. There may be enlargement of the liver, spleen and the lymph nodes, persistent diarrhoea and recurrent attacks of pneumonia. Kaposi's sarcoma, a form of skin cancer common among adults with AIDS, rarely occurs in young children.

> It is very important that older children should be well informed about AIDS. Since September 1992, information about AIDS and HIV has been included in the British National Science Curriculum for all 11 to 14 year olds. It is questionable whether this is enough. Many teachers are reluctant to go into these questions deeply with their pupils and many others feel themselves ill-equipped to do so. In some cases, they are even discouraged by their school governors from talking about AIDS. A MORI poll study of 4,000 teenagers aged 16 to 19, conducted at the request of the Health Education Authority in 1990, showed that over 30 per cent had had sexual intercourse by the age of 16 and that over 40 per cent of them did not intend to alter their sexual habits because of the risk of AIDS.

Although there is still no cure for AIDS, it is encouraging to report evidence that maternal treatment with Zidovudine may substantially reduce the risk of transmission of the infection to the baby. In addition, recent studies show that babies known to be infected with HIV may sometimes apparently clear the infection spontaneously.

Albinism

This is a genetic disorder which may take various forms. It is caused by the absence of a chemical activator (enzyme) called tyrosinase. This is needed to convert the substance tyrosine to melanin. Melanin is the one and only body colouring substance – the dark brown pigment that colours the eyes, skin and hair. If the enzyme is completely absent (the tyrosinase negative type), there is no melanin and the skin and hair are milky-white and the eyes pink, grey or blue. Such children have

wobbly eyes (NYSTAGMUS) and often have a severe defect of vision. Some of them are registered blind. This form of albinism has an autosomal recessive inheritance (see GENETICS – AN OUTLINE).

If the enzyme is present but defective (the tyrosinase positive type), the condition is usually not so severe and may be barely noticeable to the observer. The defect in pigment may be confined to the retina, at the back of the eye. In this case, the condition is known as ocular albinism and visual defect is variable. Nystagmus is always present. Albino children almost always have eye problems. The absence of pigment in the insides of the eyes reduces their optical efficiency and affected children are very sensitive to light. The acuity of vision is usually reduced, and the constant movement of the eyes (nystagmus) also interferes with vision.

The absence of pigment in the skin means that such children are seriously at risk from sunburn and must be carefully protected from the sun, especially in summer. If exposed unduly, they can suffer severe burns, and they are more likely to develop skin cancers than people with normally pigmented skin. High sun-protection factor sunscreens are necessary if they go out during sunny weather.

Alcohol effects see FETAL ALCOHOL SYNDROME.

Allergy

The body's immune system protects us against any foreign substance, not just bacteria and viruses. It does so by producing antibodies to attack the invader. Allergy is an abnormal reaction of the immune system to contact between any such substance and the skin, the lining of the nose, throat or lungs, or the lining of the digestive system.

In children with allergies, the antibodies produced become fixed to special cells called mast cells. These are full of histamine and other very powerfully irritant substances. Any substance causing allergy in a sensitive person is called an allergen. Contact between the allergen and the antibody triggers off the release of the irritating substances from the mast cells. The result may be skin weals (urticaria), ECZEMA, ASTHMA or hay fever, depending on the type of allergen and on where the antibodies are situated.

A wide range of substances can cause, trigger off, or worsen allergies in children, especially asthma. These include:

- tree or grass pollen
- ragweed pollen (especially in the USA)
- fungal spores
- kapok and feather stuffing for pillows, etc
- animal skin flakes (dander)
- house dust-mite droppings
- hair particle proteins
- a few food additives such as tartrazine
- atmospheric ozone
- smoke pollution
- atmospheric sulphur dioxide
- discharge from the sinuses
- various drugs, especially beta-blockers and aspirin
- alcohol
- nuts
- shellfish
- some fruits

In addition, a range of circumstances can bring on an allergic reaction. Some of these are:

- emotional upsets
- stress
- strenuous exertion, especially in cold air
- changes in temperature or humidity
- strong smells
- fumes of various kinds
- reflux of acid into the lower gullet (oesophagus)
- COLDS and other upper respiratory tract infections

Hay fever is rare in children under 5 years, but is common in adolescents. If possible, the tree or grass pollen causing it should be avoided, but it may be necessary to use antihistamine drugs. Severe symptoms may call for a nasal spray of beclomethasone or sodium cromoglycate.

Food allergy is much less common than generally thought, but it *does* occasionally occur in children. It is probably responsible for a small proportion of cases of eczema. The actual figures are hard to obtain because the criteria for deciding allergy are seldom strictly applied. The parents of about 8 per cent of children, however, are convinced that the child has an allergy to a food ingredient, or at least an intolerance.

Allergy to some food additives certainly occurs and these have been implicated in the production of asthma and eczema. One of the most important of these is the yellow dye tartrazine. About 50 per cent of all aspirin-sensitive asthmatics are also sensitive to tartrazine. If you suspect that this may be a problem, check for this colourant and other food additives (shown by the letter E, followed by a number) in the contents list of any foods you may suspect of triggering an attack.

> **Other additives colourings, preservatives and antioxidants that have been found to cause asthma in children and others**
> tartrazine (E102)
> quinoline yellow (E104)
> sunset yellow (E110)
> carmoisine (E122)
> amaranth (E123)
> indigo carmine (132)
> green S (E142)
> annatto (E160b)
> benzoates (E210–219)
> sodium metabisulphite (E223)
> butylated hydroxyanisole (BHA anti-oxidant) (E320)
> butylated hydroxytoluene (BHT anti-oxidant) (E321)

Trials of food sensitivity have not always been noted for their scientific rigour. But when these are properly done, they do sometimes show that suspicions are justified. Here is the result of one carefully-controlled double-blind trial of possible food hypersensitivity, duly reviewed and reported in a responsible medical journal. It should be emphasized that the children in the trial mentioned were unusual in that they were already *strongly suspected* of having food allergy. So this trial merely indicates that food allergy exists; it tells us nothing about how often food is a cause of an allergic reaction.

In this trial, neither the patients nor the people doing the trial knew, until afterwards, which of the capsules taken contained the substance thought to cause the trouble and which contained an inert dummy substance (placebo). Thirty-three children with eczema, thought possibly to be related to food, were included in the trial. When they ate an extract of the food believed to be the precipitating factor, 31 of them (89 per cent) developed itching and diffuse skin eruptions. In 19 of the children, there were also other allergic effects such as stomach upsets and wheezing. The symptoms came on between 10 and 90 minutes after the food was taken. Fortunately, there were no alarming or dangerous reactions. The foods causing the reactions in most cases were eggs, milk and peanuts. But the range of possible food allergens was wide, and some children reacted to fish, beef, wheat, rye bread and peas. Other studies have shown that seafood and nuts are also common antigens. Peanuts, even in minute dosages, can cause life-threatening reactions. Fortunately, this form of severe allergic reaction, known as anaphylaxis, is rare.

Food allergy is said to be especially important during the first two years of life. During these early years the commonest allergen responsible for promoting eczema is probably cow's milk. Many cases of infantile eczema have been cured by the elimination of cow's milk and cow's milk products from the diet. Because very small amounts of these substances can cause problems, this may be more difficult than is imagined. There are several kinds of milk-free formulas for babies:

- soya-based formulas (Isomil, Ostersoy, Wysoy, Nutrilon Soya or Prosobee)
- casein hydrolysates (Pregestimil, Nutramigen or Lofenalac)
- whey hydrolysates (Alfare Nestlé)
- comminuted chicken formula

Although the hydrolysates are made from cow's milk, this is treated with enzymes so that the milk protein is partially broken down to simpler molecules that are less likely to be allergenic. Whey hydrolysates, proteins which are made from the liquid whey that separates from the curds when the milk is curdled with renin, are less likely to be allergenic than casein hydrolysates. Casein is the other main protein of milk.

It should be emphasized that cow's milk protein enteropathy, the commonest form of food allergy in babies, is uncommon. It is unlikely that the prevalence exceeds one in 200. Affected babies fail to thrive because of malabsorption and may even have intestinal bleeding and colitis. These symptoms disappear when cow's milk is eliminated from the diet. The latest edition of the very detailed *Oxford Textbook of Medicine*, while properly sceptical about many of the claims made about food allergy, does advise that in such cases cow's milk exclusion is justified as a trial.

Surprisingly, babies' eczema can, in rare cases, be made significantly worse by cow's milk and other allergens derived from the *mother's* milk during breast feeding. Two interesting studies on this were reported in the *British Medical Journal* in July 1986. These were double blind, cross-over trials involving 37 breast-fed infants with eczema. In the cases of six of the babies, the eczema improved when the mothers eliminated cow's milk and eggs from their own diets. Significantly, the eczema got worse again when the mothers started taking milk and eggs again.

In older children, food is not a common cause of allergic conditions such as asthma and eczema. In general, dietary restrictions are seldom needed unless there are clear indications that a particular food can be implicated in causing worsening of the condition. If food allergy is suspected, a skin-prick test can be done to narrow the field of investigation. In this test, a small drop of a solution containing an extract of various food substances is placed on the skin and a small prick is made with a needle through the drop. A positive result is shown by an obvious raised, red area. Such a result does not prove that a food allergy is causing the disorder. Only about half of those with a positive skin-prick reaction to a particular food substance are found to develop symptoms after eating the food concerned.

Certain foods are more likely to promote allergies than others. It is probably wise, in allergic families (see ATOPY), to avoid giving babies certain foods altogether for the first six months of life, or even for the first year. This is especially so if there are brothers or sisters who have developed asthma or eczema. Foods that are best avoided are:

- eggs
- cow's milk
- wheat
- fish
- chocolate
- nuts, especially peanuts
- yeast
- oranges

It is easy to overestimate the importance of food allergy in causing childhood disease, such as asthma and eczema. There is no reason to believe the claims common in popular medical books – that food allergy is a common cause of a wide range of childhood problems. Even within the medical profession there has been a good deal of controversy.

So far as eczema is concerned, the great majority of cases have nothing to do with food allergy. Most are mild, and most of these respond well to simple emollients and the careful exclusion of soap, bubble baths, baby lotion, baby oil, baby moisturizer, biological washing powders and fragranced fabric conditioners.

Alopecia (Hair loss)

When this occurs in children it can cause considerable distress, both to the child and to the parents. Often, however, the latter are more affected than the former, especially if the hair loss is patchy. Common baldness is hereditary and affects males, but is not a problem in childhood. Toxic alopecia sometimes affects children, the hair loss occurring some weeks after a severe feverish illness such as SCARLET FEVER. Baldness may also be caused by disease, chemotherapy or radiation for cancer and treatment with thallium compounds, vitamin A or retinoids. Scarring alopecia may follow burns, skin atrophy, ulceration, fungus infection of the scalp (kerion) or skin tumours. Loss of hair may also follow severe physical or emotional stress.

Alopecia areata is a form of patchy baldness often affecting only one or two small areas of the scalp, but sometimes affecting all the hair of the body. There is a family history of the condition in 10 to 20 per cent of cases and it is common in children with DOWN'S SYNDROME. The cause remains unestablished, but it is thought to be an immune system upset because, prior to the loss of hair, the area to be affected attracts large numbers of lymphocytes. These cells are always massively present in any immune system reaction.

Alopecia areata almost always recovers fully within a year. Up to 40 per cent of sufferers, however, will have another episode some time during the subsequent five years or so. In a very small proportion of cases, alopecia is total and in these cases the hair loss usually starts at the back of the head and works its way forward. Unfortunately, when this happens, the likelihood of regrowth of hair is slim. In some such cases the child may best be served by being fitted with a good-quality wig.

One peculiar cause of hair loss is called trichotillomania. This is a nervous habit, often associated with severe anxiety in the child, that manifests itself by compulsive pulling at the hair. The activity can usually be observed, but confirmatory signs include stretching and corrugation of hair shafts and tiny red spots (petechiae) around the follicles of the pulled hairs. Children showing trichotillomanias badly need help and you should always report this activity to your doctor. In the meantime you can prevent too much loss of hair by oiling it.

In most cases of mild hair loss, the hair regrows spontaneously after a few weeks.

Amblyopia

This is a form of visual defect, usually affecting one eye only, and varying in severity from mild blurring to effective blindness. It is not usually due to any organic defect in, or disease of, the eye. Most cases are caused by failure of the affected eye to be used properly in early childhood as a result of SQUINT. Amblyopia is almost exclusively a childhood problem but, unless properly treated, the effects are permanent. Anything that affects vision is always potentially more serious during childhood than later in life. This is because, from birth to the age of about 7 years, the visual function is developing and remains plastic. There are two important points about this:

- normal visual development cannot occur unless the optical system of the eye is capable of forming clear, sharp images
- any failure of full development during this period cannot be corrected later in life

For these reasons it is essential that the causes of under-use of the eyes or poor early vision should be detected as early as possible and corrected without delay. During this vital developmental period – the period of neurological plasticity – nerve connections between the eye and the brain, are being made fully functional. These connections, known as synapses, are in two prominent swellings that lie on the optic nerve pathways on the underside of the brain, about half way back. Fully-functioning synapses can be made only if the right kind of complex nerve signals are sent back from the eyes along the optic nerves during the early years of life. This will only occur if the eyes are used normally.

If, as a result of any eye defect, normal optical images are not formed on the retinas, the correct nerve impulses will not be sent to the synapses, and the linkup between the eye and the brain will not be properly made. And unless something is done early to correct the problem, the outcome will be a permanent condition of defective vision known as amblyopia.

Amblyopia, literally 'blunted vision', can result from any condition that interferes with clear vision in one or both eyes. These conditions include severe REFRACTIVE ERRORS, congenital cataract (see CATARACT), opacities in the cornea, congenital drooping lid (PTOSIS), persistent internal eye inflammation (UVEITIS), and, above all, squint (cross-eye or strabismus). The term 'lazy eye' is sometimes applied to an amblyopic eye, but this may cause confusion because the same word is used to refer to an eye that turns in or out to an abnormal degree (squint). This is a common cause of amblyopia but is, in itself, much less serious than amblyopia. Because of this ambiguity, the term 'lazy eye' is best avoided.

Failure of normal visual development in one or both eyes does not lead to total blindness with no perception of light. The child always retains a varying degree of perception, but the ability to discriminate fine detail is always poor. A severely amblyopic eye may be able to make out no more than vague shapes and only distinguish various levels of brightness. In minor degrees of amblyopia the child will be unable to read print below a certain size. Many adults have one amblyopic eye and suffer no practical disadvantage; some are even unaware of the fact. The real problems arise when injury or disease affects the vision in the good eye and the child is forced to rely on the amblyopic eye.

One of the main problems with amblyopia in childhood is that the child is unaware of it. In most cases, amblyopia affects one eye only and the child manages quite happily with the other eye. It is only when the normal eye is properly covered up that the child becomes distressed. Amblyopia affecting both eyes is usually present from birth and, as the child has never experienced anything else, there is no immediate indication to the child that anything is amiss. Parents soon become aware from observation, however, if a baby has a significant defect of vision. Any suspicion of defective vision should be reported at once and the child should be seen by an ophthalmologist. Much harm has been done by the often expressed, and usually mistaken, opinion that a baby will 'grow out of' an eye problem such as a squint.

Fortunately, most cases of amblyopia, especially those caused by squint, can be reversed if the cause is detected early during the plastic period and corrected. The earlier the cause operates, and the longer it persists during the developmental period, the more serious the effect on vision. Be sensitive to the possibility of eye defects in your young children and remember that children never complain of not being able to see properly. See also CATARACT, ORTHOPTICS, SQUINT.

Anaemia

Anaemia is a reduction in the amount of haemoglobin, the iron-containing, oxygen-carrying constituent, in the red blood cells. Because a good supply of oxygen is so important to health, anaemia has widespread effects. The most important of these are:

- general misery and irritability
- poor appetite
- weight loss
- weakness
- poor muscle tone
- fatness and flabbiness
- hollow fingernails
- atrophy of the tongue
- fatigue and lack of energy
- tiredness and breathlessness on minor effort, such as climbing stairs
- pale skin
- lowered resistance to infection
- failure to thrive

There are several different kinds of anaemia that can affect children. These include simple iron deficiency anaemia; HAEMOLYTIC DISEASE, due to an abnormal rate of breakdown of red cells (see SICKLE CELL DISEASE); pernicious anaemia, due to the absence of an essential blood-forming factor; anaemia, due to folic acid or vitamin B12 deficiency; and aplastic anaemia in which the bone marrow simply fails to manufacture red blood cells. The latter is the most serious type of all. Fortunately, anaemia is rare in children, but all kinds can occur. Any suspicion that a child is anaemic should lead to medical investigation.

Iron deficiency anaemia does not occur until after the age of about 3 three months and is unusual after the age of 3 years. If it does occur, it is usually of nutritional origin and is due to an inadequate intake of iron in the diet. This is very unlikely unless the diet is severely deficient or extremely eccentric. A very few cases may be due to unsuspected blood loss from the intestine. Occasionally an intolerance to cow's milk may start up an intestinal defect that leads to iron loss. A simple blood test will show whether anaemia is present and, if so, whether it is of the iron deficiency type or is of another kind.

Folic acid deficiency is commonest in infancy. It is very rare in children fed from the breast or with a modern milk formula, but may occur if certain plain powdered milk products are used. Goat's milk is low in both folic acid and vitamin B_{12} and is not a suitable staple for infants. Certain anti-epilepsy drugs can also cause these deficiencies.

Anal protrusion

Prolapse of the rectum is a condition in which the mucous membrane lining of the anus, or the lower part of the rectum turns inside-out and passes out of the anus. In incomplete prolapse, only the lining of the anus appears, but in complete prolapse the whole thickness of the bowel protrudes as a thick cylindrical mass with the mucous membrane lining on the outside. Incomplete prolapse is common in young children and usually requires no treatment, or, at the most, strapping together of the buttocks, or perhaps a small injection to encourage internal adhesion of the lining. Prolapses are easily pushed back in but tend to recur, and complete prolapses usually require a surgical operation to tighten the anal sphincter or to carry out internal fixation of the rectum.

Anal tickle see THREADWORMS.

Anorexia nervosa

In adolescents, persistent loss of weight may be due to anorexia nervosa, which affects young girls in two peaks of incidence: between age 13 and 14 and between age 17 and 18. Up to one girl in 100 in the latter group may be affected. It is a serious and dangerous disorder of perception, causing the girl to become convinced that she is too fat, when, in fact, she may be very thin. Severe emaciation results. Anorexia nervosa occurs in early adolescence but is commoner in girls, such as models, actresses and dancers, who have a professional as well as personal interest in the appearance of their bodies. The condition appears to be becoming ever more prevalent, possibly because of the increasingly public pressures on girls to conform to arbitrary standards of appearance, especially slimness. In a minority of cases it is a symptom of a serious underlying psychiatric disorder, such as severe depression or schizophrenia. The latter condition also has a peak onset in late adolescence.

The cause of anorexia nervosa is still a matter of debate. Many anorectics come from close-knit families, and have a particularly intimate relationship with one parent. They are often obsessional in their habits. They are conformists and usually anxious to please. Some seem unwilling to grow up and appear to be trying to retain their childhood shape. Others seem to have a genuine fatness phobia, with fear of eating fats or carbohydrates. It has been suggested that the disease is due to a disorder in the part of the mid-brain concerned with the linkage between the emotions and the nervous system and with such functions as hunger, thirst and sexual activity (the hypothalamus).

Social factors are probably contributory, especially the arbitrary identification of slimness with sexual attractiveness, and can exert powerful effects.

Medically, the effects of anorexia nervosa are obvious. If calorie input is less than the energy and structural replacement needs, first the fat stores are used up and then the muscles are used for fuel. In anorexia, there is extreme thinness with loss of a third or more of the body weight. There is, inevitably, extreme tiredness and weakness, and often the effects of vitamin deficiency. The skin becomes dry and the hair falls out. The body becomes covered with a fine, infantile hair known as lanugo. There is intolerance to cold and a strong tendency to hypothermia. Early in the process there is, in almost all cases, absence of menstruation (amenorrhoea).

The psychological symptoms are also well marked. They include:

- intense hunger
- constant preoccupation with food
- indulgence in all kinds of fad diets
- depression
- anxiety
- feelings of inadequacy
- irritability
- anger
- sudden changes of mood
- extreme fatigue
- loss of concentration
- withdrawal from friends and family

Anorexia nervosa demands skilled treatment in hospital under the care of doctors experienced in the condition. Personality problems, and the persistence of the disorder can make treatment difficult. Management depends on psychotherapy and imposed re-feeding, but patients will usually make every effort to circumvent treatment, holding food in their mouths until it can be disposed of. Strict control is essential. Unless a watch is kept, food will be hidden or secretly thrown away. Often a system of rewards may be effective, in which privileges, such as visits or relative freedom, are awarded for weight gained.

Antidepressant drugs are often helpful in the early stages. Even after normal weight has been regained, girls who have had anorexia nervosa may need to remain under psychiatric care for months or years. Relapses are common and, tragically, up to ten per cent later die from suicide or starvation.

Antibiotics

These are drugs which destroy infective bacteria in the body. Sixty years ago, medicine was dominated by bacterial infection, which was the major cause of death and responsible for an immense amount of suffering, persistent ill-health and disability. Mothers used to listen with alarm to their children's coughing or contemplate with terror red streaks running up the arm and enlarged lymph nodes. Compound fractures of arms or legs often led to amputation. A squeezed pustule on the nose would cause a spreading fatal infection into the brain. Tuberculosis sanitoria were full of people coughing up blood and dead lung tissue. Lobar pneumonia was commonplace and often fatal, and osteomyelitis caused discharging sinuses for years. Childhood infections such as pneumonia, DIPHTHERIA and SCARLET FEVER were the constant fear of mothers in the era before antibiotics.

All that has changed. Antibiotics have saved millions of lives and prevented countless tragedies. These drugs have nevertheless received a bad press for doing more harm than good and being used as a 'cure-all' for busy doctors. Antibiotics have been misused, often as a result of pressure from patients, but sometimes because doctors feel they can't take chances with possible potentially serious infections but haven't time to investigate the cases as thoroughly as they might. Hospital doctors, understandably, are often more concerned with the immediate pressing needs of their patients than with the possible future hazards of antibiotic resistance, and do sometimes prescribe powerful new drugs when safer, established remedies would suffice.

Powerful antibiotics can cause undesirable side-effects and these must be balanced against the advantages. Allergies to some antibiotics, especially penicillin, are common and can be serious. A group of antibiotics, the aminoglycosides, which include streptomycin and gentamycin, can cause DEAFNESS, kidney damage and can interfere with normal blood production. The tetracyclines (Aureomycin, Terramycin) cause permanent staining of teeth if given to young children. Broad-spectrum antibiotics can destroy normal, health-giving body bacteria and allow over-growth of undesirable organisms such as the *Candida* fungus that causes thrush.

Doctors recognize that antibiotics should be used only for serious, or potentially serious, infections or to prevent dangerous conditions in especially susceptible people. There are, however, strong pressures on busy GPs to prescribe antibiotics on a 'just-in-case' basis or because of uncertainty about diagnosis. There are also some circumstances in which long-term, small-dosage, antibiotic treatment is considered to be justified in quite mild conditions. These include the use of penicillin to prevent kidney and heart damage from streptococcal infections and the use of tetracyclines in acne.

If antibiotics are used casually and in inadequate dosage – and this is not always the doctor's fault – the bacteria which are very sensitive will be killed but those which, by chance, have a natural genetic resistance may survive. When these reproduce, clones of resistant organisms result. This process of natural selection is accelerated by the short bacterial generation – only about 20 minutes, in ideal conditions. So today, we have an on-going race between the development of resistance in bacteria, on the one hand, and the development of new antibiotics, on the other. Only the development of new and more effective antibiotics will allow us to keep ahead in the race.

If you bear these facts in mind and discuss them intelligently with your doctor, your child is unlikely to come to any harm. You, too, have a part to play in the avoidance of antibiotic resistance. Ensure that you follow the doctor's instructions carefully, especially with regard to giving the child the full prescribed course. Failure to do this might result in your child becoming infected with an antibiotic-resistant strain of bacterium. Don't expect to be prescribed antibiotics for every ailment. Remember, antibiotics will have no effect on virus infections, such as colds and flu.

Antibody treatment see GAMMA GLOBULIN.

Apgar score

This scoring method of assessing the state of vitality of a newborn baby was introduced by the American anaesthetist Virginia Apgar (1909–74) in 1953 and is now used all over the world. The scoring is done when the baby is 1 minute old and, if necessary, may be repeated at 5 or 10 minutes or even later if the baby has not reached the required standard. Five qualities are checked:

- heart rate
- breathing
- muscle tension (tone)
- skin colour
- muscular response to stroking of sole of foot

Each quality may be given a score of 2, 1 or 0, so the maximum score for the whole test is 10. For heart rate, a score of 2 is given if the rate is more than 100 beats per minute; 1 is given if the rate is 100 or less; and 0 is given if no beat is detected. For breathing, 2 is given if regular and full; 1 is given if irregular or gasping, and 0 is given if absent. Muscle tension gets 2 if normal; 1 if the baby is floppy; and 0 if limp. Skin colour scores 2 if pink; 1 if blue; and 0 if white. Response to foot stroking scores 2 if the leg is sharply withdrawn; 1 if minor movement occurs; and zero if there is no response.

A baby that scores 7 or less has a significant problem and requires immediate attention and probably resuscitation. The airway is urgently checked and the mouth and nose sucked out with a soft plastic tube. The baby is placed on a board, head-down, and is ventilated with oxygen using a well-fitting mask. If this fails, an expert will pass a tube through the nose or mouth and down into the windpipe. This allows positive pressure ventilation. Various stimulating drugs may be given. If the poor state of the baby is due to narcotic drugs given to the mother for pain relief or taken by a drug abuser, a specific morphine antagonist called Naloxone may be given.

Virginia Apgar was a pioneer in establishing that anaesthetics (including resuscitation) was a speciality in its own right, calling for formal training and official recognition. Prior to her time, most anaesthetics in the USA were given by nurses. She published a book called *Is My Baby Alright?*

Appendicitis

This is inflammation of the blind-ended, worm-like appendix which hangs from the large intestine in the lower right corner of the abdomen. Appendicitis is commonest in adolescents and young adults, but occurs in children of all ages, even in the very young. It begins with pain in the region of the navel which soon moves to the lower right corner. Even gentle pressure here is very painful, often intolerable, to the child. The abdominal tenderness is such that any body movement, deep breathing and coughing may cause pain and distress. There is usually slight fever, loss of appetite, constipation, nausea and, occasionally, vomiting. Although less common than it used to be, appendicitis – or the suspicion of it – is still the most frequent reason for abdominal surgery in children.

Perforation of the appendix is especially common in infants and young children, and leads to the even more serious condition of infection to the membrane, the peritoneum, that covers the abdominal organs. This is called peritonitis. In these cases there is usually a hard, stony lump of faeces (a faecalith) impacted in the appendix. In spite of the frequency of perforation, the mortality from appendicitis in children is less than 1 per cent. Often an appendix abscess forms around the leaking organ and the mass becomes walled off by fibrous tissue from the rest of the abdomen. This is less serious than generalized peritonitis. An operation cures the condition in almost all cases. This requires general anaesthesia and usually takes about half an hour. It is one of the most familiar operations to all surgeons.

Appetite, loss of

This is common in minor illnesses and need not worry you as it resolves when the child recovers. Loss of appetite may also accompany minor emotional upsets but, if persistent enough to lead to loss of weight, you should report it to your doctor for investigation. However poor your child's appetite may seem, if there is no loss of weight, there is no cause for concern. It is common for young children to go through phases of refusing food and this often causes anxiety in parents. Even a day or two with little or no food will do no harm so long as fluid is taken. Food refusal is a normal part of child development and the child will observe, and may later like advantage of, your obvious concern.

Loss of appetite in adolescents may be due to amphetamines or other amphetamine-like drugs such as crack cocaine. Equally seriously, the appearance of loss of appetite may be due to ANOREXIA NERVOSA.

Artery disease see
ATHEROSCLEROSIS.

Arthritis

Arthritis – inflammation in a joint, usually with swelling, redness, pain and restriction of movement – is not normally associated with childhood but does occur. The two main kinds are osteoarthritis and rheumatoid arthritis and these can affect children. LYME DISEASE is commonly complicated by arthritis and this, too, can occur in children. Arthritis in childhood may follow bone and joint infections, injuries, loss of blood supply to bone, and HAEMOPHILIA. It is particularly important to be aware of these facts, as proper early treatment of these conditions can prevent the development of arthritis.

Degenerative joint problems sometimes arise in children as a result of overuse, usually in the enthusiastic pursuit of sporting prowess. Symptoms arising after strenuous athletic activity should never be ignored, especially if recurrent.

The most serious form of arthritis in children is juvenile rheumatoid arthritis, or Still's disease. This is a rare but serious disorder, often with general upset, fever, enlarged glands, joint pain, swelling and stiffness. Still's disease may be complicated by failure of growth, anaemia and serious heart and eye problems, especially UVEITIS.

Asphyxiation see
TRACHEOSTOMY.

Aspirin dangers see REYE'S
SYNDROME.

Asthma

This is an important disease of childhood in which the circular smooth muscles of the branching air tubes of the lungs (the bronchi), are liable to tighten and the lining to become inflamed so the passage of air is impeded. It is often easier for the child to breathe in than out and the lungs become inflated and cannot easily be emptied. A wheeze on breathing out is a feature of an asthma attack. The commonest kind is allergic asthma, but asthma can also be induced by infection, emotion, and exertion. One child in 10 suffers from asthma, and the condition is often a cause of serious concern to young mothers.

Asthma kills at least 2,000 people a year in Britain. If your child has asthma, you must know the signs of worsening of the condition, and of the steps to be taken to overcome them. The more you know about asthma the better. It is becoming commoner, and badly managed asthma can be dangerous. Unfortunately, children do sometimes die from asthma, often because no one was aware of the danger signs.

Asthma usually starts before the age of 5 years and often clears up completely by early adult life. It is not strictly hereditary, but the tendency to allergy, known as ATOPY is, and asthma is very much an allergic problem. People with atopy may develop eczema, hay fever, other allergies and asthma. The gene causing atopy has now been located and the nature of the condition is now much better understood.

The trigger for the tightening of the bronchial muscles is not always apparent, but in most cases it is some external substance, which may be inhaled or eaten. These substances are called allergens and the commonest are:

- grass and tree pollens and moulds blown about by the wind
- house dust
- microscopic house-dust mites and their droppings which are found every where in the house, but especially in bedrooms
- animal fur
- animal dandruff
- feathers
- various air pollutants, such as cigarette smoke, some foods, and a number of drugs, including aspirin

Asthma can also be triggered by COLDS, coughs or bronchitis, or even by exercise, especially in cold weather. Emotional factors, such as stress or anxiety, may precipitate attacks.

Asthmatic attacks vary greatly in their severity, ranging from mild breathlessness to a desperate, panicky struggle for air, or even respiratory failure. Attacks may be most frequent in the early morning. The main symptoms are breathlessness, wheezing, a dry cough sometimes brought on by exercise, and a feeling of tightness in the chest. During a severe attack, breathing becomes increasingly difficult, causing sweating, rapid heart beat, and great distress and anxiety. The affected child cannot lie down or sleep, may be unable to speak, breathes rapidly, and wheezes loudly. In a very severe attack, the low amount of oxygen in the blood may cause blue-purple discolouration (CYANOSIS) of the face, especially the lips, and the skin may become pale and clammy. Such attacks may be fatal.

Although there is no cure for asthma, attacks can be prevented to a large extent. If a specific cause is suspected, steps can be taken to avoid it. For example, if pollen is thought to be the cause, the child will need to avoid gardens, parks, and the countryside during the pollen season. If the house-dust mite is responsible, mattresses (in which the mites flourish) should be enclosed in airtight plastic covers and the home should be kept as free of dust as possible. In difficult cases, tests are available to discover whether any of the common allergens is responsible for triggering attacks.

Attacks can usually be prevented by the use of drugs such as cromolyn sodium and inhaled corticosteroids. To be effective, they must be properly taken, a number of times daily, usually from INHALERS. Once an attack has started, however, a preventive drug has limited value and a drug that relaxes and widens the airways (a bronchodilator), such as salbutamol, must be used. Most asthmatic children learn to administer the drug themselves with hand-held plastic inhaler.

The best way to take drugs for asthma is by inhalation. This way, they get to the place where they are wanted in the smallest dose needed to produce the desired effect, and with the least chance of causing general upset. Inhalers convert the drug into an aerosol of particles small enough to reach the right place. These may be liquid or a dry powder. Breath-activated powder delivery systems may be easier to use.

Unfortunately, many asthma patients don't know how to use an inhaler properly. Make sure that your child does, because the effectiveness of the treatment depends on it. Read the instructions carefully and follow them exactly or the drug may not get down to the affected bronchial muscles. It is no good just to spray the inside of the mouth. This will not help the asthma and, in the case of the steroids, it may promote a thrush infection. The idea is to synchronize a deep inhalation with the release of the aerosol of the drug so that there is a maximum concentration of the drug in the inhaled air. Note also that inhalers lose their effectiveness after a certain period (the date is marked on the container), so it is essential to renew the supply regularly.

Most attacks of asthma either pass naturally or can be controlled by the use of a bronchodilator. In some cases, however, an attack may be so severe that it fails to respond to the recommended dose of the drug. In this case, the dose should be repeated. If it has no effect, the child is in danger and should be taken to a doctor or to hospital immediately. Emergency treatment may include the administration of oxygen, a corticosteroid, and a bronchodilator by way of the air passages, or an injection of aminophylline into a vein. If these measures are ineffective (which is rare), the child will require the use of a ventilator, which forces air or oxygen under pressure into the lungs.

More than half of affected children grow out of asthma completely by the age of 21; in a large proportion of the remainder, attacks become decreasingly severe as they grow older. Monitoring of the state of the air passages is important. Here is it how it is done.

THE PEAK EXPIRATORY FLOW METER

Tests of lung function, by measuring the actual volume of air passing during forced expiration, have been in use for a long time by experts in hospital. These tests require cumbersome apparatus called recording spirometers: they are expensive, cumbersome and delicate, but the value of these tests is considerable. Research showed that the volume of air breathed out in the first second of a forced expiration, after taking the fullest possible breath, was a reliable indication of the respiratory performance for a much longer period – up to 15 seconds. This applied both to people with normal lungs and those with asthma.

Such equipment is quite impracticable for home use, but fortunately, in asthma there is a close relationship between the value of the peak expiratory volume in the first second and the maximum air flow *rate* at the beginning of a forced expiration. This maximum rate is called the peak expiratory flow rate, and you can measure peak flow rate with a very simple, portable and cheap device called a peak flow meter. This can provide asthmatics with warning of deterioration in their symptoms, and there is now a very strong case for the view that everyone using an inhaler for asthma should also be using a peak flow meter. The readings are a good indication of the severity of the airway obstruction. They can also be used to assess response to treatment.

What we really want to know is the ease with which air can pass in and out of the lungs. The peak flow meter can give us a reliable, objective assessment of this. This is very important because deteriorating performance is dangerous and may be followed by a severe, and perhaps potentially fatal, attack. This cannot be over-emphasized. Nearly all the deaths from asthma could be prevented if effective treatment could be given at an early stage to prevent sudden and severe worsening. A reducing air flow performance is a clear sign that changes in treatment are needed to improve control. Regular monitoring can, for instance, demonstrate increasing differences between morning and evening peak expiratory flow rates – a hint that control is inadequate. Properly-informed people with asthma, provided with this kind of objective indication of their air flow status, can, by themselves, make ap-

propriate changes in their treatment – such as adding or increasing steroids – or can seek medical help urgently.

Like diabetics, asthmatics should know at all times what is going on and should be clearly aware of the principles of treatment. Peak flow rate figures in asthmatics can be considered as analogous to blood sugar readings in diabetics. The main difference, however, is that oxygen lack is far more immediately dangerous than a rise in blood sugar. Many asthmatics are too young to be able to assess their own condition. In these cases, someone else – usually a parent – must do it for them.

Peak flow readings are also important in monitoring the effect of a reduction in treatment when it is thought that a patient is possibly being overtreated. Reduction in steroid dosage, for instance, can only safely be achieved if the effect of the change on peak air flow is assessed at the time.

Asthma is so potentially serious that you really cannot know too much about it. You must be able to judge the severity of your child's condition and recognise the need for action. You should understand the effects of different treatments and know the difference between short term, quick relief, drugs, which simply combat the immediate narrowing of the bronchial tubes, and longer-acting preventive drugs which reduce the likelihood or severity of attacks. You need a plan for coping with a worsening situation and should clearly understand that if an attack doesn't respond to a bronchodilator inhaler, your child is in danger and probably requires steroids. And you must understand that if, in spite of everything, his or her asthma is going out of control, you are in an emergency situation and require urgent medical attention straight away.

ASTHMA DRUGS

Short-term treatment is with drugs like salbutamol, terbutaline and fenoterol, which stimulate certain of the adrenaline receptors in your child's bronchial muscles and relax them, so allowing the air to pass freely. If attacks go on in spite of this, your child may need a mast cell membrane stabilizer to stop the mast cells producing substances that are causing his or her bronchial tubes to go into spasm. The best one is sodium cromoglycate (Intal). This cannot stop an established attack, and only works in cases of allergic asthma. Also, the drug must be present in your child's body when the pollens, dust, mites, or whatever it is that is causing the asthma, are encountered. So this is a long-term form of treatment. Sodium cromoglycate is inhaled as a powder, from a 'spinhaler' or an aerosol and should be continued for at least several weeks, as directed by your doctor. If Intal fails, your child probably need a corticosteroid such as beclomethasone (Becotide) or budesonide (Pulmicort). Children over 4 years can use fluticasone (Flixotide). These, too, are taken by inhaler, so as to minimise dosage and general effects.

Salbutamol will usually cope with flareups, but severe relapses generally require steroids in larger doses and these must be taken by mouth. So don't delay in consulting your doctor. There is much to be known about asthma and you should study one of the many popular books on the subject. Above all, you should, at all times, know about the state of your child's bronchial tubes. Ideally, you should be regularly checking, with a peak flow rate meter, the peak rates at which the child can breathe out. Keep a record of the results, and know at what point the peak flow rate has become dangerously low.

Most asthma care is given in general practice rather than in hospital, much of it by specially trained practice nurses in asthma clinics. The British Thoracic Society has published excellent guidelines for the management of asthma, based on a 'stepwise' approach.

Astigmatism see REFRACTIVE ERRORS.

Atherosclerosis

This very common condition causes more adult deaths than any other single disease. But the earliest signs are readily apparent in childhood, and the condition gets steadily worse with age. Furthermore as, diet is important in the development of the disease and dietary habits are usually formed in childhood, parents should be aware of the danger.

Atherosclerosis causes progressive narrowing of the arteries and obstruction to the vital flow of blood. Pathological examination of the arteries of children killed in accidents show that most of them already have visible fatty streaks in the lining. These are believed to be the sites of future atherosclerosis. The condition, when it develops sufficiently, is most dangerous in the coronary arteries supplying the heart muscle with blood, and the carotid and vertebral arteries supplying the brain. In adults, atherosclerosis of these two systems leads, respectively, to coronary thrombosis and stroke. Heart attacks from atherosclerosis can affect adults in their 30s. In older people, the disease also causes gangrene of the limbs by obstructing the main supplying arteries.

The prevention of atherosclerosis must start in childhood with the early establishment of a healthy lifestyle. This involves:

- eating no more than is required to maintain a normal, low-end-of-range body weight
- avoiding animal fats
- taking exercise to the point of breathlessness, at least once a day
- exercising for half an hour at least three times a week
- *never* under any circumstances smoking cigarettes

These principles should, ideally, be observed from the earliest reasonable age, so it is important for parents to be aware that atherosclerosis is the number one killer disease in the Western world.

See also EXERCISE.

Atopy

Atopy is a tendency to allergy that is inherited and runs in families. Atopy may show itself in a number of different ways. It is associated with production of antibodies in the immunoglobulin E (IgE) class, and is caused by a gene that alters the binding sites for immunoglobulin E (IgE) on mast cells. All this is explained in the article on

ALLERGY. Atopy features a proneness to ASTHMA, hay fever and ECZEMA (atopic dermatitis). These conditions are precipitated by the release, by mast cells, of irritating substances such as histamine, prostaglandins and leukotrienes. This occurs when the causal allergens, such as pollen grains, become attached to the IgE on the mast cell membrane.

Families with atopy have been studied to see whether the genetic basis of allergy can be clarified. In 1989, research scientists at the Churchill Hospital, Oxford, located a gene on the long arm of chromosome No 11 that is associated with atopy. This gene is responsible for producing the protein receptor sites on the mast cells to which the IgE molecules attach themselves. In June 1994, the Oxford research team published a paper in the journal *Nature Genetics*. In this they described how they had discovered that many families featuring atopy carry a particular variant, or mutation, of the IgE receptor gene. Not all families with atopy carried this particular gene mutation and the scientists think that there may be several other atopy genes, probably four or five. Surprisingly, the mutant atopy gene has, in every case, been found to be inherited from the mother. The abnormal IgE receptor sites produced by this gene are only very slightly different from those on the mast cells of people without atopy. Indeed, they differ by only a single protein-building unit (amino acid). But this slight difference is enough to affect the way mast cells with IgE respond to pollen grains. It seems that the abnormal IgE receptor sites simply make the mast cells much more sensitive to the triggering effect of the pollen grains or other allergens.

Autism

Although fortunately quite rare, this is a serious childhood disorder of the higher brain function which starts before the age of 30 months. Autistic children are withdrawn, self-absorbed, interested in objects but not in people, and are often unable to communicate by normal speech. They avoid eye contact. They show stereotyped, self-centred behaviour patterns, repeating the same activity, such as rocking or pirouetting, over and over again and showing rage if interrupted. General intelligence may be in the normal range, but most of them are, and remain, educationally subnormal. Some show remarkable, and often unsuspected, talent for art, music, or for mental arithmetic. Autism is believed by some experts to be a form of schizophrenia but it does not respond to medical treatment. Ten to 15 per cent of autistic children develop EPILEPSY.

Some autistic children respond to educational conditioning based on reward for appropriate behaviour. Parents need all the help they can get. In time, the behaviour problems may resolve and there may be progressive improvement in the use of language.

See also IDIOT SAVANT and HYPERLEXIA.

B

Baby breast milk see WITCHES'
MILK.

Baby doctor see
NEONATOLOGIST.

Baby reflexes

These are known as 'primitive reflexes' or
'newborn reflexes' and are automatic movements made by very young babies in response to various stimuli applied to the
body as a whole. These reflexes disappear

> **Primitive reflexes**
> * automatic closure of the hand
>   around an object such as a finger
>   (grasp reflex)
> * sudden bending up of the legs, and
>   embracing movement of the arms,
>   in response to a noise or to momen-
>   tary lack of support to the head
>   (Moro, or startle, reflex)
> * walking or stepping reflex, when
>   the baby is held upright with its
>   feet on the ground
> * turning of the head and sucking
>   actions when the cheek is stroked
>   (rooting reflex)
> * extending the arms and legs on the
>   side to which the head is quickly
>   turned, and flexing those on the op-
>   posite side, so that the baby adopts the
>   'fencing' position (tonic neck reflex)
> * The periods during which these
>   responses are present are well
>   known to paediatricians and the
>   absence or undue prolongation of
>   these primitive reflexes provides
>   valuable clinical information about
>   the health and state of development
>   of the baby.

during the first months of life, but provide
useful guidance to the health and state of
development of the immature nervous system. Most of the primitive reflexes develop
between the ages of 20 and 38 weeks of
intrauterine life (gestation). One of them –
sucking – is present as early as 14 weeks
after conception.

Balanitis

This is inflammation of the bulb (glans) of
the penis. The Greek word *balanos* means
'acorn', so the term is apt. Balanitis is
commonest in small boys with tight foreskins (phimosis) or in babies left so long in
wet nappies that the urea in the urine is
turned to ammonia by bacterial action.

Balanitis in adolescents is usually the
result of neglect of personal hygiene in
those who are uncircumcised. A white,
cheesy and nasty-smelling material called
smegma accumulates under the foreskins of
boys who do not wash there regularly and
this eventually becomes an irritant and
causes inflammation.

In older boys, other causes of balanitis
include thrush (candidiasis) and trichomo-
niasis, both of which commonly infect the
vagina. If sexual intercourse is likely to
continue, it is useless, in such cases, to treat
only one partner, as infection readily
spreads either way. Various other sexually
transmitted infections can cause balanitis.

Ballooning of foreskin see
CIRCUMCISION.

Barking at print see
HYPERLEXIA.

Bat ears

'Bat ears' are common and may be a serious
matter for a young child, whose appearance

may evoke the merciless taunts of peers. Happily, an operation to correct unduly prominent ears can turn a butt into a hero, for the idea of surgery is fascinating to children. Children's ears are three-quarters grown at the age of 3 and almost fully grown by 8, so any unusual prominence is much more obvious than in an adult.

Cosmetic surgery for bat ears is highly effective. The skeleton of the ear is a single piece of gristle (cartilage) of complicated shape, and this is covered with skin which is firmly stuck to the front surface but more loosely attached behind. This is convenient, because, to conceal the scars, the surgeon wants to do the operation on the back of the ear. Great care is taken to ensure that any cuts made on the back do not come right through to the front where the skin would be marked.

If the prominence is due to a folding outwards of the cartilage, the principle is to thin or weaken it along an almost vertical line so that it can easily be bent backwards towards the head. The surgeon makes a vertical cut through the skin on the back of the ear and exposes the cartilage. The weakening can be done in various ways. Some surgeons actually cut a thin vertical strip out of the cartilage, but this is apt to cause rather sharp bending, when the cartilage is folded back, with a very prominent ridge. Others prefer to weaken the cartilage by making a large number of fine cuts with the point of a sharp scalpel. Alternatively, the line of bending can be thinned by the use of a tiny rasp, or file, or the line can be carefully pared thin.

Once the cartilage is thinned in the right place, it will bend back easily and, to keep it back, the surgeon removes a vertical ellipse of skin from the back of the ear and then sews the edges together. Because there is now less skin on the back of the ear, the edges of the incision can only be brought together if the cartilage folds back. The degree to which it will bend back will, of course, depend on the width of the ellipse of removed skin, and this must be skilfully judged to get the amount of bending just right. Quite often there is a difference in the prominence of the two ears and, in such a case, the width of the ellipse will have to be varied accordingly.

If the ear prominence is due solely to a large angle between the ear and the head, a different operation is necessary. In this case, the skin removal behind the ear is more extensive, and it is necessary also to take away some skin covering the adjacent mastoid bone of the head. When this is done, the bared area includes the angle between the ear and the head. When the free edges of this area are sewn together, vertically, the ear will be brought close against the head and will be less prominent. In very severe cases, where both angles are large, both procedures may have to be combined.

BCG

BCG is not quite the same as other forms of immunization and should not be thought of as a vaccine against tuberculosis in the way that polio vaccine protects against polio. The bacille Calmette-Guérin, is a French variant of the tubercle bacillus, the cause of tuberculosis. It is obtained by repeatedly growing the organism to form a culture of colonies, and then regrowing one small sample of one of these. The aim is to produce a form that does not cause infection but that still prompts a protective immunological response. Léon Calmette (1863–1933) and Camille Guérin, working at the Pasteur Institute, Paris, started the process in 1906 and for 13 years they patiently grew one subculture after another, until they had recultured the organism 231 times and were satisfied that the strain was safe. The vaccine, prepared from this strain, came into use in 1921.

Most people acquire a useful degree of immunity to TB by early contact with the organism followed by an inapparent 'primary' infection. The healed and calcified resultant scar can be seen on the chest X-ray films of most adults. But people who have not had a primary infection don't have antibodies against TB and are particularly susceptible to it. Because the organisms can be found almost anywhere, such people are liable to develop the disease, especially in the lungs (pulmonary tuberculosis). The risk is greatest for immigrants from parts of the world where prevalence is high, and for people intending to travel to these areas.

BCG is now established as a valuable method of conferring a measure of immunity on people susceptible to the disease. It reduces the likelihood of acquiring tuberculosis by about 80 per cent. Before considering BCG vaccination, a simple tuberculin test, the Heaf test, is always used to determine the immune state of the individual. BCG is never given to those who give a positive reaction to tuberculoprotein.

Bedwetting

This usually occurs at night or during sleep. The normal child develops adequate control early in life, but one in 10 still wets regularly at the age of 5. Most infants will, by the age of 18 months, be able to let others know that they have urinated. By 2 years many children will indicate that they want to urinate. By 2 years 6 months, the majority of children can attend to their own urinary needs and many are usually dry throughout the day. The situation during sleep is somewhat different because the bladder must be able to hold about eight hours' worth of urine before the child can be expected to be dry all night. The bladder does not usually develop to this extent until the age of about 3.

With all children, accidents will occasionally happen, especially in times of stress, but persistent bedwetting after 5 is considered abnormal. Unfortunately, a large number of children fall into this category. About 15 per cent of children over 5 regularly urinate in bed and about 7 per cent of 10 year-olds also do so. Most bedwetters are merely slow in developing full nerve control and, unless there is some underlying disease, such as urinary infections, kidney trouble, DIABETES, SICKLE-CELL ANAEMIA or emotional disturbance, bedwetting nearly always stops before puberty. Bedwetting runs in families.

Training to pass urine regularly during the day is helpful as is a simple, battery-operated electrical bed alarm which rings as soon as urine is passed. Don't let your child have drinks last thing at night and insist on a visit to the toilet before bed. Persistent bedwetting should always be medically

investigated. If no organic cause is found, counselling by a child psychologist is often helpful.

Behaviour problems see AUTISM, CONDUCT DISORDER, HYPERACTIVITY, JUVENILE DELINQUENCY, MANIPULATIVE BEHAVIOUR, MISBEHAVIOUR, NAIL BITING, PICA, SLEEP PROBLEMS, TICS. See also introductory section (especially 1 to 3 years).

Bereavement

The effect of the loss of a parent, whether by death or by abandonment, is, in general, the more serious the younger the child at the time of the parent's departure. This will not surprise anyone with even a basic understanding of the nature of the child-parent relationship (see introductory section) and its importance for the vital early conditioning – consider it as programming, if you like – of the child. Much has been published on the subject, and there is good evidence that children who lose a parent, at an early age, quite often grow up into adults with a low opinion of themselves; they may also be chronic worriers who regularly suffer strong guilt feelings and are given to depression and anxiety.

This kind of personality damage is obviously one of the worst things that can happen to anyone and it is important to consider whether anything can be done to reduce the effect. Unfortunately, in most cases, the only person available to help the child is the bereaved adult. If you are in such a position, you are likely to feel that knowledge of this kind is just too much of an additional burden for you to bear. But it is worth remembering that there is at least a possibility that accepting this responsibility might provide you with some comfort.

Bereaved children are apt to regress in their educational development. A 2 year old with a growing vocabulary might stop talking altogether and might say nothing for a year. When they do talk, they are likely to ask where the absent parent is. How does one respond to such a question? It is difficult enough to try to find an answer without having to translate it into terms an infant can understand. For many, the immediate impulse is to lie – to find some comforting formula to help one out of the difficulty. 'Daddy's gone away.' Something of that sort.

These responses, although very common and understandable, are neither helpful nor desirable. If Daddy decided to go away, it means that he didn't care, and this could play havoc with a child's confidence and self-image. It might also raise the possibility that Mummy might also decide to 'go away'. And it is not likely to assist a child's spiritual development to ask him or her to believe that God has taken away one of the two most important people in his or her life.

The first thing to remember is that your young child sees itself as the centre of the universe and frequently believes that anything that goes wrong is his or her fault. Most children are thoroughly familiar with the concept of blame long before they can possibly understand the concept of death. They get this idea from you, for you would be less than human if you had never, at least occasionally, expressed disapproval. In the midst of many mysteries, children try desperately to make some kind of sense of cause and effect and regularly postulate magical connections. So you must assume the definite possibility that the child will blame him or herself for the death. This is a distressing thought, but one you should recognise and handle. And you will not handle it by telling lies.

But talking about death to children need not be as difficult as you think. Probably, your instinct will be to shy away from discussion of death. A sympathetic woman recounted how, when she was about 10 years old, she once saw that the much younger children from next door were looking curiously at a dead bird. They asked her why it was unable to move, so she tried to explain to them what death was. She told them that it happened to everyone, 'but not for a long time – not until they were old'. The children were very interested and the discussion led to their playing games in which they pretended to be dead. There was no content of horror or

distress, only a pleasing frisson of half-alarm.

Unfortunately, the sequel to the episode was a sharp note of protest from the parents of these children requesting that she should not frighten them with such morbid matters. To children, there is nothing morbid or unhealthy in the idea of death; it was the response of the parents that was unhealthy.

So you should not, on that account, be inhibited from talking frankly to your child about the real reason for the absence of the beloved parent. Children readily accept authoritative statements, so you must be careful what you say. To the best of your ability and the child's understanding, you must make it perfectly clear that the death was involuntary, unwished, and in no circumstances the responsibility of any living person. You must emphasise that the dead parent did not wish to go and was very sorry to leave the family, but had no choice in the matter. But you must also try to mitigate distress on behalf of the deceased by explaining that the dead person cannot now feel grief. Perhaps, above all, you must show, by word and deed, that the event has in no way diminished your love and concern for the child.

None of this will be easy, and you may feel that you already have enough to cope with. But it is important. Careful studies by experienced psychiatrists have shown that the effects of the death of a parent on the social and educational development and happiness of a child can be markedly affected by the way the child is handled immediately afterwards. And one of the most important factors in avoiding these unhappy effects is open and frank discussion of what has happened.

Dr Dora Black, a psychiatrist who has specialised in this subject, has reported that when parents were counselled on how to handle this situation, the effect on the children was that there were fewer and briefer behaviour problems, that there was less trouble with sleeping and restlessness, that their general health was better and that they had fewer problems at school. Interestingly, and significantly, such children found it easier than others to cry over, and to talk freely about, the dead parent.

Here is what a girl of 16 wrote about her father, who died when she was 11. 'The only thing that I find difficult is the way other people react . . . Really I would love to talk about my Dad for hours on end, but I never have, because nobody wants to know. They seem to think that it is wrong'.

Bile duct narrowing see
CONGENITAL BILIARY ATRESIA.

Birth defects see CONGENITAL MALFORMATIONS.

Birthmarks

These affect about one-third of all babies at birth or soon after. They are harmless tumours of skin blood vessels, and are of cosmetic importance only. They take various forms. The strawberry naevus is a small, bright red, raised tumour which grows to its full size during the first six months of life and then subsides. In most cases it disappears altogether by the age of 5 years. No treatment is needed.

The port-wine stain, or capillary haemangioma, is a flat tumour of the smallest blood vessels. It is present at birth and is permanent. It usually occurs on one side of the face and is often a conspicuous blemish. Even worse is the cavernous haemangioma which is raised, lumpy and highly coloured and consists of a mass of medium-sized blood vessels and blood spaces. It, too, is permanent.

Haemangiomas, if small enough, may be removed and the skin edges brought together with stitches. Larger haemangiomas may require a skin graft. Lasers and freezing may also be used with some success. See also STORKBITE.

Birthweight

The average weight of a baby at birth is about 3.3 kg (7 lb). There is, however, much natural variation and many babies are heavy because their mothers are obese. Abnormally high birthweight tends to occur if the mother is diabetic. Very low birthweight may sometimes be due to infection in the womb or to genetic defects.

See also PREMATURITY.

BIRTHWEIGHT AND LATER DEVELOPMENT

Since the middle 1980s many babies born with a birthweight of less than 750 g have survived, and it is now possible to assess the effects of such low birthweights on development. Regrettably, it has been found that, as they develop, such children, on average, suffer a marked disadvantage compared with those of normal birth-weight. They have a substantially higher incidence of learning difficulties, CEREBRAL PALSY, visual defect and reduced physical skills. They do less well academically, have inferior social skills and suffer from attention and behavioural problems. About 20 per cent of such children have below-normal mental abilities and almost half of them require special educational attention.

Doctors are now beginning to appreciate that it is not enough to be concerned only with saving the life of a fetus; the avoidance of extreme prematurity at birth is also of critical importance for the future well-being of the individual.

See also PREMATURITY.

Bites and stings

Children are no more susceptible to bites and stings than older people but are often affected more seriously by them. Most bites and stings have only a local effect and the trouble is limited to pain, redness, swelling, persistent irritation and annoyance. Annoyance from multiple mosquito, midge or sandfly bites can, however, be extreme. Some areas are, in fact, rendered uninhabitable by mosquitoes, but these do not feature in the travel-agents' brochures.

Most of the million or so known species of insects are entirely harmless, but a few, such as bees, wasps, hornets and horseflies, will sting you or your child if you provoke them by panicky attempts to brush them away. Just let them crawl on the skin and try to avoid getting them under the clothing.

If your child has been stung by a bee, the insect usually departs, leaving the sting protruding from the skin. Try not to be too upset by the child's howling. Explain that you have to get the sting out. *Never* use tweezers. If you do, you are sure to inject more venom by squeezing the venom sac. The idea is to remove the sting by a scraping action in an appropriate direction, using the edge of a credit card or a fingernail. Remember that the bite can give access to infective organisms, so wash the area well, but gently, with soap and water. An ice-cube in a handkerchief can be applied to produce narrowing of the local blood vessels and decrease venom absorption. Some kind of soothing lotion can then be applied with lots of tender loving care. Antihistamines by mouth can be very helpful in relieving symptoms.

Multiple bee, wasp or hornet stings can be more dangerous to children. Many species inject a combination of formic acid and a powerful neurotoxin and the effect can be very painful, causing much local swelling, redness, burning and itching that lasts for as long as two or three days. Swelling is of rapid onset and may be associated with FEVER, HEADACHE, muscle pains and cramps, drowsiness, and, in severe cases, even loss of consciousness.

Do everything you can to reduce absorption of venom. Carefully remove stings, as described. Remember that tweezers could fatally increase the dose of venom. Cold compresses should be applied. Unless the child has been so unfortunate as to receive some hundreds of stings, there is little risk to life. Medical attention should, however, be sought without delay and a close watch kept for the signs of acute allergic reaction. This is known as a anaphylaxis and, although rare, is the real danger. *If a child has had a previous sting and is known to have become allergic to insect venom, a single further sting can be disastrous.* In a severe anaphylactic reaction, the main danger is from ballooning of the mucous membrane lining of the voice box (laryngeal oedema) and tight contraction of the circular muscles of the air tubes of the lungs (bronchospasm).

These effects can be so severe as to cut off the air supply completely, leading rapidly to collapse and, if the airway obstruction is unrelieved, death. Every year, in Britain, a few people die from this cause. In the USA About 100 people die in this way each year – more than from snake bites. In America, the common stinging insects are wasps,

bees, hornets, yellow jackets, bumble bees and fire ants.

Life-threatening allergic reactions
Beware of the following:
- severe swelling in parts of the body remote from the bite, especially in the face
- raised, purplish areas on other parts of the skin (urticaria)
- severe itching
- wheezing
- coughing
- obvious difficulty in breathing
- blueness of the skin (CYANOSIS)
- nausea and vomiting
- abdominal cramps
- dizziness
- severe anxiety
- collapse
- loss of consciousness

The priority in such a case is the maintenance of the child's air supply. You may have to use mouth-to-mouth artificial respiration. If the appearance of these effects is obviously associated with a sting on an arm or a leg and there is a known history of severe reaction to insect stings, you may consider tying a handkerchief tightly around the limb just above the sting. *But this must never be so tight as to eliminate an arterial pulse below it.* Such a measure could be life-saving, but places a heavy responsibility on you to ensure that it does not cause loss of the limb from cutting off the arterial blood supply. It should be briefly loosened every five minutes.

If the child is fully conscious and can swallow normally, an aspirin tablet can help to counter the release of irritating substances from damaged cells. Aspirin is not normally given to children but this is an emergency. Ice-cubes in the mouth can sometimes help to reduce swelling in the larynx. You will be in little doubt when urgent medical attention is needed, so lose no time in getting the affected child to a hospital or other facility where he or she can receive adrenaline, intravenous antihistamine and steroids, perhaps TRACHEOSTOMY and cardiopulmonary resuscitation.

Bites, animal

Children are commonly bitten by domestic dogs and occasionally by other animals. These bites should always be taken seriously, mainly because of the risk of infection. The mouths and teeth of animals are teeming with infectious organisms, some of which are very dangerous. You should thoroughly clean wounds with plenty of soapy water and encourage free bleeding so long as it is not spurting. Thorough wound cleansing markedly reduces the risk of infection, including rabies.

Cover the wound with a clean dressing and take the child to a doctor. If surgery is necessary, any damaged tissue will probably have to be removed. The wound may be left open for a time, as early closure can encourage infection. Antibiotics and anti-tetanus immunisation will probably be given.

Rabies must always be considered. So it is important that the biting animal should be kept under restraint for observation. If the animal remains apparently well for 10 days, the risk of rabies is eliminated. A rabid animal will die within 10 days. If the animal dies or is killed, its head should be sent, as soon as possible, to a public health laboratory so that the brain can be examined for signs of the characteristic rabies virus colonies found within the nerve cells.

Bites from free-ranging wild animals pose problems. If the animal can be killed, its head should be sent for examination. If it escapes, and if the area is one in which rabies has occurred in the previous 10 years, human rabies immunoglobulin can be given, followed by a course of vaccination. This usually involves five intramuscular injections in the arm or the thigh, on days 0, 3, 7, 14 and 28. Human diploid cell vaccine, made from viruses grown in human cell cultures, is now preferred. Some 500,000 people receive rabies vaccination each year.

Blackheads see ACNE.

Bleeding

You can always control bleeding from minor injury simply by pressing something on the area. It also helps if you elevate the wound. Press firmly on the wound, preferably with a sterile compress until the bleeding stops. Even spurting from a cut artery can always be stopped by firm pressure. You must always do this at once if blood is spurting, so as to avoid dangerous loss of blood. Use your hand immediately, then any clean material, such as a folded handkerchief. Just press firmly and maintain the pressure. Tie on the pad if necessary. Send for help. Tourniquets are dangerous and should never be used to control bleeding.

NOSE BLEEDS can almost always be controlled by pinching the nostrils. Apart from nose bleeds, which are usually harmless, any bleeding without apparent cause should always be reported to your doctor.

See also introductory section (**Safety and First Aid**).

Blepharitis

Blepharitis means inflammation of the eyelid. Although the inflammation is usually confined to the lid margin, it is often very persistent. The lid edge is reddened and sometimes thickened and the skin at the roots of the lashes becomes scaly and is often greasy. Many fine flakes of skin may be seen stuck to the lashes. Blepharitis is often associated with DANDRUFF or SEBORRHOEIC DERMATITIS of the scalp and treatment of this is an important part of the management of the condition. Scales on the lids should be carefully removed with moistened cotton buds. Your doctor may prescribe some mild steroid ointment, from time to time, to control the inflammation.

Blindness in infancy see
RETROLENTAL FIBROPLASIA.

Blocked nose see NASAL
OBSTRUCTION.

Blood deficiency see ANAEMIA.

Blue baby

This is a common term for a relatively uncommon condition – a baby born with a heart defect which prevents blood from taking up its full complement of oxygen. Normally, all the blood returning to the heart from the body is immediately passed to the lungs to pick up more oxygen. If the heart defect prevents this, some of this blood is returned to the tissues in its low-oxygen state. Blood fresh from the lungs is bright red, but after it has given up its oxygen to the body tissues it is a bluish-purple colour and gives a blue tinge to the skin. This is called CYANOSIS. When this is constantly present, it is a clear indication of a major circulatory problem.

The normal heart has two sides which do not communicate with each other. The right side receives used blood from the head and body and pumps it to the lungs for re-oxygenation. Freshly oxygenated blood from the lungs returns to the left side of the heart to be pumped to the whole body. In several forms of CONGENITAL HEART DISEASE, the two sides of the heart do not remain wholly separated, and blood returning to the right side can mix with blood returning from the lungs. The condition of HOLE IN THE HEART refers to an opening in the central wall which divides the two sides, internally. Because the pressure on the left side is usually higher than on the right, the blood is adequately oxygenated and cyanosis may not be a feature. But in some of these conditions, the right side of the heart enlarges in response to an increased load, and there is a right to left shunt, bypassing the lungs, with severe lack of oxygenation of the blood.

Boils

A boil is a bacterial (staphylococcal) infection of hair follicles that has progressed to abscess formation. Children with boils on the face or neck usually have permanent colonies of staphylococci in their noses. Those with boils on the lower part of the body have resident staphylococci in their armpits or groins.

Several factors encourage recurrent boils. These include poor standards of personal hygiene with insufficient body washing, SCABIES and obesity, especially where there is resulting rubbing and dampness between layers of the skin of the neck, buttocks and armpits. ECZEMA is another causal factor. Because a boil implies enormous numbers of staphylococci locally, boils commonly occur in crops in the same general area. When several closely adjacent hair follicles are affected, the resulting large multiple boil is called a carbuncle.

If crops of boils are to be avoided, the heavy bacterial contamination of the skin in the area around the boil must be treated by frequent, thorough washing, preferably with a good antiseptic soap. In severe cases ANTIBIOTIC treatment, with a drug such as flucloxacillin by mouth, may be necessary. Antibiotics have little or no effect on an established boil which must take its course. STYES are small boils in eyelash follicles. Recurrent or frequent boils should arouse the suspicion of possible DIABETES.

Bonding see introductory section (Birth to 1 year).

Bone cancer

Primary bone cancer in young people takes two principal forms, although, happily, both are rare. The most frequent bone cancer in children is the osteogenic sarcoma (osteosarcoma). This usually appears at the lower end of the thigh bone. Fortunately, the disease affects only about two young people in a million, but when it does happen it is very serious. The average age of occurrence is 12, when growth is most rapid.

The first indication is bone pain, especially at night. Such pain, occurring for no obvious reason in an adolescent, should never be ignored for there are few other indications that a cancer is present until a late stage. By then the chances of cure are remote. Often, the next sign is COUGH, FEVER and chest pain, suggesting pneumonia, but actually caused by secondary spread of the cancer to the lungs. The tumour forms a swelling in the bone and the X-ray often shows radiating spicules of bone in the ominous 'sun-ray' pattern known to all doctors.

The other form of bone cancer is Ewing's tumour. This is a highly malignant cancer affecting children up to the age of about 15 years. The tumour causes areas of bone destruction, and the body responds by surrounding these with layers of new bone, giving a characteristic 'onion skin' appearance on X-ray. The affected area is swollen, tender and painful and the child often has a fever, so the condition is apt to be confused with bone infection (OSTEO-MYELITIS). Unfortunately, in spite of the most energetic treatment, even amputation and radiotherapy, the outlook is often un-favourable.

A major advance in the treatment of both of these forms of bone cancer has occurred in recent years and this has improved the five-year survival rate from about one young person in five to better than one in two. The drugs adriamycin, cisplatin and methotrexate, in conjunction with amputa-tion and radiotherapy have greatly im-proved the outlook. In addition, recent immunological studies have shown that the tumour has antigenic properties which can be attacked by specific antibodies. Loss of the limb has been avoided in some cases by a bone graft from a dead donor. Second-ary spread to the lungs can sometimes be effectively treated by surgery.

Bone inflammation see
OSTEOMYELITIS.

Bone distortion see RICKETS.

Bottle-feeding see introductory section (Baby care).

Bowel obstruction see
CONGENITAL PYLORIC STENOSIS, INTUSSUSCEPTION.

Bow legs

Bow legs, bandy legs or genu varum, are common and normal in healthy toddlers, and the condition usually rights itself by about 18 months. It is not caused by bulky nappies. If you find that the bowing is still present after this time, and particularly if it gets worse, your child needs attention. The problem may be the condition of osteochon-drosis of the tibias – the main bones of the lower leg. Another possibility is RICKETS, from vitamin D deficiency, which causes softening of the bones. In this case, inspec-tion will show that the bowing does not occur at the knees, but at the upper ends of the tibias.

If treated early, bow legs can be readily straightened using night splints. Neglected genu varum, in addition to causing adult deformity, usually leads to later osteoar-thritis in the knee joints. See also KNOCK-KNEE.

Brace, dental

The extent to which teeth can be moved, by applying steady pressure in one direction, is remarkable. Bone in the tooth socket actually is absorbed on the side opposite to that on which pressure is applied to the tooth, and regrows on the same side, so that the new position of the tooth is permanent. This principle is the basis of ORTHODONTICS, in which a wide variety of appliances are used to apply sustained pressure in appro-priate directions.

Dental braces may be supplemented by an external wire structure, usually worn only at night, or may be wholly internal. Sometimes small metal anchorage points are cemented to the teeth so that pressure can most effectively be applied via attached wires.

Children, of course, hate these appliances and strong encouragement is often neces-sary. They will need to be regularly re-minded that the treatment is for a limited period only and that the results will be permanent.

Brain inflammation see
ENCEPHALITIS.

Brain tumour

Brain tumours are rare in children. Those originating within the skull may arise from several different sites such as the brain coverings (meningioma), the neurological supportive tissue (glioma), the blood vessels (haemangioma), the bone (osteoma) or the pituitary gland (pituitary adenoma). Some are present at birth (CRANIOPHARYNGIOMA and teratoma) and are due to abnormal development.

The symptoms of a growing tumour within the skull are due to a progressive rise in the internal pressure, either from the growing mass or from interference with the normal circulation of the fluid that surrounds the brain and fills the cavities within it. The symptoms include:

- severe, persistent headache
- vomiting which is sometimes sudden, unexpected and projectile
- fits, either major seizures or local twitching
- loss of part of the field of vision
- hallucinations
- drowsiness
- personality changes
- abnormal and uncharacteristic behaviour

HEADACHE is probably the commonest of all symptoms and it is important to appreciate that only a tiny proportion of even severe headaches are due to brain tumour. But if a child complains of a new, persistent and severe headache, without any obvious cause, you should certainly seek medical attention without delay. A key point in the examination, in such a case, is the inspection of the optic nerve heads within the eyes, using an ophthalmoscope. In one quarter of cases of brain tumour and in most of those with raised pressure within the head, the parts of the optic nerves visible within the eyes are obviously swollen.

An especially important sign of brain tumour is actually caused by the raised pressure in the skull. This is sudden, unexpected projectile vomiting, often without NAUSEA. Such a sign, especially if associated with recent headache, is an indication for immediate and urgent medical attention.

In doubtful cases the diagnosis can usually be made by computed tomography (CT) or magnetic resonance imaging (MRI) scanning. The outcome depends on the location, type and degree of malignancy of the tumour. Many common brain tumours are not malignant. Treatment is by surgical removal, often supplemented by radiotherapy.

Brain jaundice see
KERNICTERUS.

Brain lining inflammation see
MENINGITIS.

Breast enlargement in boys see
GYNAECOMASTIA.

Breath-holding attacks see
introductory section (1 to 3 years).

Breathing difficulty see
RESPIRATORY DISTRESS SYNDROME, ASTHMA.

Bruising without obvious cause

Most bruises are caused by an obvious injury, and children are naturally prone to these. Bruises result from the release of blood into the tissues from small blood vessels (veins and capillaries), and over the course of a week or two, the blood is gradually absorbed and the bruise turns from black to yellow and then disappears. Bruising can be minimized by applying a cold compress as soon as possible after the injury. This temporarily shrinks the bleeding vessels and hastens sealing by blood clotting so that the amount of blood released is less.

A bruise that appears *without* injury is a different matter and suggests a disorder of small blood vessels or of blood clotting. This should always be reported to your doctor for investigation. One must be alive to the possibility that this may be an indication of LEUKAEMIA.

The commonest bleeding disorder of childhood, however, is not leukaemia but a less serious condition called acute idiopathic thrombocytopenic purpura. This mouthful is not so difficult to explain as you might imagine. Purpura is a group of bleeding disorders which cause haemorrhages into the tissues from small blood vessels. These may often be seen under or in the skin either as the tiny pinhead petechiae or as larger 'black and blue' bruises called ecchymoses. Purpura arises in two ways – from damage to small blood vessels or from a shortage of blood platelets (thrombocytes), which are necessary for normal clotting. Platelets are small cell fragments normally present in the blood in large numbers. 'Thrombocytopenia' just means that there is a shortage of platelets; and 'idiopathic' means that the doctors don't know what causes the problem. Idiopathic thrombocytopenic purpura can be passed from mother to child.

Some causes are known, however. Thrombocytopenia in children also commonly follows virus and other infections, and, like many other conditions, is probably due to an anomaly in the functioning of the immune system. Other cases are due to the platelet type of the baby being different from that of the mother, much along the lines of rhesus factor disease. Some may be due to bone marrow abnormality or prescription drugs, such as tolbutamide or thiazide diuretics, taken by the mother.

Platelet deficiency interferes with normal clotting and the result is an abnormal tendency to bleed anywhere in the body. The skin shows tiny red spots (petechiae) and bruising, there may be nose bleeding, bleeding into the bowel, urinary system, vagina, brain, spinal cord and joints. Such haemorrhages cause effects varying with the site, but, in addition, the persistent blood loss tends to lead to anaemia with fatigue and weakness. The condition is very variable in severity, showing, at the one extreme, only a few petechiae, and at the other, severe and barely controllable bleeding. This degree of severity is very rare in children and the condition usually clears up spontaneously within a few months.

Another type of purpura that affects children is allergic purpura, or Henoch-Schönlein purpura. This often follows a streptococcal infection in children and is due to damage to the lining of small blood vessels by the resulting immune complexes (antibody linked to the material causing the reaction). In addition to the signs of bleeding, the skin may show redness and urticaria. This form of purpura causes local inflammation and itching and may affect a wide range of organs, especially the kidneys, the joints and the bowels. There is a pinkish skin rash. Kidney disease occurs in about 10 per cent of cases. There may be swollen and painful joints, abdominal pain and sometimes blackening of the stools from altered blood (melaena). Sometimes there is bleeding into the brain, causing HEADACHES, dizziness and confusion.

Most cases recover spontaneously but about 5 per cent of cases of Henoch-Schönlein purpura go on to develop severe kidney damage.

Bruxism see TEETH GRINDING.

Bullying

For many children this is a desperate matter that can seem to make life hardly worth living. Bullying is one of the obvious examples of the corrupting effect of power. It is a repetitive process that inflicts on a child a variety of injuries, humiliations, threats, insults and other damage. As a rule the bullied child refuses to talk about the matter either to teachers or to parents and simply suffers miserably in silence. This is because of shame, embarrassment and, perhaps most important, fear of recrimination and an exacerbation of the bullying. In a desperate attempt to avoid it, children will play truant, deliberately simulate various illnesses, or find other excuses for not attending school. Occasionally a child will commit suicide to escape from it.

Bullying is commonest in children, because those who bully have not yet matured to the stage at which empathy with the victim is possible. Some never do. There is good evidence that many confirmed bullies continue aberrant social behaviour in adult life. Many bullying children, however, simply have no conception of what it is like to be bullied and are unaware of the harm they are doing. Some are simply repeating a pattern of behaviour they have learned from their own parents.

The long-term effect of bullying on victims can be serious. Because it causes children to perceive themselves as inadequate and incapable, many of them never completely get over it. It is not at all fanciful to suggest that many adult neuroses, depressions and inter-personal relationship problems may stem from childhood bullying.

The activity is widespread in schools and, because of the conspiracy of silence, its prevalence is greatly underestimated. Research in Sheffield has shown that more than a quarter of junior and middle school pupils and one-tenth of secondary school children had been bullied in recent weeks. Ten per cent of juniors reported that they were being bullied at least once a week.

Various factors encourage bullying. Peer identity is one. A child who, for any reason, seems to the majority to be different-it may be no more than a 'posh' accent or better quality of clothes – is liable to be bullied. Again, a child who is small for age, naturally quiet or retiring, or whose interests do not seem to conform to those of his or her peers, is at risk. Some children are bullied simply because they are conspicuously better at schoolwork than average. One little-known factor is the faintly perceptible odour of bacterially-altered urea that clings to a bedwetting child.

Parents need to be alive to the possibility of bullying and should be alerted at once if a child shows a sudden inexplicable reluctance to attend school. One of the first questions to be put frankly to the child is whether this might be happening. For the reasons already given, denial should not necessarily be accepted. If there are any real grounds for a suspicion of bullying, the matter should immediately be taken up with the school authorities, quoting the facts mentioned in this book.

Research has shown that an effective school intervention programme can reduce greatly bullying and with it truancy.

Burns and scalds

Put the fire out and cool the burned area as quickly as possible. Heat destroys tissue, and immediate cooling is the only thing that can help. So get the part under the cold tap and keep it there. Chemical burns need prolonged washing. You cannot over-do this.

Do not burst blisters. Do not apply any medication, grease, oil or anything else to a severe burn. Burns rapidly lead to loss of fluid from the blood and this has to be replaced. A burned *conscious* child is the only kind of casualty who should be given plenty of fluids by mouth.

See introductory section (**Safety and First Aid**).

Burping see WIND.

C

Café au lait patches

These are oval or leaf-shaped, milky coffee-coloured patches or freckles on the skin, and may be as long as 6–8 cm. They are usually of cosmetic significance only. But if they occur in childhood and six or more large ones are present, or they are present in areas, such as the armpits, not normally exposed to the sun, the affected child may have the rare disease neurofibromatosis (von Recklinghausen's disease). In this case, multiple skin bumps – benign tumours of the sheaths of skin nerves – may be expected to develop in adolescence or early adult life.

Neurofibromatosis has a prevalence of about one case in 3,000 people. It is a genetic disorder with dominant inheritance, but about half the cases occurring result from a new mutation. The disease varies in severity from a few minor skin features to severely disfiguring and dangerous involvement of other parts of the body, including the nervous system. In the fully established condition, the fibrous sheaths of numerous nerves in the skin and elsewhere develop soft tumours called neurofibromas. In most cases these are confined to the skin and have cosmetic significance only. But in about 20 per cent of cases, serious complications arise from massive skin involvement or involvement of the central nervous system.

The tumours can involve the brain and spinal cord; the eye sockets, leading to increasing protrusion of the eyes; the bones, leading to spontaneous fractures; and the spine, causing severe deformity and sometimes paralysis. LEARNING DIFFI-CULTY, usually mild, occurs in a proportion of cases.

People with neurofibromatosis need support and help and, in Britain, this is supplied by such organisations as LINK (Let's Increase Neurofibromatosis Knowledge). Similar organisations exist in other countries.

Caput

Latin for 'head'. The term is used as an abbreviation for caput succedaneum, to describe the soft boggy swelling which forms on the top of the scalp of a baby as a result of prolonged pressure of the head on the partly opened neck of the womb (cervix) before birth. The caput corresponds to the area of the scalp overlying the opening. The rest of the scalp is compressed, and congestion of veins occurs with leakage of fluid (serum) into the unsupported part, causing a swelling (oedema). The caput disappears in a few hours or days after birth and, in spite of the temporary odd appearance, need cause no concern.

Car sickness see MOTION SICKNESS.

Cataract

Cataract is an opacification of the internal (crystalline) lens of the eye. In children, cataracts may be caused by injury, but the great majority are present at birth (congenital) and are due to factors operating during the development of the lenses, early in the pregnancy. Congenital cataracts are not particularly common and many are of minor degree and are non-progressive and require no treatment. Opacities that significantly interfere with image formation, however, will cause severe AMBLYOPIA and may require early treatment. Such cataracts will usually cause discernible whiteness in the pupils.

Cataract in children is almost always the result of a discoverable cause, and there are many of these. Congenital cataract is often caused by maternal rubella (German measles) early in pregnancy, or less often, by the effects of drugs taken by the mother during the early weeks when the eyes of the fetus were developing. DOWN'S SYNDROME is commonly associated with cataract as are various rare hereditary conditions. A number of severe skin problems, all fortunately rare, or severe childhood diabetes, with high blood sugar levels, may cause cataract. GALACTOSAEMIA is a genetic condition in which the infant is unable to break down galactose into simpler sugars so that it accumulates in the body. Unless a galactose-free diet is given, cataract is inevitable.

There is a major problem with dense, one-sided congenital cataracts – such a serious one, in fact, that, until quite recently, ophthalmic surgeons simply refused to operate on them. The point is that, so long as the good eye can see normally, the deprivation of the image in the eye with the cataract has a devastating effect on the development of vision in the cataractous eye. A great deal of clinical experience showed that, in spite of later attempts at treatment, full vision never developed in these eyes. And if the one-sided cataract was dense, the best that could be hoped for was a very poor standard of vision indeed. It seems that the brain simply latches on to the good eye and entirely ignores the other.

We now know, however, that if the cataract is removed at a very early stage and the baby is provided with an optical correction in the form of a contact lens, it is possible to make this eye work by careful occlusion of the other. There is no denying that this involves all kinds of difficulties and that the outcome may not be very good, but some potential vision can be saved in the affected eye. The child concerned may never use this eye and may well never suffer any disadvantage from a monocular existence, which will, for him or her, be normal. The real point of it all becomes apparent only in the unlikely event of loss of vision in the good eye by injury or disease.

Injury to the eye is an important cause of cataract. A concussive force such as that caused by a flying stone or high-speed squash ball, a sharp poke from a finger or a severe blow to the face, may cause cataract even without any external injury to the eye. Penetrating wounds of the eye are even more likely to cause cataract, especially if the lens capsule is penetrated or torn. In such cases, water immediately enters the lens substance and, within a matter of hours or days, a dense cataract will develop.

Opaque lenses in young children are soft and easily removed by a relatively simple suction procedure. But this leaves the eyes severely unfocused and this, in itself, will result in severe amblyopia. So if cataracts are treated in early life, strong optical correction is necessary and this, at present, is best done with contact lenses. See CONTACT LENSES. Some surgeons will insert plastic lens implants in children but many are reluctant to do this in babies.

Cats, diseases from

The most important diseases transmitted from domestic cats to humans are two comparatively uncommon parasitic disorders of similar names but quite different character – TOXOPLASMOSIS and TOXOCARIASIS – both of which are carried in in cat faeces.

Toxoplasmosis is caused by a microscopic organism called *Toxoplasma gondii* which usually infects people before they are born, gaining access to the fetus by way of the placenta during pregnancy. Toxoplasmosis can have serious effects if this occurs early in pregnancy and may cause abortion or severe congenital abnormalities. Later in the pregnancy, the fetus has more resistance, but the nervous system and the eyes are commonly infected.

Toxoplasmosis of the choroid of the eye, acquired in this way, is commonly seen in ophthalmic departments but the real prevalence is comparatively low. The organisms tend to lie dormant for many years, but later, in adult life, often cause a flare-up of patchy, spreading inflammation (choroiditis) which may severely damage vision.

Toxocariasis is quite different. It is caused by a small round worm, *Toxocara cati*, a similar species of which, *Toxocara canis*, is common in puppy dogs. The infestation is acquired by children, whose fingers become contaminated by worm eggs in the anal fur, or by touching cat faeces. These eggs are then transferred to the children's mouths and the cycle is started. Toxocariasis causes a brief, feverish illness as the hatched worm juveniles pass around the body, but generally causes little harm unless a tiny worm happens to enter the eye. In this event a damaging reaction occurs that may destroy the vision in that eye.

Other diseases caused by cats include:

- tinea, a fungus infection of the skin
- ASTHMA from cat skin scales
- cat-flea bites, which are common and very irritating and may become infected
- cat scratch fever

The latter is an uncommon condition that may follow about two weeks after a scratch. It causes marked enlargement and tenderness of a group of lymph nodes ('glands'), usually in the neck or armpit, and a few days of fever, headache and sore throat. The lymph node enlargement may persist for months, but eventually settles.

Mange is a mite infestation caused by mites of the same variety that cause scabies and these mites may be transferred to humans, causing scabies. Rabies can be contracted and transmitted by domestic cats, but at present the risk in Britain is negligible. See also DOGS, DISEASES FROM.

Cephalhaematoma

This is a collection of blood between the skull and the overlying membrane (the periosteum), usually resulting from unavoidable injury sustained in the course of a difficult forceps delivery. The haematoma forms a soft, boggy swelling on the baby's scalp which disappears over the course of the first few weeks of life.

Cephalhaematoma appearing later in life must be accounted for, because it is an indication of a head injury, sometimes of a fractured skull. Non-accidental injury (child battering) will have to be considered by the doctors if no satisfactory explanation is forthcoming.

Cerebral palsy

Also called spastic paralysis, this is a non-progressive, non-hereditary disorder of the brain control of movement. It affects about one child in 500, appears early in life and varies considerably in degree, from slight to almost total disability.

There is stiff 'spasticity' of the muscles, lack of coordination and sometimes involuntary jerks and movements. There is almost always some difficulty in walking. Commonly the legs press tightly together, causing a characteristic 'scissors gait' on walking. Often speech is affected. About half of the affected children have some degree of LEARNING DIFFICULTY. About a quarter also have seizures.

Causes of cerebral palsy
- birth brain injury, especially oxygen lack during delivery
- physical malformations
- RHESUS INCOMPATIBILITY with severe brain JAUNDICE
- infections such as ENCEPHALITIS and MENINGITIS
- head injury early in life
- smallness for age before birth
- poor fetal blood supply from the placenta (placental inadequacy)
- separation of the placenta before birth
- bleeding within the womb (antepartum haemorrhage)
- fetal poisoning
- compression of the umbilical cord during birth
- prolonged or difficult labour
- premature birth
- low blood sugar (hypoglycaemia) early in life
- respiratory distress syndrome early in life
- hypothermia
- early brain haemorrhage

In over one-third of cases the cause remains unknown. About three-quarters of children with cerebral palsy have spastic paralysis. Fifteen per cent suffer from walking problems (ataxia) without muscle spasm and about 5 per cent have constant writhing movements of the limbs (athetosis) or of the whole body (chorea). In most cases the legs are more severely affected than the arms and it is quite common for only the legs to be involved. Typically, the legs remain outstretched and permanently crossed. Normally, when one muscle group contracts, the opposing group relaxes, but in spastic paralysis relaxation does not occur. Sometimes only one side of the body is affected and occasionally only one limb is involved. In the more severe cases, all four limbs may be affected.

In addition to these difficulties, children with cerebral palsy may have:

- visual problems
- DEAFNESS of varying degrees
- speech difficulties, either in articulation or comprehension or both
- various problems with perception or understanding
- any combination of the above

About half of the children with cerebral palsy are mentally normal. One-quarter are retarded to a moderate degree and one-quarter are severely retarded. There is usually, but not necessarily, a close relationship between the degree of retardation and the severity of the muscle paralysis.

In almost one-third of cases of mild cerebral palsy the problem with walking has resolved by the age of 7. In general, the outlook depends on the degree to which mental function is affected. Many children with average or near-average intelligence can live reasonably normal happy lives. In children with severe cerebral palsy, especially those with frequent epilepsy and learning difficulty, the outlook is less good. Up to half of these die before the age of 10, usually from infection.

Severe spastic paralysis can impose a terrible burden on parents but attitudes should always be as positive as possible. Much can be done to help children to control muscular action and to prevent deformity from muscle shortening (contractures).

Chest deformities

These are much less common than they used to be but still occasionally occur. They may take several forms. In pigeon chest the breastbone (sternum) projects rather sharply, like that of a bird. This may be a natural shape, present from birth or it may be the result of nutritional deficiencies, especially a shortage of vitamin D that has led to childhood RICKETS. Nutritional rickets is now almost unknown in Western societies and, if present, may arouse the suspicion of neglect.

In funnel chest the breastbone is depressed so as to produce a distinct hollow which may be quite deep. This, too, can be either natural or the result of rickets. As a rule, neither pigeon chest nor funnel chest causes any real harm, apart from the aesthetic disadvantage.

Asymmetry of the chest is usually due to a twisted spine of the type known as kyphoscoliosis (see SPINAL PROBLEMS). It may, however, be the result of serious lung problems such as collapse of the lung, tuberculosis or pleurisy. Chest asymmetry should always be investigated and the cause corrected, if possible. If the child is entirely well, the condition need not, in itself be harmful.

Chickenpox

This highly infectious disease of childhood is caused by the same virus that causes shingles in adults. Chickenpox, or varicella, is usually trivial, a minor event of childhood which often passes almost unnoticed. It generally occurs between the ages of 2 and 8, and is often picked up at school and then passed round the other susceptible members of the family. It is spread by the aerosol of infected droplets coughed out by another child in the early stages of chickenpox.

Chickenpox is commonest in the winter and spring and occurs in epidemics, once every three years or so as enough new and susceptible children accumulate. The signs appear 10 days to three weeks after infection. There is a slight FEVER and a feeling of unwellness and there may be HEADACHE and aching in the muscles. At this stage, tiny blisters, full of virus, form in the mouth and throat, and these ulcerate to provide the source of infection to others.

The rash begins as tiny, flat, intensely itchy red spots, mostly on the body, which quickly become small blisters. These soon turn milky, dry to crusts, form scabs and drop off. The sequence, from spot to scab, takes only 12 to 24 hours and successive crops occur for one to six days, so the spots are seen at all different stages of development. In many cases, they are so few and scanty that they may hardly be noticed.

The varicella-zoster viruses acquired in this way, settle in certain collections of nerve cells called ganglia, mainly on the spinal nerves. There they remain dormant for the rest of the child's life. Often, some 60 years or more later, a drop in the efficiency of the immune system may allow these viruses to become active again. They do not, however, become generalized to cause another attack of chickenpox. Instead, their activity is confined to the nerves in which they lie, causing the distressing condition of shingles. In recent years, shingles, long thought a disease only of elderly people, has been occurring in young adults and, very rarely, even in children and babies.

Chickenpox is generally said never to recur, but numerous cases of second attacks have been recorded. It can even occur for a third or fourth time and there is reason to believe that the virus is mutating over time to defeat the immune system. Chickenpox in adolescents or adults can be very severe and these cases may need urgent treatment. The new antiviral drug famciclovir is said to be highly effective.

Chilblains

These are raised, red, round itchy swellings of the skin of the fingers and toes occurring in cold weather. This condition, together with other related disorders, is known medically as 'perniosis' but this gets us no nearer to an explanation and the cause remains obscure. Chilblains can be avoided by keeping your children's hands and feet warm with woolly gloves and stockings and fur-lined boots.

Child development see introductory section.

Child differences

Why are children so different from each other? This is not just an academic question. If the variations, especially in intelligence, are entirely due to heredity, then many of us are condemned from birth to a lifetime of inferiority. Educational effort and special educational programmes intended to improve performance are likely to be a waste of time and money. But are these variations simply a matter of the genes?

This question, put in different ways, has been argued for centuries. Mostly it has been put in terms of 'nature' (genetics) and 'nurture' (environmental influences). One or other – or both – is responsible for determining the human characteristics we call intelligence, personality, abilities, academic performance, and so on. In spite of advances both in genetics and in our understanding of psychology, those who would seem to be best qualified to pronounce on the matter still appear to be as divided in their opinions as ever.

Historically, most people have plumped for heredity as the main determinant of human behaviour and have cited families in which succeeding generations have shown high levels of achievement in particular spheres. In support of this view are numerous citations of families of poets, scientists, judges, statesmen, literary men, musicians, painters, and even oarsmen and wrestlers. The conclusion was that outstanding abilities of these kinds are transmitted in proportion to the closeness of descent.

The view that intelligence is mainly a matter of genetics has had some support from the psychologists, but opinions of this kind have often been formed with scant regard to the effects of the environment on the growing child. In the past, a few discerning individuals – people like the Jesuit founder Ignatius Loyola – clearly understood the enormous effect environmental influences could have on the young: 'Let me have the child until it is seven,' he said, 'and I care not who has it after. In the early part of the 20th century scientists quickly ranged themselves on one side or the other. Some eminent geneticists seriously contended that there were genetic grounds for people becoming artists, poets, scientists, actors, servants or farmers. Those impressed by the extent of environmental influences tended to take a diametrically opposed view. Some took an extreme position, claiming that any healthy baby, taken at random without regard to the parents' abilities, could be trained to become a specialist of any type – a doctor, lawyer, artist – or even a genius.

Because identical twins have identical genes, they offer ideal experimental subjects for studies into the nature-nurture problem. Such twins normally share the same general environment, so the chief interest is in twins who have been reared apart. Unfortunately, identical twins are seldom reared apart, and even if they are, the environments are usually not sufficiently different to make the observations worthwhile. There have, however, been a few remarkable instances in which such twins have grown up with extraordinary similarities in tastes, interests and activities.

Studies have been made of deprived children who were adopted by affluent families soon after birth. When the adopted children were compared with their siblings who had not been adopted, the former showed consistently higher IQ scores. The adopted children averaged an IQ of 111; their non-adopted siblings averaged 95. It can, of course, be argued that variations of this kind might be due to factors such as differences in nutrition, rather than to educational differences. We know that young children who are severely nutritionally deprived often suffer permanent loss of intellectual ability.

Nowadays, most psychologists take some kind of a compromise position. They accept that the two major elements – nature and nurture – are essentially interdependent. Few genetic traits of importance can operate without some environmental contribution, and this contribution may be highly significant. Consider, for instance, a purely genetic inborn metabolic error in which a gene necessary for the normal breakdown of the amino acid phenylalanine is deficient (see GENETICS – AN OUTLINE). If a child with this error consumes a normal diet containing the amino acid phenylalanine, a toxic product will accumulate in the blood and the brain; the child will have the disease known as PHENYLKETONURIA and will suffer learning difficulties. But if the condition is detected early and the child given a phenylalanine-free diet, he or she will grow up normally. This is but one of many examples that could be given of the interaction of heredity and environment.

A helpful, if limited, analogy is that of the personal computer. One might consider the role of heredity as providing the hardware and the role of the environment as providing the software. One might inherit hardware of high or low quality, but the achievements realized will depend equally on the quality of the input (software).

Child guidance

When a child develops problems such as solitariness (withdrawal), obvious anxiety or phobias, serious LEARNING DIFFICULTIES, late and persistent BEDWETTING, sleep disturbances or persistently aggressive behaviour, skilled attention is required. This is best provided under the overall guidance of a child psychiatrist who will be able to distinguish the extremes of normal behaviour from the abnormal.

In some cases there is an actual physical disorder, possibly neurological, and sometimes unsuspected learning difficulty. Often there are psychological problems relating to earlier emotional or physical trauma; abnormal behaviour in children is often a reflection of a psychologically unhealthy family situation. So careful and accurate diagnosis of any possible organic disorder, or of a possible external causal factor, is a first priority. This may involve referral to other specialists, such as a paediatrician or a neurologist, and the psychiatrist may wish to investigate the family setting and interview both parents and, possibly, other members of the family. A psychologist specializing in the measurement of mental performance (psychometry) may be needed.

Much can be achieved by attention to these factors, but in some cases psychiatric treatment may be necessary. There is comparatively little interest, in Britain, in the use of classical Freudian psychoanalysis in such cases, but a greater emphasis on counselling, family discussion therapy, the judicious use of drugs and, sometimes, behavioural therapy.

Childhood medicine see
PAEDIATRICS.

Children and violence

Emotions often run high when considering violence in relation to children. Even the issue of SMACKING is liable to arouse strong feelings.

Mention of the subject immediately raises the question of whether the amount of violent activity witnessed by children on TV is harmful. This is not an easy question. Short of banning their children from watching TV altogether, there is no way that parents can avoid children being exposed to scenes of violence. It must also be acknowledged that a great deal of violent crime is committed by juveniles – people under the age of 18. In such contexts it is worth considering American experience which points to potential trends in Britain, some years later. There are already some indications that this is exactly what is happening. In the decade 1981 to 1990, in the USA, there was a 60 per cent rise in the number of juveniles arrested for murder and manslaughter. The rise in all those over 18 was only 5 per cent. There was also a 28 per cent rise in the numbers of juveniles arrested for rape; a rise of 54 per cent for car theft; and a rise of 57 per cent for those arrested for aggravated assault.

Certain factors are known to be associated with violent behaviour in children. Research has shown that the following, present at the age of 8, tend to predict future violence:

- parental violence or severity
- lack of parental discipline
- lack of parental care and affection
- parental separation
- poverty
- HYPERACTIVITY
- impulsive behaviour
- low level of parental education
- being the victims of BULLYING

The question of the effect of television has never been resolved. Over 1,000 different research studies have shown that there is an association between watching TV violence and the level of aggression in children. The principal conclusion to be drawn from this is that children with a higher than average level of aggression watch more violent TV than other children. This may be a consequence of lowered parental control, or of the fact that aggressive children are keener on watching violent television. The real difficulty is to show that watching violence on TV or video is the cause of the aggression in children, and this has never been done. The general medical view is that, on its own, it does not. Other factors, such as those mentioned above, are believed to be more important in causing aggression.

It has to be remembered that what is seen by adults as obvious and shocking violence is not likely to be perceived as such by most normal children with an emotionally healthy background. Killing the 'baddies', however brutally, is, for these children, a source of satisfaction that has little or no connection with real life. It is a different matter if violence has been directly experienced or is observed being used on others in the home. Children with that kind of genuinely violent background will be liable to process TV violence in a different way. They may, for instance, use it as a basis for wish-fulfilment revenge on those who have hurt them.

Some TV and, in particular, video recorded material, is so oppressively disgusting that it may be difficult to think calmly about its possible effect on children. Clearly, every effort must be made to shield children from the products of conscienceless people concerned only to make money. The Video Recording Act, 1994 goes some way to achieve this, but the mere existence of 'video nasties' means that some children will contrive to watch them. Nevertheless, there is little or no evidence that young offenders are driven to crime by a diet of horror films. Studies suggest that the viewing habits of young delinquents differ little if at all from those of well-behaved children.

It is clear, however, that disturbed children may react to these films in a different way from normal children. One idea is that the films release the children from inhibitions and so promote greater violence. They may lower the threshold of what the child takes to be acceptable to him or her. Some psychiatrists consider that violent TV is at least a risk factor in the development of aggressive behaviour. Children who watch violent programmes exclusively might come to regard what they see as normal behaviour. Moreover, an addiction to such films deprives the child of other, and better, formative experiences. At the very least they are wasting a great deal of time. Almost all TV has at least some useful educational elements in it; this kind of thing has none.

Simply banning nasty videos and imposing censorship on TV films might suggest that the government is doing something positive to combat juvenile crime; there is very little reason to think so. Such actions certainly do not get to the root of the matter.

Another growing aspect of violence and children is the increase in the number of handguns and automatic weapons used in Britain The pattern is beginning to follow that which has long been established in the USA so it is important for us to be aware of what has been happening there. In the USA, an increasing number of children are involved in shooting incidents and accidents.

A study of children and adolescents involved in one type of shooting incident in Los Angeles in 1991, showed that in that year there were 1,548 drive-by shootings during which 2,222 people were shot at. Nearly 700 of them were children or adolescents under the age of 18. Of these, 429 had gunshot wounds and 36 of them died from their injuries. Most of the shootings occurred in public streets and mostly after dark. One-third of the guns used were semi-automatic, capable of firing up to 17 rounds without reloading. The figures showed that children and adolescents involved in any way with street gangs were 60 times more likely to die from homicide than those not involved. Admittedly, Los Angeles is an exceptional case and the incidence of violent street gangs is much higher there than in most cities. But it is easy to visualize how the present trend in Britain might develop.

The domestic situation in the USA is equally worrying. Increasing criminal violence has led to an enormous increase in the private ownership of hand guns, ostensibly for the purposes of protection. There are about 120,000,000 privately owned guns in the USA and about half of all the homes contain one or more firearms. Most are kept for sporting purposes but at least one-fifth of owners give 'self-defence' as the reason for possessing a gun. Studies have shown that keeping firearms in the home carries a substantial risk of accidental injury or death and greatly increases the likelihood that domestic quarrels will end in tragedy. Suicide impulses, too, are more likely to have a fatal outcome if a gun is to hand.

Almost two-thirds of gunshot deaths occur in the home and few of these involve self-protection. Less than 2 per cent of homicides are deemed legally justifiable, over 80 per cent occurring in the course of arguments or altercations. In cases of assault, people tend to reach for the most deadly weapon readily available and if this happens to be a gun, this is that is likely to be used. Ready access to firearms is clearly a major danger in households given to violence. In the home, handguns are about three times as often the cause of death as shotguns or rifles combined.

The gun culture is, of course, perpetuated and fostered by the natural interest children show in these objects. But in the light of the tragedies at Hungerford, Dunblane in Scotland, and Port Arthur in Tasmania, there are indications that governments are beginning to see the need for a review of gun legislation.

Children from other countries

Children of ethnic minorities may have health problems that are relatively uncommon in Britain. Many members of these groups have been born in Britain, but this does not necessarily eliminate these special risks, some of which are genetic or cultural in origin. If you are a member of an ethnic minority there are certain medical points you may find worth reading about, even if you are already familiar with them. The most important of them are of genetic origin and you will find it helpful to read the article GENETICS – AN OUTLINE for explanations of the homozygous and heterozygous state.

Afro-Caribbean people are far more likely to suffer from SICKLE CELL DISEASE than Europeans. This is a recessive genetic disorder in which part of the haemoglobin in the red blood cells is abnormal. The sickle cell trait – the heterozygous state, in which only one of the pair of genes is affected – usually causes no symptoms. But it is present in 40 per cent of East African, 20 per cent of West Africans, and 20 per cent of people from the West Indies. In view of these frequencies, it is fairly common for two people with the recessive trait to marry so that any child may have both genes. Statistics show that about one Afro-Caribbean child in 400 is homozygous and will have the disease. Because of this risk, every Afro-Caribbean woman should have a blood test for sickle cell trait. Your newborn babies should also be tested. Blood can be taken for this purpose from the umbilical cord and will cause no pain or ill effects.

If you have sickle cell disease, you should know all about it and how it can affect you. You should certainly be under the care of a hospital haematology department who will give you all the information you need. You must wear a bracelet or amulet indicating the problem.

Another group of haemoglobin disorders affecting ethnic minorities are the thalassaemias (see THALASSAEMIA). These feature a persistence of the fetal type of haemoglobin. This, unfortunately, has a shorter life than the normal 120 days, so ANAEMIA is common. Babies and infants fail to thrive and may suffer other undesirable effects: The thalassaemias are commonest among people from Cyprus, Turkey, Italy and parts of China and Asia. There are two kinds, thalassaemia major (homozygous form) and

thalassaemia minor (heterozygous form) and the significance of these is very different.

About 17 per cent of the Cypriots living in North London have the minor form of thalassaemia. If two such people marry, there is a one in four chance that they will produce a child with the very serious major form.

There are various other much less common haemoglobin abnormalities, some of which are combinations of sickle cell disease and thalassaemia. In general, these are less serious than the homozygous forms of either of these disorders. They may affect some people from Asian, Arab and Far Eastern countries.

Vietnamese and Chinese people may suffer from the condition of glucose-6-phosphate dehydrogenase deficiency. The cause is an X-linked gene mutation, so is largely confined to men. The shortage of this enzyme means that when certain drugs are taken the blood partially breaks down (haemolysis). This can happen with anti-malarial drugs and with sulphonamides and other drugs. There is also a Mediterranean form of the disease in which the blood problem occurs when broad beans are eaten. This is called favism. A very mild form can affect some African people.

A number of non-genetic disorders have been found, in general, to be commoner in certain ethnic minority groups than in the general population. Iron-deficiency anaemia is especially common among Asian and West Indian infants, probably because of prolonged breast-feeding. Rastafarians may also be at risk from anaemia.

Vitamin D deficiency may arise in some groups as a result of inadequate exposure to sunlight because of the cultural necessity to cover up the body. In some cases, this, together with the use of cow's milk on weaning, has led to RICKETS.

Umbilical hernia is especially common in Afro-Caribbean babies. The traditional method of treating this well-known condition – by binding a coin over it – it more likely to make things worse than better. The condition is usually self-correcting.

Children arriving in Britain from other countries, or children who have been on an extended visit to their countries of origin, may be suffering from, or incubating, a number of diseases. These include:

- malaria
- amoebic dysentery
- chronic DIARRHOEA
- roundworms
- hookworms
- typhoid
- unexplained fevers

Most of these will occur only in children who have been exposed to poor hygiene.

Children's concept of death

A child's idea of death comes from observation of how grown-ups react to death. This is how children acquire emotional reactions. Logic has nothing to do with it. The child draws inferences, which may be very powerful, simply from seeing how we react. This is an important point for those dealing with older children who are dying. Such children may be terrified by seeing that we are horrified or even severely distressed.

Children between about 3 and 5 years have no concept of the finality of death. They see death as a departure, probably temporary, and, unless they have been frightened by thoughtless adults, have no sense of the gravity of the situation. They do, of course, suffer exactly the same kind of pain as anyone else, from the loss of someone precious to them. But they do not anticipate their own deaths in terms of loss, as adults often do.

Around the age of 8 or 9, children come to an adult understanding of death and an awareness that it comes to all of us. But exposure of a child, of any age, to the grief or distress of others, or allowing a young child to attend a funeral without a full explanation of what is happening, can be damaging. So, too, can refusal to discuss the subject of death. The child cannot understand what has happened but will always be acutely aware that something very important is going on. Refusal to discuss it, or even deflection of the child's questions, establishes a strong taboo – a sense that the subject is forbidden, mysterious, pro-

hibited – which will remain with the child for the rest of its life.

Children, like adults, need to be allowed to express their distress and sense of loss when a parent dies. Shared mourning is best, but you may find this difficult if you are not prepared to face up to the need for a frank and open discussion on what has happened. This, as we shall see, is an essential part of the handling of a child's grief. You should understand that if the grief is not allowed to show itself in the normal and natural way, it will come out in other ways – in moodiness, aggressive or resentful behaviour, sometimes lying or stealing, and in physical symptoms.

Mourning must be worked through and completed. But the 'stiff upper lip' syndrome, may prevent this. And even in a child, the failure to complete mourning may result in persistent depression and other ill effects. Children mourn naturally and will do so if allowed. But the blunting of emotion, which you may experience for a long time after the bereavement, and your own difficulty in expressing your grief, may confuse them – perhaps lead them to think that you do not care. This is just one of the many difficulties you have to face when left with young children.

You are likely to feel that very young children are too young to understand what you say to them. This may be so, but something is likely to get through. If the child does not understand, no harm is done, but the very act of talking about the death is valuable and if the child observes your grief, he or she will share it.

See also BEREAVEMENT.

Choking

This is what happens when any solid or liquid material obstructs the air passages, especially at the opening to the voice box (the larynx). This is especially likely if solid material is inhaled, as may occur if a sudden, unexpected breath is taken during eating. Laughing with the mouth full is not a good idea. Children commonly choke on small objects they have put in their mouths.

If a small quantity of solid or liquid is inhaled, coughing occurs and the resulting repeated blasts of air usually drive out the unwanted material. Total blockage is uncommon, but a large foreign body, and the resulting swelling of the surrounding tissues may cause this. Death from suffocation is then inevitable unless the obstruction can be overcome. Attempts to dislodge the obstruction should be made by suddenly and forcibly squeezing up under the ribs in a bear hug from behind or rapid upper abdominal thrusts from the front (Heimlich manoeuvre). If this fails, the only hope of saving life lies in boldly cutting an opening into the windpipe, in the midline, on the front of the neck just above the notch on the top of the breast bone (see TRACHEOSTOMY, and **Safety and First Aid** in the introductory section).

Chromosomal disorders see
GENETICS – AN OUTLINE.

Circumcision

If you are the mother of a baby boy you may well be worried about whether or not he needs circumcision. Very likely, much of what you have read on the subject has served only to increase your confusion. Here are the basic facts.

Circumcision is the removal of the male foreskin, the loose fold of skin which encloses the head, or glans, of the penis. It is probably the oldest recorded surgical procedure and dates back at least 4,000 years. Two of the great religions, Judaism and Islam, require ritual circumcision – for orthodox Jews on the eighth day of life and for Muslims before the age of 12. All males converted to Judaism must submit to circumcision, and the practice is so well ingrained that many Jews who have abandoned all other religious beliefs and practices will still opt for circumcision for their children. To the orthodox, the procedure is of high religious importance.

Circumcision is a controversial subject at international medical conferences and it is interesting to note that the operation is widely practised in societies in which surgery has to be paid for and quite rare in those in which surgical treatment is free. In spite of the published opinion of the American Academy of Pediatrics that routine circumcision was unnecessary, the practice has continued in the USA. There are no problems in arranging for circumcision in Harley Street, but NHS surgeons are rightly reluctant and usually require medical rather than purely social reasons. As a result, comparatively few British boys suffer this fate. In the 1970s, the British Medical Association condemned routine circumcision.

It is normal for the foreskin to be attached to the head of the penis, by fine strands of tissue, during the early months of life, and it is normal not to be able to pull it back. Whatever anyone may tell you, the fact that you can't do this is certainly not a reason for having your baby circumcised. The opening at the tip of the foreskin is normally quite small, but will almost always stretch in time.

Quite rarely, the opening is a mere pinpoint, so small that the foreskin balloons out when the baby is urinating. This is called phimosis and can lead to later trouble. This is the one unquestioned justification for circumcision. Back-pressure of urine is undesirable and can cause urinary tract infection and kidney damage. Circumcision eliminates this risk, but the risk exists only if the outlet is extremely narrow, tight and, usually, scarred.

Some time ago there was a report in the *American Journal of Pediatrics* claiming that uncircumcized boys were 10 times more likely to develop urinary tract infections than circumcised boys. This was widely reported in the public press and helped to strengthen the opinion of the American public that nature has somehow got the human anatomy wrong.

You will want to know what to do about a tight foreskin. Don't try to pull back the foreskin in babies or infants, but it will do no harm if you occasionally try gentle retraction in little boys. This will help to stretch the skin. Later, towards puberty, it does become important that the foreskin can be pulled right back so that the cheesy-looking and smelling material, smegma, which collects under it, can be washed away every day. Don't be in a hurry, and particularly don't force it back, as it may stick in the groove or neck behind the head of the penis. Full retraction should be achieved gradually and may take months. It should be possible by late adolescence to pull it right back without difficulty. If not, you should seek medical advice about circumcision.

One of the arguments put forward as a reason for universal circumcision is the suggestion that smegma can cause cancer of the penis and of the cervix in women. This idea is based on very dubious evidence, but, like most good stories, has been widely quoted and widely believed. It is not disputed that married Jewish women have a much lower incidence of cancer of the cervix than married Gentile women. We now know that the difference can be accounted for on the basis of the virus which causes cervical cancer – the human papillomavirus – which is known to be sexually transmitted. Jewish sexual laws and family tradition, and other factors, can partly explain the reduced incidence in Jewish women.

So far as cancer of the penis is concerned, it is true that this is almost unknown in circumcized men. But it is also almost unknown in uncircumcized men – only about 100 cases occur each year in Britain. Cancer of the penis nearly always starts under the foreskin in men with poor standards of personal hygiene. There is every reason to believe that normal standards of hygiene will prevent it.

American enthusiasm for circumcision remains undiminished. The latest American attack on the foreskin comes in the form of a suggestion, in a letter in the *New England Journal of Medicine*, that uncircumcized men are more likely to acquire HIV than the circumcized. Informed opinion in this country simply does not agree. Professor Lewis Spitz, Nuffield professor of paediatric surgery, states that if there is an increased risk, which is by no means proved, it relates merely to long exposure to material trapped under the foreskin, a risk easily avoided by normal daily washing.

Cleft lip and palate

During the early development of the fetus, the face forms by the fusion of a number of finger-like processes that grow out from the front end of the primitive tubular structure of the body. Cleft lip or cleft lip and palate is a developmental defect caused by the failure of these processes fully to fuse together. It occurs in about one baby in a thousand.

The cleft lip is a gap in the upper lip, which may be no more than a small notch, or which may extend right up to join one nostril. Cleft palate is a gap in the roof of the mouth, which may partially or completely divide the palate. Sometimes there are two gaps in the upper lip, extending up to both nostrils and these may be associated with partial or complete cleft palate. Cleft palate may occur on its own, without cleft lip.

The surgical management of these conditions has improved immeasurably in recent years and it is now rare to see obvious residual deformity (HARE LIP) from cleft lip. Babies with cleft palate cannot breast-feed and must be fed from a bottle. Although good surgical repair is possible, usually around 1 year of age, there may be a long-term problem with speech articulation. Speech therapy is often necessary.

Club foot

This rare deformity, present at birth, affects the shape or position of one or both feet. The commonest type is called talipes equinovarus and in this the entire foot, including the heel, is twisted inwards, so that the plane of the sole is almost vertical. The arch of the foot is also greatly exaggerated.

Talipes is thought to be caused by a lack of balance in the muscles which stabilise the foot, and the condition has a definite familial tendency. Treatment must begin at, or as soon as possible after, birth, and consists of repetitive deliberate manipulations in which the inturn and the high arching are gently but positively corrected, followed sometimes by the application of a splint. If started during the first week of life, splintage may not be necessary and you may, after careful instruction, be able to continue the manipulation yourself. If the start of treatment is delayed for three weeks, splintage will probably be required. Longer delay means greater difficulty in correction. Failure to achieve full correction at 6 months of age means that surgery will be needed.

Coarctation of the aorta

This is a rare condition, present at birth, in which a short section of the main artery of the body, the aorta, is severely narrowed. The usual site for the narrowing is just beyond the point at which the arteries to the head and arms branch. As a result, there is high blood pressure in the upper part of the body and low blood pressure in the lower parts. Other congenital heart defects may accompany coarctation.

Babies with coarctation may suddenly develop heart failure and collapse and may require urgent supportive treatment and then surgery to open up the narrowed segment. In lesser degrees of coarctation, surgery, if necessary, may be deferred until the age of about 6. Some cases develop severe high blood pressure. Surgery for coarctation is usually very successful but the condition can recur. The operation carries a small risk of paralysis, but the same small risk exists if the operation is not done.

Coffee patches see CAFÉ AU LAIT PATCHES.

Colds

There are many superstitions about the common cold. The outdoor life builds up resistance, so do cold baths; colds are less common in dry climates; 'feed a cold and starve a fever'; whisky and lemon juice cures a cold; colds are caused by exposure to cold air, by getting our feet wet, by wearing wet clothes; and so on. All wrong. Colds are certainly much commoner in winter than in summer, but this has nothing to do with the lower external temperature or with wet extremities. The efficiency of the immune system may be compromised by exposure to cold. The feeling of cold during the incubation period of the infection is due to a higher resetting of the body thermostat by substances produced by the immune system in response to the cold viruses.

Most surprising of all, to most people, is that the old saying 'coughs and sneezes spread diseases' is a myth. This is certainly true of diseases like chickenpox, which are predominantly spread by aerosol, but it is quite misleading in connection with the common cold. Colds are caused by viruses spread, not primarily by coughs and sneezes, but mainly by hand to hand contact. The route of transfer of cold viruses is from the nose of the sufferer to his or her hands; from there, directly or indirectly, to the hands of a susceptible child; and from there to the new victim's eyes or nose. The mouth is not an effective means of entry.

We do not acquire useful resistance to cold viruses because there are over 200 of them and they are constantly changing (mutating). But you can cut down the number of your colds, and those of your children, by acting on your new knowledge. Watch how a person with a cold contaminates his or her environment by face-to-hand-to-surroundings contact. Don't touch anything touched by the sniffler. But if you can't avoid touching or being touched, keep your hands away from your own face until you have washed them thoroughly. If you have a cold yourself, remember the route of spread and spare your children the misery you are currently suffering.

There is no practical treatment for a cold. Drugs called interferons, which are actually natural body substances, can cure some colds, but they are very expensive and have some side-effects such as nose bleeds. Colds can often be aborted at the earliest stage by taking about 1500 mg (1.5 g) of the antioxidant vitamin C (ascorbic acid). This 'mops up' the damaging oxygen free radicals caused by the viruses. Doses of vitamin C smaller than about 1000 mg don't work.

Incidentally, if you are into antioxidant preventive treatment it is important to remember that the other major antioxidant vitamin, vitamin E, can be seriously toxic to babies and small children in large doses. The white cells that combat infection (phagocytes) use free radicals to kill germs; if you overdo the mopping up in babies, a severe bowel infection may result.

Cold sores see HERPES SIMPLEX.

Colic

This is the pain caused by stretching of any tubular structure in the body. The intestine is very sensitive to stretching, and when the normal process (peristalsis) by which the contents are passed along, is impeded, segments become ballooned and stretched. The result is colicky pain which peaks, as the bowel is stretched, and then passes off, as it relaxes. The same effect can be caused if the intestine contracts strongly around a hard object, such as a lump of undigested food.

Bowel colic is usually caused by inadequately chewed food, but may occur in genuine intestinal obstruction. In biliary and renal colic the pain is caused by contraction of the bile duct or kidney-to-bladder tube (ureter) around a stone.

Children are quite susceptible to colic, especially if they gulp down their food without chewing it properly. Unripe apples are a common cause of colic. The term 'colic' is often applied wrongly in the case of children (see COLIC, INFANTILE).

Colic, infantile see introductory section (Baby care).

Colour blindness

Complete colour blindness, with no perception of any colours, is almost unknown, so the term is misleading. Difficulty in identifying some colours is, however, common, especially in males. There is variable difficulty in perceiving one or more of red, green or blue. This defect is almost always inherited, the gene concerned being recessive and residing on the X chromosome (see GENETICS – AN OUTLINE). Males have only one X chromosome; females have two. Males suffer the defect if their solitary X chromosome carries the gene; females have a colour problem only if *both* of their X chromosomes carry the gene. So, although almost 10 per cent of males have some degree of colour perception defect, the condition is rare in women, less than 0.5 per cent being affected.

Colour perception defect can also be acquired and is a fairly common consequence of optic nerve fibre damage from any cause, such as multiple sclerosis, DIABETES or drug or chemical toxicity. In cases of one-sided damage, a comparison of the intensity of colour of an object, as viewed by each eye, will show an obvious difference. Colour perception defect from such causes is very rare in children.

Colour perception can be tested in various ways. The Ishihara, multidot test is a quick and useful screening test. People with normal colour vision see one sequence of numbers, those with colour problems see another. Colour matching is also a sensitive test of perception, as is placing in sequence a large series of discs of gradually changing colour value.

For certain occupations, normal colour perception is needed and boys with ambitions to join the Armed Forces should be tested well in advance. Colour perception defect is not an absolute bar to recruitment, but denies entry to certain occupations and trades. Commercial flying calls for good colour perception.

Compulsive reading see HYPERLEXIA.

Comforters see SECURITY OBJECT.

Conduct disorder

This article is not concerned primarily with behaviour disturbances in young children, but with established delinquency in adolescents. For information on the former, see AUTISM, HYPERACTIVITY, JEALOUSY, MANIPULATIVE BEHAVIOUR, MISBEHAVIOUR, NAIL BITING, PICA, SLEEP PROBLEMS, TICS. See also introductory section.

'Conduct disorder' is an arbitrary term for a persistent pattern of behaviour that consistently violates the rights of others or the accepted norms of society. Activities typical of conduct disorder include theft, repeatedly running away from home, firesetting, breaking and entering, destroying property, cruelty to people or animals, a tendency to initiate physical aggression and the use of a weapon in a fight.

Conduct disorder results mainly from defective early programming of the child by parents and others whose own problems and upbringing have prevented them from forming socially acceptable values. Many such adults have, through life disappointment and frustration, developed strongly antisocial values. Alcoholism, marital strife and crude machismo attitudes expressed in physical violence often feature in their backgrounds. Tragically, their own bitter experience is all too often repeated in their children.

The affected children tend, unconsciously, to accept and act out their parents' antisocial attitudes, and this early programming becomes built-in, and is very influential and very difficult to displace. Other factors known to cause conduct disorder include rejection by parents, harsh institutional treatment and frequent changes of guardianship.

The treatment of conduct disorder is difficult, but a major advance has resulted from the proper recognition that this is not a matter of inherent wickedness, but rather a question of defective early conditioning. Life experience will often, in time, bring a realization of the advantages of social conformity, and conduct disorder is less prevalent in the middle-aged and elderly than in adolescents and young adults. Psychoanalysis is of little value. Skilled and enlightened counselling can often help. But the greatest success, at least in the United States, has been achieved by group therapy based on reformed delinquent peers to whom young people with conduct disorders are willing to turn for understanding, advice and emotional support.

See also JUVENILE DELINQUENCY.

Congenital

Any feature that is present at birth can be said to be congenital. A congenital disorder need not be hereditary or of genetic origin, although many are. Conditions acquired during fetal life are congenital and these include defects caused by infections passed on by the mother or even those acquired during the process of birth.

Congenital artery narrowing see
COARCTATION OF THE AORTA.

Congenital biliary atresia

This is a condition, present at birth, in which the bile ducts are abnormally narrowed so that bile has difficulty in escaping from the liver. It is important to make the diagnosis as early as possible as this affects the outcome. The condition must not be confused with other and commoner causes of JAUNDICE in newborn babies. If necessary, a sample (biopsy) of liver may have to be taken to confirm the diagnosis.

Treatment is to re-establish bile drainage by surgical operation. If this is done within two months of birth the outlook is usually excellent.

Congenital cataract see
CATARACT.

Congenital dislocation of the hip
see HIP, CONGENITAL DISLOCATION OF.

Congenital heart disease

This means any heart abnormality present at birth. About seven babies in every 1000 are affected, sometimes very mildly, sometimes severely. Usually the cause is unknown, but the commonest known cause is maternal RUBELLA occurring early in the pregnancy. There may be an opening in the inner wall of the heart (see HOLE IN THE HEART), a narrowing of the heart valves or of the outlet arteries or abnormal shunts of blood between different parts of the heart. There may also be a combination of defects (see FALLOT'S TETRALOGY).

Heart disease interferes with the normal supply of properly oxygenated blood to the body. Because poorly oxygenated blood is bluish, the result may be blueness of the skin (CYANOSIS). There may be breathlessness, poor growth, poor muscular development, thickening of the finger-tips (clubbing) and limitation of exertion. Nowadays, surgical correction is available for nearly all types of severe congenital heart disease and the outlook is usually good. See also EISENMENGER'S COMPLEX, PATENT DUCTUS ARTERIOSUS.

Congenital malformations

These are bodily malformations present at birth, caused by interference with normal development. This commonly occurs at the early embryo stage, but may occur later. Congenital malformations are not necessarily obvious at birth. Some do not become apparent until later in life. They may be single or multiple, but many of them are minor and of little or no importance.

Major malformations commonly occur at the earliest stages, even at the time of conception, and experts estimate that as many as 15 per cent of fetuses have major abnormalities. Very few of these survive to be born live and are aborted early in the pregnancy. In many such cases the woman concerned may not even be aware that she has been pregnant. Many factors can cause congenital malformations. These include genetic abnormalities, illness in the mother, infection of the fetus, especially with certain viruses, radiation, drugs and alcohol (see FETAL ALCOHOL SYNDROME).

Congenital malformations should be distinguished from congenital deformations. These are abnormalities, often temporary, caused by restriction of freedom of movement of the fetus so that its body is pushed out of shape. Deformations include CLUB FOOT, congenital dislocation of the hip, sideways bending of the spine (scoliosis), WRY NECK (torticollis), distortion of the skull and asymmetry of the jaw. Deformations are usually correctable by suitable manipulation and sometimes splintage immediately after birth. See HIP, CONGENITAL DISLOCATION OF.

Congenital pyloric stenosis

This is a rare condition, present at birth, in which the outlet of the stomach – the muscle ring or sphincter known as the pylorus – is abnormally thick, strong and tight. The condition affects about one baby in 3,000, boys more often than girls. In about 10 per cent of cases there is a known family history. As a result of the obstruction food cannot readily pass from the stomach to the small intestine and the baby fails to gain weight. When the obstruction is severe there is forceful VOMITING starting two to six weeks after birth. In addition, the baby tends to be totally constipated or to pass only a few loose stools and is often dehydrated. Often the upper part of the abdomen is distended and careful observation may show visible movement of the bowels under the surface of the abdominal wall.

Any baby under 2 months of age who shows constant vomiting, and not just the normal regurgitation after feeds, should be considered to have pyloric stenosis. An expert paediatrician can usually feel the thickened pylorus, known as the 'olive'. Happily, the treatment of this condition, although involving a simple surgical procedure known as Ramstedt's operation, is highly successful. First, fluid loss is corrected and the stomach is emptied. Then a small incision is made through the thickened muscle ring, but not through the inner lining. The results are excellent.

Conjunctivitis see RED EYES.

Constipation

Genuine constipation is a disorder of civilized societies and is unknown among peoples whose diet is largely vegetable in content, with a high fibre intake. Such people are free from many of the colonic disorders suffered by those of us who enjoy more expensive diets containing a high percentage of refined foods.

There is a widespread belief that the failure to empty the bowels at least once a day is dangerous. This is untrue. Constipation causes symptoms, but they are not the result of the absorption of 'toxins' from the bowel. These symptoms – a sense of fullness, headache, furred tongue, loss of appetite, depression – can be produced by packing the rectum with sterile cotton wool. The toxin fallacy is often imposed by anxious parents on their children.

Fastidious parents may feel that it is essential to get rid of 'unclean' excreta every day, and inevitably transmit this anxiety to their children, who are often dosed with laxatives. This can turn an imaginary disorder into a real one. The way to cure constipation is to ensure that the child has adequately bulky stools by replacing refined carbohydrate, in the diet, with foods containing much vegetable fibre such as fruit, vegetables and bran-containing cereals. This will produce bulky, soft stools and regular motions. See also Potty training in **Baby Care** (introductory section).

Contact lenses

Clear vision during the first few years of life is essential if the eye/brain function is to develop normally (see AMBLYOPIA). There are some cases in which only contact lenses will provide sufficiently clear vision to allow this. These include:

- very high degrees of short sight (myopia)
- large differences in the focus of the two eyes
- irregularities of the outer lens of the eye, the cornea
- the severe focusing error resulting from removal of a congenital cataract (see CATARACT)

Close supervision and regular ophthalmic examination are essential and, in most cases, as soon as the visual system is mature – around the age of 8 – glasses can be used instead.

After the age of 8 years, contact lenses are worn in cases of severe aversion to glasses or for cosmetic reasons. It is seldom justified to fit contact lenses as a replacement for normal glasses in a child below the age of about 14. Such young children cannot be expected to remove their contact lenses simply because they are causing discomfort, fogging or misting of vision. But these are symptoms which might indicate sight-threatening corneal damage. Such fogging, coming on after a period of clear vision, is never the result of a wrong prescription or a defective fit. By about 16 year, a responsible child can usually be trusted to wear contact lenses safely, but close supervision is necessary to ensure that the rules about wearing time and high standards of hygiene are maintained. Such children should be reminded that trouble arising from overwear and insufficient care with cleaning of lenses and containers are the commonest causes of having to revert to glasses.

Convulsions

A fit may involve the whole, or part of, the body and may be followed by loss of consciousness. In the major fit of EPILEPSY (grand mal), there is a sudden violent contraction of most of the voluntary muscles of the body (tonic contractions), followed by relaxation and then a succession of smaller jerky contractions (clonic contractions), persisting for a minute or so.

Convulsions occur in many brain conditions, of which epilepsy is only one. In children, the commonest type are FEBRILE CONVULSIONS and these do not imply epilepsy. They are caused by fever, especially prolonged high temperature, and they should be prevented, if possible, by bringing the temperature down by treatment of the cause and by sponging the body with tepid water. There is reason to believe that repeated febrile convulsions might predispose to epilepsy later in life. ABSENCE ATTACKS sometimes involve minor convulsions and may progress to major epilepsy.

Corneal softening see
KERATOMALACIA.

Coronary artery disease in
children see KAWASAKI DISEASE.

Cot death see SUDDEN INFANT
DEATH SYNDROME.

Cough

A cough is an automatic reflex to rid the lungs of potentially dangerous semi-solid material or liquid in the air tubes (bronchial tubes) or voice box (larynx). In coughing, a deep breath is taken and the vocal cords are pressed tightly together. The diaphragm is then forced upwards, compressing the air in the lungs, and the vocal cords are sharply released so that a blast of air passes upwards from all parts of both lungs. This usually carries out any material, such as excess mucus, sputum or small foreign bodies. Many persistent (chronic) chest disorders feature regular coughing because of the production of excessive bronchial secretions.

Coughs should not automatically be checked, as the cough is part of the defence mechanism of the respiratory system. But tiring and distressing coughing in children over 1 year, not otherwise unwell, may helpfully be relieved by a mild antihistamine expectorant mixture such as Galenphol.

Craniopharyngioma

This is a rare brain tumour affecting mainly children. The craniopharyngioma arises from a group of primitive cells in the region of the pituitary gland, which are present in the early embryo and which, instead of disappearing, have persisted and developed into a kind of non-malignant cyst-like swelling. Because pressure rises within the skull and damage may occur to the pituitary gland, the affected child may have HEADACHES and visual loss and may show delayed physical and mental development. As the tumour grows, the neurological effects become more marked. Sudden, projectile VOMITING, often without NAUSEA, is common.

A Computed Tomography (CT) scan or Magnetic Resonance Imaging (MRI) easily shows up this kind of tumour. The only effective treatment is surgical removal.

Cricothyrotomy see
TRACHEOSTOMY.

Cri du chat syndrome

This sad but very uncommon genetic disorder is caused by the absence of the short arm on chromosome number 5. Affected babies are small with very small brains (microcephaly), have round faces with downward-sloping eyes, low and abnormally shaped ears, short necks and often heart defects. They usually have severe LEARNING DIFFICULTY and most of them die before reaching adult life. The condition is characterized by a peculiar, high-pitched, mewing cry, very like that of a kitten.

Croup

This is an inflammation of the main air tubes to the lungs. The disease is known to doctors as laryngo-tracheo-bronchitis. It affects young children and causes swelling of the lining of these passages. The result is a partial obstruction to air flow through the voice box (larynx) so that breathing and coughing are difficult, harsh and painful. Breathing in is often more difficult than breathing out, causing the characteristic crowing sound known as 'inspiratory stridor'. There is often a typical 'barking' cough.

Croup was common in the days of DIPHTHERIA but is now rare and is usually caused by a parainfluenza virus infection, causing inflammatory swelling of the mucous membrane lining of the voice box (larynx) and the windpipe (trachea). The child, usually 6 months to 2 years of age, may become very restless and alarmed, with a fast pulse rate, heaving of the shoulders, and even some blueness of the skin (CYANOSIS).

Severe croup may lead to life-threatening airway obstruction and, in such a case, it may be necessary to make an artificial opening into the trachea, just below the larynx (TRACHEOSTOMY). More often, the condition requires no more than inhalation of humidified air and other general medical measures. In an emergency you can put the child in a closed, warm bathroom with all the hot taps running, while waiting for the doctor or ambulance.

Crowing cough see CROUP.

Crying in infancy see
introductory section (Baby care).

Cryptorchidism

This exotic-sounding word just means 'undescended testicle'. Literally, it means 'hidden testicle' and it affects about one boy in 40. The testicles develop in the abdomen and should pass down temporary canals (the inguinal canals) into the scrotum by the time of birth. If either testicle fails to descend, or to be brought down, before puberty, the higher temperature in the abdomen interferes with normal sperm production and the testicle will be permanently sterile. Testicles retained in the abdomen are also more likely to develop cancer later. For these reasons you should always seek medical advice if you cannot feel two testicles in the scrotum. Feel gently: boys of any age don't appreciate having their testicles squeezed.

Curvature of the spine see
KYPHOSIS, LORDOSIS.

Cuts and grazes

Minor injuries of this kind are inevitable in childhood, and sympathy and loving comfort are far more important in their management than medical expertise. Careful cleansing and removal of any foreign material by gentle dabbing with cotton wool soaked in warm water, with a drop of Dettol or Cetavlon, careful drying, an Elastoplast dressing and, above all, lots of fuss, are all that is usually required. Any sign of persistent inflammation should, of course, be reported to your doctor.

Cyanosis

This is blueness of an area of the skin due to the presence of blood that is not carrying enough oxygen. Fully oxygenated blood is a bright red colour and imparts a healthy pinkness to the skin. Blood whose oxygen has been used up is a dark reddish-blue colour and, through the skin, looks a dusky blue.

Cyanosis may occur because the blood is stagnant and is not being returned quickly enough to the lungs for re-oxygenation, or it may be due to inadequate oxygenation from asphyxia or lung disease. Cyanosis is a common feature of some forms of CONGENITAL HEART DISEASE in which blood is shunted away from the lungs. BLUE BABY is so called because affected babies have cyanosis. In rare cases, cyanosis may be due to poisoning with substances that interfere with the oxygenation of the blood.

Cyanosis must never be ignored. It is a clear sign that something potentially serious is wrong, in most cases either with the heart or with the lungs, and must be put right. Delay in reporting cyanosis to your doctor is never justified.

Cystic fibrosis

his is a genetic disease that occurs in about 1 white child in about 2,000 live births. The condition is recessive and does not occur unless both parents contribute a defective gene (see GENETICS – AN OUTLINE). It is much less common in non-white children. Cystic fibrosis affects the millions of tiny mucus and water secreting glands of the lining surfaces of the body. The salivary glands, the glands of the intestine, the pancreas, the gall bladder, the lungs and the skin either produce excessive quantities of secretion, or a thick, sticky mucinous discharge which clogs them or obstructs the passages into which they normally open.

Babies with cystic fibrosis often get early bowel blockage from sticky contents (meconium). Others have swollen abdomens and pass frequent oily stools. Appetite is very good but growth is slow. About half have lung complications due to blockage of the bronchial tubes with excessive mucus secretions and plugs of thick muco-pus. There is a troublesome cough, wheezing and difficulty in breathing and the chest becomes barrel-shaped from the effort of breathing. Sinusitis and nasal problems are common. The sweat contains excessive salt and the skin may be powdered with dried sweat. This is a common early sign of cystic fibrosis.

Children with cystic fibrosis suffer growth retardation and delayed puberty and cannot participate normally in games and sport. They may suffer collapse of a lung, heart failure, cirrhosis of the liver, pancreatitis and DIABETES. Medical management involves skilled and comprehensive care and much-needed psychological support, both for the child and the parents.

In 1989 the gene for cystic fibrosis was found on chromosome number 7 and cloned. Since then over 230 different mutations of the gene have been identified. There is a simple test, involving only a mouthwash, by which carriers of the condition can be detected. If a woman is pregnant and both she and the father test positive for the gene, there is one chance in four that the baby will inherit both positive genes and have the disease. Whether this has happened can be determined, early in the pregnancy, by the chorionic villus sampling test. If the misfortune is confirmed at that stage, the option of terminating the pregnancy arises.

Dandruff

This condition features scaliness of the scalp from flakes of dead skin, the scales being most conspicuous when loosened and separated by combing or brushing the hair. Significant dandruff represents an increase in the normal rate of scale shedding, often because the skin is mildly inflamed and itchy from various causes.

One of the commonest forms of dandruff is known as SEBORRHOEIC DERMATITIS. The cause of this condition is unknown, but some dermatologists believe it may be due to a yeast fungus *Pityrosporum ovale*. It is usually worse in winter and is often so mild that little is seen except scaling. It may, however, be severe, with yellowish-red, greasy, scaly patches along the hair-line and spreading to other areas of skin such as the eyelids, causing BLEPHARITIS, or the external ears. In babies, mild seborrhoeic dermatitis is very common and is known as 'cradle cap'. It usually responds well to a mild baby shampoo.

Dandruff in older children responds well to the use of medicated shampoos, especially those containing selenium. Selsun shampoo is a popular remedy. Seborrhoeic dermatitis responds well to corticosteroid ointments and, in some sufferers anti-yeast drugs are effective.

Deafness

Hearing difficulty can be a matter of critical importance for young children, because so much of their mental and educational development depends on information obtained by hearing. A child severely deaf from birth will never learn to speak unless the condition is detected early and special efforts are made to compensate. So early diagnosis of deafness is of critical importance if irremediable developmental loss is to be avoided. All babies should be screened for deafness at the age of about 8 months by a family doctor or at a 'well baby' clinic. Those failing the routine test should be referred to a specialist at an audiology clinic for fuller investigation.

But if, even before that age, you have reason to believe that your baby's hearing is below normal, you should report the matter at once and insist on specialist attention. Experienced doctors have learned always to take seriously a parent's claim that the baby is deaf and, in such cases, to assume that the parent is right until the matter is proved otherwise. No one has a better opportunity to assess a baby's hearing than the parent.

Deafness in childhood may be due to one of a number of causes. In rare cases, the external ear canal or the small bones in the middle ear fail to develop. More often, the problem is in the deeper part of the ear – the cochlea – or in the acoustic nerve. These part may also suffer a defect of development. Sometimes the defect is hereditary. The commonest cause of congenital deafness is infection of the fetus, especially with the RUBELLA virus, early in the pregnancy, when the inner ear system is developing. This is complete by the fourth month of pregnancy. RHESUS INCOMPATIBILITY, in cases in which a rhesus negative mother is carrying a rhesus positive baby, can also lead to deafness. If severe, the resulting jaundice can damage the acoustic nerves.

The period of a few days from immediately before to immediately after birth, is especially dangerous and babies may be at risk from various causes that can lead to deafness. These include:

- severe maternal toxaemia of pregnancy
- PREMATURITY

- oxygen lack before and during birth
- birth injury

Deafness acquired after birth, although commoner than congenital deafness, is often less severe. It is generally due to middle ear infection that has led to the condition of secretory OTITIS MEDIA or GLUE EAR. In this condition, a sticky secretion in the middle ear interferes with the free movement of the tiny bones that convey the sound vibrations from the ear drum to the inner ear. Such acquired deafness in young children can also have serious effects on mental and speech development and must be detected as early as possible.

> Severe deafness in a baby is nearly always suspected by the parents within the first year of life. Deaf babies often seem unusually placid and do not respond to loud noises. Up to the age of about 6 months, babies who can hear will react to an unexpected loud noise by the 'startle' or Moro reflex – a sudden jerky extension of the limbs and spine, followed by a quick folding movement of the arms across the chest. After this age the child simply turns his or her head in the direction of the sound. Toddlers may be tested by observing their response to speech or to musical sounds from a xylophone. Children born partially deaf can often partially understand speech by lipreading. This can mislead you. But such children will show unusual concentration on the lips of the speaker, and this can give a clue to what is happening.

Once a suspicion of deafness has been aroused you must see to it that the child is seen by an expert in an Ear, Nose and Throat or specialist audiology department, so that the cause can be discovered and remedial action taken. Early diagnosis, treatment of 'glue ear' by the insertion of grommets, and of other conditions when possible, and the use of hearing aids, often for both ears, can do much to prevent the harmful effects of early deafness in children.

Death of a child

No one who has not experienced it can ever know what the death of a child means to the bereaved. For many, it is the most terrible loss suffered in the whole of their lives. Others seem to be able to assimilate it and live on, apparently unchanged. The overall response seems to differ in different countries and cultures. In North America, for instance, the loss of a child is regarded as a less serious blow than it is in Israel, where the death of a child is considered by many to be more serious than the death of a spouse. Studies done at the Hadassah Medical Centre in Jerusalem have shown that bereaved parents, even five years after the death of the child, often continue to suffer emotional disturbance.

There is some comfort in the knowledge that young children do not think of their own deaths. The stage of development of the higher brain functions makes it impossible, in the early years of life, for them to have any realistic concept of death. And even up the age of 8 or 9 they are not able to grasp the idea of the permanent ending of their own lives. So when young children die, although the loss and the grief may be dreadful to the bereaved, at least there is the consolation that the child suffered none of the fears and terrors which some older people have to face. We, all of us, at the very last, die easily, in exactly the same way as we fall asleep, but in the case of young children there is the additional fact that, even well before the final stages, they have no idea of what is happening. So we need not be distressed on their account, unless we are unable to hide our own distress from them.

The real burden falls on you the bereaved parent, and a grievous burden it is. We know that, for many, the loss of a child is a more severe blow and has more serious emotional consequences than the loss of a husband, wife or parent. We know that, while the death of a child may bring the grieving parents closer together, it may often have the opposite effect, and that separation is not uncommon. The gravity of the loss, of course, varies and we must recognise that some children are more precious than others.

Miscarriage and stillbirth, too, are in every sense bereavements, although those who have not experienced it may not think so. Almost all women who suffer stillbirth, miscarriage, or even, to a lesser extent, early abortion – loss of the fetus in the first few weeks of pregnancy – go through a period of mourning. This is easy to understand in the case of loss of a baby late in pregnancy. In that case, the baby is already an individual who may have been given a name, who has been felt moving, both by the mother and the father and who, quite often, has been ascribed a personality of its own. The parents' feelings of possession and kinship are already strong and their expectations, for the future, bright.

But even in the case of a much smaller fetus, emotional factors connected with one's attitudes to life and relationships are often stronger than one might expect and very few women are able to contemplate the loss of a tiny baby – even if the abortion has been deliberately sought – with indifference.

The effects of miscarriage and, particularly, stillbirth are often severe and may last for a very long time. It is common for the mother to mourn for over a year. In the case of the father the period of mourning is usually less – generally about six months. The loss of a baby often puts a heavy strain on the relationship of the parents and this is usually because the couple fail to share their grief. Quite often, the father seems to think that he should be very controlled and unemotional, and this leads the mother to think that he is uncaring. The death of a baby is the apparent cause of marital separation in about 6 per cent of cases. The evidence suggests, however, that in such cases there are usually other problems. Happily, for most, such an event has the opposite effect and serves to bring couples closer together.

Unfortunately, the situation is often made worse by the well-meaning but misguided behaviour of medical and nursing staff at the time of the event. There is, for instance, a widespread belief that it would be unnecessarily distressing, and perhaps even damaging, to the parents to see the dead baby. As a result, the baby is taken away and disposed of without the parents knowing what has happened to him or her. The causes of death, too, are often thought to be too painful to disclose. Strangulation by the umbilical cord, displaced placenta, diabetes in the mother, acquired congenital abnormalities, hereditary diseases, rhesus incompatibility – whatever the cause, a full explanation is thought by some medical people as likely merely to add to the grief of the parents.

These views are mostly wrong. When parents have never seen or touched their baby, they tend to feel he or she has never existed. They have feelings of great emptiness and commonly suffer prolonged depression because of their inability to grieve for a 'real' infant. Informed medical opinion is now in favour of encouraging parents to hold the dead baby and for them to ask detailed questions about the cause of death. Inappropriate guilt feelings about the latter are very common and these can only be finally put to rest by a full medical explanation.

A careful study of this problem was made in 1978 by a group of medical and nursing specialists. The group included midwives, obstetricians, paediatricians and psychiatrists, and the result of their study was to make some clear recommendations. They agreed that parents should see and hold the dead baby, that the baby should be named, that a formal funeral should be held in which the parents should take part, that the causes of death should be fully discussed and explained, and that any implications for future pregnancies should be made entirely clear. It was believed that if these recommendations were followed, the normal bereavement reactions would be possible and that, in time, full recovery would result.

Most women who have had a miscarriage or a stillbirth experience a strong desire to have another baby and about half of them are pregnant again within about a year. But there is plenty of evidence that women suffer much anxiety about, and sometimes adverse reactions to, the 'replacement baby'. If you are in this situation, it is imperative that you have good and understanding medical advice. Even in the case of an elective abortion, in spite of the circumstances, the element of bereavement is not necessarily negligible. Although, for most, the element of loss in abortion is quite a minor matter compared with the loss of a baby or a late miscarriage, women are often surprised by the strength of their own reactions.

Dehydration

This is a potentially dangerous state in which the normal water content of the body is reduced. Dehydration is usually due to excessive fluid loss which is not balanced by an appropriate increase in intake, but it may be due to intake deficiency alone. In children, it commonly results from prolonged DIARRHOEA and VOMITING and excessive sweating, as in long fevers.

Dehydration leads to an alteration in the vital balance of chemical substances dissolved in the blood and tissue fluids, especially sodium and potassium. The function of many cells is critically dependent on the maintenance of correct levels of these substances, and serious and often fatal effects result from any change. The risk is especially great in babies and infants whose high mortality, from conditions such as gastroenteritis, is largely attributable to dehydration.

The signs of dehydration are:

- a low-volume, concentrated urine
- dry, flushed skin
- sunken eyes
- dry mouth
- furred tongue
- confusion
- irritability
- loss of skin elasticity
- depression of the FONTANELLES
- lethargy

Dehydration can almost always be prevented, or its ill effects avoided, by ensuring an adequate fluid intake, preferably by mouth. In the early stages, water or other normal drinks will suffice. Severe dehydration is an emergency in small children and requires urgent treatment in hospital where suitable tests can be done and appropriate fluids can be given by intravenous infusion.

Delinquency

Children who habitually engage in criminal behaviour have been described as having psychopathic personalities, sociopathic disorders, or, more recently, antisocial personality disorder. None of these terms is satisfactory for they all imply that criminal behaviour is a form of mental disorder. Current psychiatric opinion tends to dismiss this. While it is true that antisocial behaviour can result from mental disorder, most young criminals do not have a mental or psychiatric disorder. Criminal behaviour is not now regarded as a disease.

Young people with an antisocial personality have a history of repeated acts which violate the rights of others. Other main features are:

- truancy from school
- habitual lying
- a poor work record
- low tolerance for boredom·
- addiction to reckless and dangerous activity
- early drug and alcohol abuse
- drug dealing
- promiscuous sexual behaviour
- prostitution
- aggressive family behaviour
- fighting and other forms of violence
- persistent stealing
- a lack of anxiety, guilt or depression in relation to offences
- a failure to be deterred by punishment

These young people do not have delusions, hallucinations, signs of irrational thinking or other manifestations of psychiatric disorder and their intelligence may be high. Educational levels vary widely. They may be charming to those who do not know them well. Closer acquaintances, however, especially those of the same sex, often find such people manipulative and excessively demanding.

Some psychiatrists make a distinction between antisocial personality disorder and common criminality, suggesting that people with an antisocial personality disorder are unable to conform to social norms while criminals are able to do so but choose not to. There is, however, little support for this view. Most people who engage in criminal behaviour have complete insight into their conduct and are perfectly aware of social norms. Their decision to breach these norms is based on their perception of their chances of getting away with it.

Peer pressure to conform, by engaging in criminal activity, often to 'prove oneself' to the gang, is an important cause of delinquency, and there is often a keen awareness of the conflict between the received values of the delinquents and those of the more prosperous members of society, against which much hostility may be felt. Educational or financial advantages are often resented, as a rationalization of the delinquent's personal failings and disadvantages.

Delinquents usually have a poor school record, with much truancy and resentment of authority. They leave school at the first opportunity, but seldom find good jobs. They are often impulsive and unable to defer immediate gratification. Interestingly, most delinquents learn, in due course, to conform to acceptable social patterns of behaviour.

The arguments about the causes of criminal behaviour have never been settled, but we know that a major factor is the nature and quality of the early childhood experience. In general, children who, from the beginning, have been loved and respected, have been made to feel secure in the affection of their parents, and who have been trained in patterns of conduct acceptable to society, such as honesty, truthfulness and respect for the rights and property of others, are very unlikely to become habitual criminals. On the other hand, those who have found that they are unwanted, who have been neglected physically and emotionally, who have been abused in various ways, and who have never been guided in acceptable conduct are forced to look out for themselves and to seek satisfaction in the only ways that seem available to them.

Such children commonly show early criminal behaviour and are in danger of embarking on a life of crime. Fortunately, for most of them, the peak of criminality is reached in late adolescence, after which life itself supplies the programming necessary to teach better ways of living. Those who do not amend their ways become a real danger to society. Most remain minor criminals engaging in car thefts, burglaries, robberies with violence, and so on. Some become confidence tricksters relying on their charm, persuasiveness and manipulative skills to talk the unwary into parting with their money.

Because the patterns of behaviour are established early and are correspondingly strong, correction is very difficult. Prison sentences or other forms of punishment seldom have any useful effect. Self-help groups, however, consisting of small numbers of people willing to acknowledge that they have a problem and ready to talk together about their difficulties, have been much more successful. Therapeutic communities have been established to try to correct these deficiencies. In these, antisocial young people can sometimes be rehabilitated by a process of analysis followed by social therapy in a stable, supportive and disciplined environment. All those participating have to share decisions and, at regular group meetings, discuss unacceptable behaviour and its consequences. Some of the results have been encouraging.

See also CONDUCT DISORDER, CHILD GUIDANCE, FAMILY THERAPY, MANIPULATIVE BEHAVIOUR.

Dental abscess

A dental abscess is a collection of pus around the root of a tooth. This results from infection and destruction of the pulp that fills the central cavity of the tooth. Infection usually follows tooth decay (dental caries), which destroy a small area of the hard outer enamel and the inner dentine, allowing bacteria to reach the pulp. This can happen very rapidly in young children and is especially common in those given sweetened comforters or neat syrups in feeding bottles. The carbohydrates are converted by bacteria to acids and these attack tooth enamel.

A dental abscess causes great pain and the gum around the tooth is tender, red and swollen. There may also be severe swelling of the face. Untreated, an abscess will work its way through the bone of the jaw to the gum surface, where it forms a gumboil (swelling). This may burst, discharging the pus into the mouth and relieving the pain. A child with a dental abscess should always be seen, without delay, by a dentist. ANTIBIOTICS may be needed. Permanent teeth can often be saved by skilled dental care.

Dermatitis

This is a general term meaning inflammation of the skin from any cause. Different kinds of dermatitis may have a similar appearance, but the causes can be very different. They include:

- infection by viruses, bacteria or fungi
- allergy to metals, plants, cosmetics, drugs, foodstuffs, etc
- chemical irritants
- solvents
- defatting agents
- poisons
- injury by insects, such as the scabies mite, or lice

Most of these forms are commoner in adults than in children. ECZEMA, or atopic dermatitis, is very common in children. It runs in families and is commonly associated with hay fever and ASTHMA.

The appearance of most forms of dermatitis is similar, with redness, blister formation, swelling, weeping and crusting. There is itching and burning and a strong impulse to scratch, which often makes the condition worse and may, in itself, keep it going.

In babies, the commonest form of dermatitis is NAPPY RASH, from ammonia formed from the urea in urine by bacteria. This is usually easily managed. Seborrhoeic dermatitis, or 'cradle cap' is a layer of greasy, brownish scales on the scalp or behind the ears of babies, which can be

removed with oil or shampooing. Persistent dermatitis calls for skilled medical attention.

Dermoid cysts

These are benign tumours occurring fairly commonly as skin swellings in the region around the eyes of children. They occur as a result of the abnormal infolding, early in embryonic life, of a small quantity of the surface tissue known as ectoderm. This is the outer of the three primitive layers of the embryo. Ectoderm develops into skin, hair, bones, teeth and nerve tissue and if some early ectoderm is buried in this way, a cyst will form which may contain any of these structures. The dermoid cyst is commonest on the face, around an eye, but may occur elsewhere.

Dermoid cysts are usually harmless and most of them, being near the surface, can easily be removed by a simple surgical operation. When such a cyst is opened it will usually contain horny (keratinous) material, such as is produced by skin, and a tight bundle of hairs. Sometimes rudimentary teeth and spicules of bone are found.

Development see introductory section (Child Development).

Diabetes

Diabetes affects one child in 500 below the age of 16. Untreated, it is a wasting disease in which sugar, the normal fuel of the body, cannot be properly used and is passed in large quantities in the urine. There is a great increase in the volume of urine produced and corresponding severe thirst. Fat and muscle protein are converted to sugar, so there is severe loss of weight. The disease is due to a shortage of insulin, the hormone produced by the pancreas. In the type of diabetes that affects young people (Type I diabetes), the damage to the pancreas is believed to be related to a virus infection that alters pancreatic tissue so as to render it unrecognizable as 'self' to the immune system. The insulin-producing pancreas cells are then attacked by the immune system and destroyed. A few cases, caught at this stage, have been cured by immuno-suppressive treatment, but almost always, the damage has been done before the problem is suspected.

A young person with Type I diabetes must be aware of the need to balance diet, exertion and insulin. At present, the latter can be given only by injection. He or she must also be well aware of the effects and dangers of a relative excess of insulin (hypoglycaemia). Diabetes requires lifelong treatment with insulin, constant checking of the level of sugar in the blood and in the urine, and regular medical checks for eye, kidney, and other complications.

Diabetes, like ASTHMA, is special among diseases in that so much responsibility for its control and management falls on the affected person, or, if he or she is too young, on the parents. Effective management of diabetes calls for an education in the subject. It is impossible to know too much about it and the earlier the child diabetic starts learning, the better. There is far more to be known than can be covered in a book of this kind, but a few general and practical points for young diabetics will not go amiss. A good book devoted entirely to the matter is, however, essential.

GIVING INJECTIONS

Insulin is always given half to three-quarters of an hour before meals, as time must be allowed for its absorption. Beginners may have some difficulty in drawing up insulin into the syringe. The secret is to inject some air into the bottle before withdrawing the piston of the syringe. If this isn't done, the removal of fluid leaves a partial vacuum in the bottle so that it gets harder and harder to get the solution out. Care should be taken to ensure that the needle point doesn't touch anything hard – it is easily blunted and this will make injections more painful.

It is often necessary to mix two insulins in the same syringe – a rapid and a medium or long-acting insulin. This means two different bottles and it will not be possible to inject air into the second one once insulin has been drawn up from the first. So the secret is first to inject air into the second

bottle, then pull out the needle and inject and withdraw insulin from the first bottle. Then push the needle into the bottle already pressurised and withdraw the required amount. Users must avoid getting any long-acting insulin into the bottle of rapid insulin or it will no longer be rapid and this could cause trouble.

WHERE AND HOW TO INJECT

The injections should not be done successively in the same place, as this may make the area hard and lumpy from fibrous tissue formation and, worse still, may lead to inadequate absorption from the site. There are plenty of places to chose from and the user should be taught to move from one to the next in a strict routine. Use the upper and outer parts of the arms and of the thighs, the outer parts of the buttocks and anywhere on the abdomen. Assuming the skin is clean and dry, no skin preparation is necessary. Thin diabetics may have to pinch up the skin; fat ones should stretch it. The needle must be firm on the syringe so that it will not come off while injecting. The metal part of the needle must never be touched as this will contaminate it and may possibly carry germs deep under the skin and cause infection. In fact, this is very uncommon, so long as standards of cleanliness are reasonable.

The needle should be inserted with a quick jab, vertically into the skin, almost as if throwing a dart. It should not be put in at an angle, as this may result in an injection too near the surface. The piston should not be drawn back before injecting insulin. If the needle is in a blood vessel, the insulin will simply be absorbed a little more rapidly than normal. The user should inject slowly, wait for a few seconds, then pull the needle out quickly. If there is bleeding, pressure with a dry cotton ball for a minute or two will check it. An occasional bruise should be ignored. These will be absorbed in two weeks. Frequent bruising should be reported to the doctor who will check whether the blood clotting system is working properly.

Most insulins now used are made by bacteria that have been persuaded to produce human insulin by recombinant DNA technology (genetic engineering). This insulin is, in every respect, identical to insulin produced by the human pancreas. Trade names for human insulin include Humulin S, Humulin M1 to M5, Humulin Lente and Humulin Zn.

BLOOD GLUCOSE MONITORING

Urine testing is much less valuable than direct blood sugar testing. A casual urine test for sugar does not always indicate the state of the blood sugar at the time of the test, because the urine being tested may have been produced by the kidneys quite some time before. This is why it is important to empty the bladder, then wait until a little more fresh urine can be produced for the test. Even then, the result, as an indication of the blood sugar, will be somewhat out of date. The real way to know what is going on is to perform blood glucose measurement and keep the results in a book.

Blood glucose testing is far more important and useful than urine testing as it gives the facts wanted – the precise level of blood glucose at the time of testing. All insulin-dependent diabetics should be able to check their blood glucose quickly and easily. Ask your doctor to prescribe the necessary equipment and a supply of strips and be sure you are quite clear about the instructions. Checking is simple but you have to do it right. If you are in any doubt, or if you get results that seem improbable, ask your doctor to advise. The trouble you take is well worth while. Aim to keep peaks below 10 mmol/l and not to let levels fall below 4 mmol/l. Don't panic if occasional readings are outside these limits.

GENERAL POINTS

Any sort of major illness, or any illness lasting for more that three days, is definitely a matter for the doctor. Even colds, influenza, stomach upsets and other minor or short-term illness can sometimes be quite important, especially if there is vomiting or diarrhoea. Fluid loss from these two should *always* be reported to the doctor.

The normal routine should be modified as little as possible. Diabetic children may occasionally not feel like eating, but must be encouraged to maintain the normal intake and balance it with the normal dosage of insulin. If the child can't be persuaded to take normal food, try to replace it with liquid carbohydrates like fruit juices, milk shakes, jellies or even fizzy drinks. Half a cup of orange juice or ginger beer is equivalent to 10 g of carbohydrate.

An insulin injection should never be omitted for fear of a 'hypo' (hypoglycaemic attack). It is always important to drink plenty of fluids. This is especially important if there is abnormal fluid loss, as from sweating, vomiting or diarrhoea, but a watch must be kept on the carbohydrate content of the fluid drunk. Remember, also, that some medicines contain a considerable quantity of sugar. All diabetics are, or should be, extremely sensitive to the sweetness of anything taken by mouth. Care may be needed with things like cough mixtures, linctuses, elixirs, medicinal syrups, antibiotic suspensions, and so on. These could provide an unexpected glucose boost and cause changes in the test results.

HYPOGLYCAEMIA

All young diabetics and their parents or carers need to know about hypoglycaemia. Hypoglycaemia is a dangerous condition in which, for various reasons, the levels of glucose in the blood drop below a required minimum. Glucose is the main body fuel and the brain is very sensitive to a drop in the supply. Low blood sugar causes a release of adrenaline into the blood, which forces the liver to give up its glucose rapidly and to manufacture new glucose. This adrenaline has important effects. Here is a list of most of the effects that can happen in hypoglycaemia:

- anxiety
- hunger
- rapid pulse
- skin over-sensitivity
- sweating
- shakiness
- 'sinking feeling'
- double vision
- NAUSEA
- sense of unreality
- pallor
- 'drunken' behaviour
- belching
- yawning and tiredness
- rapid breathing
- unsteadiness

- weakness
- lightheadedness
- muscle twitching
- regular muscle spasms
- fits
- loss of consciousness
- abnormal deviation of the eyes
- enlarged pupils
- deep coma
- shallow breathing
- slowing of the pulse
- death

The causes of hypoglycaemia must be clearly understood. They are extremely important. They are:

- too much insulin
- insufficient calorie intake, eg missed meals
- excessive exercise *in relation to calorie intake* and insulin dosage
- illness, especially infections
- beta-blockers, monoamine oxidase inhibitors, sulphonamides
- certain liver diseases

The latter two are unlikely to affect young diabetics but they should be known about. The first four are those that really matter. Some diabetics on long-acting insulin, whose dosage is too high, have less obvious effects and tend to show the brain deprivation signs rather than the adrenaline signs. So they may seem to have developed a change of personality with lowered standards, apparent laziness, deterioration in work performance, loss of memory and irrational behaviour. All these effects may result from long-lasting hypoglycaemia, or from inadequate carbohydrate intake. It can also happen if a diabetic deliberately takes less food than is required.

Hypoglycaemia can occur during sleep and parents of young diabetics should be aware of the indications of this. The possibility of this happening often causes diabetics great concern. Many fear that they will go into coma and never wake up. Happily, this is almost unheard of, but lesser degrees of hypoglycaemic effects during sleep are quite common. Again, the danger is more likely with people using long-acting insulin, as this may actually

have its maximum effect after the person has gone to sleep.

Here are one or two signs which may give you a clue to whether this is happening:

- disturbed sleep
- NIGHTMARES
- sleeping in unusual positions
- crying out during sleep
- sleepwalking
- BEDWETTING
- HEADACHE on waking

The new occurrence of any of these should alert you to the possibility and you should report them to your doctor. Some modification of insulin dosage, or type, may be necessary, or it may be sufficient just to increase the size of the late-night snack a little.

The overall aim in the management of diabetes is always for the person concerned to lead a normal life. Young diabetics should be encouraged, not to adjust their lives to the disease, but to manage the disease in such a way as to do everything they want to do, including high-level athletics. A thorough understanding of the condition is essential and parents should ensure that this is achieved. Good diabetic control minimizes the risk of complications, and this is possible only with the full cooperation of the patient. Much research is in progress to improve on the current methods of controlling diabetes, and there is a real prospect that some form of insulin-producing implant may be possible. Automatic monitoring of blood sugar with appropriate continuous dosage of insulin is feasible but still impracticable for wide usage. The outlook is good.

Diarrhoea

Because of the ever-present risk of dehydration, diarrhoea in babies should never be taken lightly. Breast-fed babies are much less likely to suffer intestinal infection, a common cause of diarrhoea, than those on the bottle, but normally pass very soft stools. If the faeces are very watery and runny and if there is any sign of general upset, such as fever, vomiting or failure to feed, then the baby needs urgent medical attention. Babies with gastroenteritis can become seriously ill very rapidly.

Diarrhoea can be caused by lactose intolerance due to deficiency of lactase, the chemical activator (enzyme) that splits milk sugar. Unsplit milk sugar attracts fluid into the intestine, causing diarrhoea, abdominal distention, bowel noises and failure to thrive. The same problem may occur if excessive sugar is added to the feed or if fruit juices are given in too concentrated a dilution. They should be diluted as instructed. Even sugary-based medicines can cause diarrhoea. The move to solid food (weaning) can also cause diarrhoea because of the unaccustomed bowel irritation. In such a situation, formulas of low lactose, easy-to-digest carbohydrate, with adequate vitamin content, may be useful, for a short period.

Diet see introductory section.

Diphtheria

Diphtheria is a serious and highly infectious, disease, now, happily, very rare in developed countries, because of IMMUNISATION. Diphtheria can progress to serious illness within a day of the appearance of the first symptoms. These are FEVER, sore throat, HEADACHE, difficulty in swallowing and enlarged lymph nodes in the neck. The organism produces a powerful poison (toxin) which is released into the surrounding tissues, causing severe damage and the formation of a greyish-white membrane which can obstruct the upper air passages, causing asphyxiation. This may necessitate an emergency artificial opening into the windpipe (TRACHEOSTOMY).

The toxin enters the bloodstream and is carried throughout the body, where it may cause serious damage to the heart, the nervous system – causing permanent muscle weakness – or the kidneys. Many children have died from severe heart damage within a few days of onset. Even today, the death rate from diphtheria is about 10 per cent. In underdeveloped parts of the world, it is much higher.

Because of the success of the immunisation programme, a generation of mothers has grown up with no knowledge of the horrors of the disease. There is a risk that immunisation may be neglected. Have your children been immunized?

Discharging ears see OTITIS EXTERNA, OTITIS MEDIA.

Dogs, diseases from

The most common diseases transmitted to children from dogs are the parasitic worm infestations. The commonest of these is TOXOCARIASIS, from the puppy worm *Toxocara canis*. The eggs of this parasite are commonly plentiful in the fur around the animal's anus and in the excreta, and children's hands can acquire them by patting and stroking. The soil of all parks, where dogs are allowed, is heavily contaminated with *Toxocara* eggs. Toxocara larvae can penetrate the intact skin of a human and pass into the bloodstream. This worm may, rarely, lead to loss of sight in an eye if the migrating larval stage of the worm should pass by way of the blood to the layer of the eye behind the retina. A tiny worm dying in that site will set up an acute and destructive inflammation and produce a mass resembling an eye tumour.

The tapeworm eggs, from dogs, can lead to hydatid disease – large fluid-filled cysts in any part of the body including the brain. These can cause EPILEPSY. Dog mange, which is a parasitization with mites of the SCABIES family, can lead to scabies in children. Various other mites and ticks can cause minor skin problems.

Animal skin or hair scales (dander) commonly cause allergic ASTHMA and skin fungus infection in dogs (tinea). This is commonly, but inaccurately, called 'ringworm' and can be passed to children. In common with many mammals, dogs may, in endemic areas, be affected by rabies. The effect of this disease on the brain of the animal (mania) makes rabid dogs especially dangerous.

See also CATS, DISEASES FROM.

Dosage of childhood medicines

Because teaspoons are of widely varying capacity, the dosage of medication in mixture form has always been notoriously inaccurate. Fortunately, this has seldom caused problems because most paediatric mixtures have a considerable margin of safety. But it should be remembered that the claimed safety of much modern medication, containing pharmacologically active ingredients, is based on the assumption that the recommended dose will not be exceeded.

The standard 'teaspoon' dose is 5 ml and you can easily obtain children's plastic medicine spoons calibrated so as to deliver accurate dosage. Although it is possible to make rough adjustments to dosage on the basis of the child's size (rather than age) for over-the-counter medications, you should be very careful not to modify dosage in the case of prescribed drugs. Children are not just little adults. There are many other factors that determine the appropriate dosage. Follow your doctor's instructions carefully.

Children hate swallowing tablets or capsules and should be given mixtures if possible. Medication spat out or vomited should be replaced. If the medicine tastes too pleasant, guard against the risk of overdosage.

Disclosing agents

These are stains that conspicuously reveal dental plaque on the teeth with the aim of ensuring more effective toothbrushing and flossing. Plaque is the mixture of dried saliva, bacteria and food debris that collects around the necks of neglected teeth and promotes TOOTH DECAY.

Down's syndrome

Formerly called 'mongolism', Down's syndrome is a major genetic disorder caused by the presence, either in the egg (ovum) or the sperm, of an extra chromosome. The cells in the body of a person with Down's syndrome have 47 chromosomes instead of the normal 46. There are three copies of chromosome number 21. This is called trisomy. For young mothers, the incidence is about one in 2,000. For older mothers (35 and above), the incidence is about one in 40.

The higher incidence in older women is due to the fact that all the eggs are preformed in the ovaries by the time of the mother's birth, so those released and fertilized late in the reproductive life have had up to 50 years to acquire defects. In about a quarter of the cases, the extra chromosome comes from the father.

A child with Down's syndrome has oval, down-sloping eyelid openings and a large, protruding tongue. The head is short and wide and flattened at the back, and the ears are small. The nose is short, with a depressed bridge, and the lips thick and turned out. The hands are broad, with short fingers, and the skin is often rough and dry. Physical development is slow. Heart and inner ear defects are common and there is a special susceptibility to LEUKAEMIA. There is always some degree of LEARNING DIFFICULTY, but this need not be severe and many children with Down's syndrome benefit from normal education and are later able to engage in simple employment. Children with Down's syndrome are usually happy, friendly and lovable.

Those without major heart problems usually survive to adult life, but the processes of ageing appears to be speeded up and many of them develop a form of Alzheimer's disease in their 40s or 50s.

Not all children with Down's syndrome have 47 chromosomes in all their cells, and some cases are so mild as to be almost normal (see MOSAICISM).

Down's syndrome is easily diagnosed by amniocentesis or chorionic villus sampling at an early stage in the pregnancy. Amniocentesis is often offered to pregnant women over the age of 35. If the trisomy is detected, the question of terminating the pregnancy can be considered.

Drooping eyelid see PTOSIS.

Drowning

Drowning implies death from suffocation as a result of exclusion of air from the lungs by fluid, usually water. Drowning results most commonly from submersion in water, but any liquid may exclude air. The need to breathe is so powerful that when the nose and mouth are immersed in a fluid, that fluid will eventually, in spite of the efforts of the child concerned, be inhaled into the lungs. Drowning may also occur in fluid produced within the lungs themselves (pulmonary oedema) as a result of the inhalation of irritants or as a result of lung or other disease.

The exclusion of air from the lungs, and, consequently, of oxygen from the blood, soon leads to loss of brain function and loss of consciousness. Within five to eight minutes, in most cases, permanent damage is caused to the higher centres of the brain so that, even if the affected child is resuscitated and breathing maintained, return of normal brain function, or even of consciousness, is unlikely. Notable exceptions to this rule have, however, often occurred, especially in very cold conditions. In these, the body metabolism is slowed and the oxygen requirement is reduced. Children have been rescued and restored to apparent normality after immersion in water, under ice, *for half an hour.*

The so-called 'diving reflex' is another protective mechanism which is believed to have saved many. The effect of this is to slow the heartbeat and constrict the arteries in the limbs, intestinal tract and other areas remote from the heart, so as to confine the circulation largely to the heart and the brain. In this way, the small amount of precious oxygen in the blood is conserved for the most vital functions and recovery is possible after a longer period under water. Eating shortly before swimming interferes with this reflex.

Inhaled fresh water is more dangerous than inhaled sea water, and often gives rise to a sharp increase in the total volume of the blood, with general rupture and dilution of the red cells and alteration in the chemical constitution. Death may occur from this cause alone. But in every case of apparent drowning, mouth to mouth artificial respiration and, if necessary, heart compression should be done.

See also introductory section (**Safety and First Aid**).

Drug abuse

Parents have much reason to be concerned, these days, over the possibility that their children, even those of pre-teen age, may be getting involved in the use of illegal drugs. Without direct evidence in the form of actual drug possession or the finding of drug equipment among the young person's belongings, it is seldom that parents and others can be quite sure that a young person is abusing drugs.

Because young people do not use drugs at home, parents will seldom directly observe the effects. But these should be known. Here is an outline.

AMPHETAMINE ('SPEED')

This is an 'upper' and is taken for its effects in causing a mental 'high'. This state of artificial euphoria is associated with other effects, including:

- shakiness
- trembling of the hands
- fast pulse
- a rise in the blood pressure
- headaches
- palpitations
- anxiety
- sweating
- difficulty in sleeping

In some cases there may be psychiatric symptoms such as false beliefs (delusions) and false perceptions (hallucinations). Occasionally fits (seizures) occur. Long-term amphetamine use may lead to drug dependence.

ECSTASY (METHOXY-METHYLENE-DIOXYAMPHETAMINE OR MDA)

This drug is a hallucinogenic amphetamine derivative similar in chemical structure to the natural hallucinogenic drug mescaline. In low doses it acts like amphetamine and in higher doses it acts like LSD. It is, however, more toxic than mescaline in increasing doses and may cause death. The effects are:

- behavioural excitement
- sensory hallucinations
- hyperexcitability
- hyperactivity
- tremors
- convulsions
- dehydration
- prostration

Because there is no commercial preparation of ecstasy, there is no official standardization either of dosage or purity. Ecstasy is a designer drug, produced purely for profit by people concerned only with profit and who have no regard for the safety or well-being of the young. Many tragic deaths have resulted from the use of this drug at 'rave' parties. Some of these deaths result from dehydration, some from drinking excess water in an attempt to avoid dehydration.

Ecstasy can cause an acute hepatitis that can progress to acute liver failure. In some cases, the stimulant effect on the brain and the resultant hyperexcitability may be so severe as to lead to bleeding within or around the brain. Irregularities of heart action may occur, and these, too, can be fatal.

Other names for ecstasy include XTC, Adam and E.

LSD (LYSERGIC ACID DIETHYLAMIDE)

This drug was first produced in 1938 from ergot of rye. It acts in almost infinitesimally small dosage – only a few micrograms – and has major effects on the mind, but relatively minor effects on the body. The effects are:

- restlessness
- difficulty in concentration
- laughter or sadness, or both simultaneously
- loss or distortion of the sense of time
- marked distortion of visual imagery
- out-of-body experience
- distortion of sound perception
- emotional withdrawal
- hypervigilance

The drug starts to take effect between 30 to 60 minutes after an oral dose and the effects persist for 10 to 12 hours. These effects vary considerably with the personality of the user and with his or her expectations of what the drug will do. Tolerance is readily acquired with usage and the dose has to be increased. There are no withdrawal symptoms.

LSD can have a serious effect on the psychological state of the user and can induce a confusional, panic or frankly psychotic reaction. Sometimes the perceptual distortions are prolonged and there may be long-term inability to control the emotions.

'Flashbacks' to the drug-induced state may occur spontaneously at intervals for several years after using LSD. About 15 per cent of users experience flashbacks. There is reason to believe that the drug can cause permanent damage to the brain.

COCAINE

The abuse of this widely used drug can be dangerous to health. The commonest serious physical effects are:

- epileptic-type fits
- loss of consciousness ('tripping out')
- unsteadiness
- sore throat
- running and bleeding nose
- sinusitis
- pain in the chest
- coughing blood
- pneumonia
- severe itching ('the cocaine bug')
- irregularity of the heart
- loss of appetite
- stomach upset

The nose and sinus disorders are due to the constricting effect of cocaine on the blood vessels in the nose linings. This is followed by rebound swelling, but is sometimes severe enough to destroy part of the partition between the two halves of the nose, leaving a perforation.

Crack cocaine, like amphetamine, can lead to a short-lived, acute form of mental illness. This is called a cocaine psychosis. The symptoms include:

- severe depression
- agitation
- delusions
- ideas of persecution
- hallucinations
- violent behaviour
- suicidal intent

People with a cocaine psychosis often have 'lucid intervals' in which they seem normal and will often deny using the drug. Cocaine psychosis usually follows long binges or high doses.

There are several indicators that should arouse strong suspicion that a child is taking drugs. Remember that the maintenance of a drug habit is expensive and that the young person must be getting the money from somewhere. Warning signs, that should never be ignored, include:

- unexplained losses of money or valuables from the household
- possession by the young person of unexplained sums of money
- secretive behaviour
- apparent personality changes
- unexpected mood swings
- deterioration in personal appearance and grooming
- sudden reduction in school or college performance
- loss of interest in former activities such as sport
- acquisition of new acquaintances and rejection of old friends
- inability to account for activities during regular periods of time
- memory loss
- accident proneness

Many young people, unable to obtain the money they need for drugs, turn to drug-dealing. In this case, they may have more money to spend than can plausibly be accounted for. Remember, however, that most of these signs may have an innocent or alternative explanation. Schizophrenia and other psychiatric disturbances commonly develop during adolescence, and this is also a period when young people commonly have severe, but often temporary, behaviour problems. An aggressive response to these is inappropriate and unproductive and a major effort at sympathy and understanding is often required by older people. It may often be best openly to discuss the possibility of drug abuse.

MARIJUANA

Also known as cannabis, pot, weed, grass, reefer, hashish, hash, bhang, ganja, kif, dagga, this is one of the most popular of the drugs of abuse among young people. It is taken as a relaxant, and to produce euphoria – easy promotion of laughter or giggling – often for reasons that seem silly or childish to the observer. Under the influence of the tetrahydrocannabinol all the senses are heightened especially sight. Colour intensity and contrast are increased, and there is distortion of the dimensions of objects and of the perception of distance. The perception of time, too, is distorted, or sometimes seemingly eliminated. Usually, passage of time is experienced as being slower than reality, so that estimates of periods past are greater than clock time and those of future periods less.

One of the much-valued properties among some devotees is the sense of deep philosophical insight conveyed by the cannabinoids. There is a conviction of omniscience, of knowing all the answers to the riddles of the universe, and this is often accompanied by a feeling of calm superiority, so that one hardly bothers to bring the great accessible truths to mind. For those of genuine philosophical bent, however, the inability to retain these insights, as the effects of the drug wear off, is a bitter disappointment. In fact, intellectual performance is impaired during the period of the drug action. Mental arithmetic is less accurate than normal and short-term memory defective. The affected person often forgets the beginning of a sentence before reaching the end.

Controversy continues in medical circles as to whether the cannabinoids cause organic brain damage. This has been demonstrated in rats and monkeys, but not objectively in humans. Neither computed tomography (CT) scanning nor electroencephalography (ECG) have shown changes. There is, however, plenty of indirect evidence of brain dysfunction in persistent heavy users. Such people can develop the *amotivational syndrome* and show apathy and loss of interest and concern. Students stop working, suffer a drop in academic performance and give up courses. This effect is to be expected because the cannabinoids are concentrated in the limbic system – the motivational centre of the brain – and because of the effects on memory and reasoning.

Cannabis withdrawal produces quite severe symptoms, including anxiety, irritability, HEADACHES, sleeplessness, muscle twitching, sweating and DIARRHOEA, but these will pass and, in most cases, the amotivational syndrome will eventually resolve.

Other possible effects include:

- reddening of the eyes
- a fall in blood pressure
- mild engorgement of the genitals
- a rise in the heart rate
- panic attacks
- acute anxiety
- precipitation of schizophrenia, mania, or a confusional psychosis
- depersonalization

The effects on the cardiovascular system can be dangerous. In most cases, the severe psychological effects arise in young people with personalities predisposed to them – people who might have developed the disorders, in due course, without cannabis. But sometimes they occur in people with no apparent psychiatric problem. Young teenagers, especially those under social or other stresses and those suffering emotional disturbances, are especially at risk. Psychiatric patients controlled on drug treatment often suffer severe recurrences on using cannabis.

Reefer smoke has been shown to be as capable of causing lung cancer as tobacco smoke. Some studies have suggested that it may be more so, but total exposure to marijuana smoke is less than with tobacco. It also causes chronic bronchitis. Oddly enough, the cannabinoids reduce the appetite and can control severe NAUSEA and the drug has some effect on preventing epileptic fits.

Concern has been expressed about the probability of progress from cannabis use to that of harder drugs. Only a small proportion of casual users progress, but it is clear that heavy users commonly do. Nearly all heroin addicts have had previous experience of cannabis. It is unnecessary to propose any pharmacological reason for this, but undoubtedly the cannabis experience in certain predisposed individuals does, for psychological reasons, cause progression to drugs such as heroin. This was accepted by the Canadian Commission of Inquiry into the Non-Medical Use of Drugs, in their 1972 report on cannabis.

ALCOHOL

Increasing concern has been voiced about the rising consumption of alcohol by children and young people. This problem is not helped by the marketing of low-alcohol 'soft' drinks specifically targeted at young people.

Alcohol is damaging to the growing child in two ways: it is a poison capable of harming the child, possibly to the extent of interfering with full mental and physical development; and early habituation increases the probability that alcohol will be abused throughout life. In France, it is common practice to allow children a regular intake of dilute wine. The incidence of alcoholic liver cirrhosis and other alcohol-related diseases in France, however, is substantially higher than in countries where children are not encouraged to drink alcohol.

See also SOLVENT ABUSE.

Dwarfism

A distinction needs to be made between dwarfs and midgets. Most dwarfs have relatively large heads and short arms and legs; midgets are of normal proportions but very small. Some people are dwarfs because of an inherited genetic defect, others because of nutritional deficiency or a glandular defect.

Most dwarfism results from one of two conditions: ACHONDROPLASIA and growth hormone deficiency. Growth hormone is produced by the pituitary gland, a protrusion from the underside of the brain. If, during childhood, normal amounts of this hormone are not produced, the result will be an overall reduction in body growth which may be very severe. Growth hormone production may fail because of a nearby tumour or because of unexplained underaction of the pituitary gland. It may also result from radiation or injury to the gland or from infection of it (meningoencephalitis).

Other causes of dwarfism include:

- severe undernourishment or starvation
- DOWN'S SYNDROME
- trisomy 18
- TURNER'S SYNDROME
- cretinism (thyroid gland malfunction) from severe iodine deficiency early in life
- precocious puberty with premature closure of the bone growth zones (epiphyses)
- early adrenal gland overaction with resulting excess production of anabolic male sex hormones and premature puberty
- various metabolic disorders

The metabolic disorders are rare and hereditary and include TAY-SACH'S DISEASE, Gaucher's disease, Hurler's syndrome and Niemann-Pick disease. These conditions tend to result in both a short spine and short limbs.

Once suspicion has been aroused, careful serial records of growth of the child will confirm or deny the diagnosis of dwarfism. Remember, however, that children of small parents also tend to be small. Ninety-five per cent of normal people will be within 8.5 cm (3½ in) of the average of the heights of the two parents. The different forms of dwarfism are readily recognized by experts. In cases of doubt, chromosomal or biochemical tests can confirm the diagnosis.

There is no treatment for metabolic dwarfism, but the condition can be diagnosed before birth by amniocentesis and the option for termination of the pregnancy can be considered. Growth hormone deficiency can be treated by daily bedtime injections of growth hormone. This hormone is now being produced by genetic engineering so there is now no possibility of the hormone causing Creutzfeldt-Jakob disease, as has happened in the past when it was obtained from cadaver pituitary glands.

You can easily detect precocious puberty by observing the premature growth of the sex organs. This condition is treated with synthetic hormones (gonadotrophin releasing hormones) to improve the prospects for adult height and avoid the physical and mental problems.

Dyschondroplasia

This is a rare progressive disease of the growing parts of bone, affecting children and causing growth retardation. Bones are abnormally, and often unequally, shortened and show nodular swellings. The arms, legs and fingers are commonly affected but the skull, spine, ribs and pelvis are usually spared. The process continues until early adult life, but by then, severe deformity may have resulted, with limbs of unequal length. Disability from finger deformity may also occur.

Dyslexia

Many parents, concerned about a child's slowness in reading, wonder about dyslexia. This condition is defined as an inability to achieve an average performance in reading or in understanding what is read, in a child of normal or high intelligence and of normal educational and socio-cultural opportunity and emotional stability. Dyslexia has nothing to do with defects of vision or speech. It may range from a very minor reading problem to an almost total inability to read. It is commoner in males, tends to run in families, and persists into adult life. There is much greater than normal difficulty in the use, meaning, spelling and pronunciation of words.

Figures for the prevalence of dyslexia are seldom to be found, largely because the condition is hard to distinguish from other causes of reading difficulty or illiteracy. Not all dyslexic children are illiterate and by no means all illiterate children are dyslexic.

In practice, the child appears to have difficulty in visual perception and discrimination. Letters and words are perceived as being reversed, so that 'd' becomes 'b' and 'was' becomes 'saw'. Complete mirror writing occurs. Children affected in this way seem to show an absence of the normal dominance of the left side of the brain and are neither obviously right- nor left-handed, as in the case of those with normal cerebral dominance.

In spite of major advances in psychology, neurology, brain function studies and linguistics, the experts continue to argue about dyslexia. There are even those who deny that it exists and claim that the problems are purely educational or emotional. Most authorities, however, recognize the condition and many are convinced that it is a disorder essentially of the language function of the brain.

Some scientists have claimed that dyslexic people have an abnormal symmetry in the size of the areas in the temporal lobes of the brain that contain the association areas for hearing. These are normally larger on the left side. The evidence for these views is, however, conflicting.

It seems possible that dyslexic children are anatomically less well equipped than others to recognize sounds presented to them in rapid succession. An interval of about 100 milliseconds is required to separate sounds. This is greater than the interval that separates the component sounds in many common syllables. Phonetic reading is the major problem in dyslexia.

You can do a lot to help dyslexic children. The first thing to do is to accept that the condition is a specific difficulty and not the result of inattention, laziness or perversity. You must not add to the child's anxiety by over-emphasizing the problem. You should be ready and willing to read to the child, or to encourage the use of recorded books, long after the age at which he or she would normally be able to read fluently. Cooperation with a specialist teacher or educational psychologist can be most helpful. Some educational authorities have been willing to allow dyslexic children extra time during examinations.

E

Earache

This is especially common in children, in whom it is usually caused by a change in the air pressure in the middle ear due the inability of air to move freely in and out of the middle ear. This occurs because of blockage of the eustachian tube – the short tube that connects the middle ear to the back of the nose. This blockage is usually due to ADENOIDS or inflammation and swelling of the nose lining. Earache caused in this way can be relieved by correcting eustachian obstruction by means of decongestant drops or inhalants. ADENOIDECTOMY or TONSILLECTOMY may sometimes be necessary.

Eustachian obstruction also interferes with fluid drainage of the middle ear and may lead to infection of the middle ear (OTITIS MEDIA), another common cause of earache. Earache may also be caused by infection in the external ear passage by viruses, bacteria or fungi (OTITIS EXTERNA). A small boil in this area is exquisitely painful because the skin is bound down to bone and cannot stretch. Discharge of the boil brings wonderful relief.

Ear discharge see OTITIS EXTERNA, OTITIS MEDIA.

Ear disorders see BAT EARS, EARACHE, EAR, FOREIGN BODY IN, GLUE EAR, HEARING PROBLEMS, OTITIS EXTERNA, OTITIS MEDIA.

Ear-drum surgery see MYRINGOTOMY.

Ear, foreign body in

Children's fascination with their bodily orifices inevitably leads to the introduction, of anything small enough, into mouths, noses, navels and ears. Beads, pebbles, peas, beans, seeds or ball-bearings commonly become impacted in the external ear passage. Organic objects which swell with moisture are especially troublesome. This common childhood incident is usually compounded by frantic attempts by parents to remove the foreign body by means of various improvised instruments. Such attempts may be relied upon to push the foreign body further in. Contact with the eardrum causes pain, a noise like thunder, and a notable worsening of the situation.

This is a job for an ENT (ear, nose and throat) specialist. A surgeon skilled in child psychology will often succeed without an anaesthetic, for the problem is not so much one of mechanical difficulty as of securing a non-moving operating field. But in many cases, unfortunately, a brief general anaesthetic, or the use of a quick-acting tranquillising drug, may be necessary. Foreign bodies can easily be removed with fine hooks, if the child is safely still.

Ear plastic surgery see OTOPLASTY.

Eating dirt see PICA.

Eczema

Unless you are unusually well-informed the chances are that you think that eczema is a single specific condition, like impetigo or chickenpox. This is understandable because the term is commonly used, even by doctors, as if eczema *were* a single condition. In fact, eczema is the response of the skin to a wide variety of damaging influences and is a feature of many different skin disorders. It is a very general term meaning 'inflammation of the skin', without implying any particular cause. For practical purposes the terms 'eczema' and DERMATITIS mean the same thing.

Eczema features scaly, red, itchy patches which cause scratching, leading to thickening and shiny areas with deepened skin markings. Often, there are small, fluid-filled blisters which leak serum, so that the skin becomes 'weepy'. Exuded serum quickly clots to form crusts. The damage to the skin surface may allow germs access to the deeper layers where they can flourish, causing more severe inflammation and pus formation. This is called secondary infection and is a complication of the eczema, not a basic feature.

Eczema may affect any part of the skin. Adolescent eczema commonly occurs on the hands as a result of allergy to substances such as washing-up liquid; on the groin, from contact with biological washing powders; on the wrists, back or ears from contact with nickel watch-straps, name-bracelets, bra fasteners or spectacle frames; or anywhere else where there is contact with materials to which allergy has developed. Contact dermatitis may also occur in babies and children, but this is less common than in older people.

In babies and young children, the common type of eczema is called atopic eczema. This word simply means that, unlike contact dermatitis, the effect does not occur at the same place as the cause. The word comes from the Greek *topos*, a 'place' and *a*, 'not' (see ATOPY). In atopic eczema the allergic tendency is hereditary and the condition often appears in the first year of life. Affected children, or other members of the family, often have other allergies, such as ASTHMA or hay fever. Eczema is not contagious or infectious unless secondary infection occurs. Even then, infectivity is low.

Atopic eczema usually affects babies between the ages of 2 and 18 months. There are thought to be many causes in babies but these are often inapparent. One known, but uncommon, cause is allergy to protein in milk, wheat or eggs. The rash appears behind the knees, in the creases of the elbows, behind the ears and on the face. It is usually mild but very itchy, rather scaly

and with small red pimples. It is almost impossible to prevent the baby from scratching, and soon the pimples begin to ooze serum and the affected parts may join to form large weeping areas. Infection may occur, particularly in the nappy area.

If you think your baby has eczema, you should always consult your doctor, and he or she will try to discover the cause and, if possible, remove it. Because prevention is better than cure, local treatment to the skin is always secondary to finding and removing the cause. Obvious possibilities such as soap, detergents, baby oil, baby skin moisturizers, and so on, must be considered. Avoidance of these often results in a cure.

Local treatment can be effective in removing the irritation and preventing scratching which prolongs the condition and encourages infection. If the condition is mild, it may be sufficient to apply a protective and softening cream; but care must be taken not to add to the possible causal factors. If there is any question of secondary infection, ANTIBIOTICS may be given, either in an ointment or by mouth. Antibiotics are of no value in uninfected eczema. Antihistamine drugs help to reduce itching and are especially useful if your baby is being kept awake at night by irritation. Don't let the baby get too hot, as this simply makes the irritation worse. And be careful about the kind of material coming in contact with the skin. There is nothing like cotton. In more severe cases, the doctor may prescribe an ointment containing a steroid. Steroids are powerful hormones. They are very effective against inflammation and can work like magic even in quite severe eczema.

Like many parents you may, quite rightly, be unhappy about the use of steroid drugs on your child, but you have to get this into perspective. Steroids applied to small areas of skin in moderation do not involve the risks of steroids given in large dosage by mouth or injection – stunting of growth, reduced resistance to infection, breakdown of healed conditions, such as peptic ulcers, TB lesions, & healed scars, and other effects. Even so, they should be used with reasonable caution. Although very effective against eczema and other allergic conditions, they can encourage the spread of infection by bacteria or fungi. If used for long periods, they can cause atrophy of the skin, local loss of skin colour, and even disfiguring purplish 'strain lines' called striae. These are much the same as those occurring in pregnancy. Sometimes when steroids are stopped there may be 'rebound' worsening of the eczema. Experienced dermatologists use them in careful moderation and avoid them if they can. Simple, bland remedies are often preferred.

Atopic eczema often clears up, even without treatment, as the child grows, and although it may come and go over the years, it usually settles completely by early adolescence.

> **Warning**
> The most dangerous complication of atopic eczema is secondary infection with the herpes simplex virus. This can produce a widespread condition, known as Kaposi's varicelliform eruption, or eczema herpeticum, which may prove fatal.
> The commonest way for children with eczema to acquire this condition is kissing people with cold sores. This can literally be the kiss of death, and frequently was before anti-herpes drugs like acyclovir were developed.

Seborrhoeic eczema is a form that often affects very small babies, causing patches of brownish, greasy scales on the scalp and in areas in which skin surfaces come into contact with each other. Apart from the scalp, seborrhoeic dermatitis is common in the armpits, the groins or behind the ears. It may also affect the neck or the face. If you see these patches, ask your doctor's advice. Mild seborrhoeic eczema will usually clear up if you carefully wash and dry the affected areas, but some soaps and baby lotions may make it worse. You can safely use olive oil or a bland emulsifying ointment to clean away the seborrhoeic patches on your baby's skin. If in doubt, consult your doctor.

See also NAPPY RASH.

Eisenmenger's complex

This is a CONGENITAL HEART DISEASE that starts with a HOLE IN THE HEART or a failure of closure of the fetal blood vessel, which bypasses the lungs, before birth (PATENT DUCTUS ARTERIOSUS). These defects are associated with, and may possibly cause, a serious condition of the lung blood vessels. Once the Eisenmenger's complex has developed, the outlook is unfavourable and little can be done to help.

If a 'hole in the heart' allows a large shunt of blood from the normally high pressure left side to the right, the raised pressure in the lung circulation will, eventually, cause permanent damage to the lung blood vessels. The effect of this damage is to make it harder for blood to get through the lungs. Eventually, the pressures on the right side exceed those on the left. At this point, a proportion of the reduced-oxygen blood returning from the tissues fails to pass through the lungs but is shunted through the hole to the left side of the heart, or through the patent ductus to the aorta. It is then pumped around the body without having had the chance to pick up more oxygen from the lungs. As a result the blood haemoglobin, instead of being the bright red, highly oxygenated colour, is a bluish-purple, and the affected child looks blue (CYANOSIS). To try to increase its oxygen-carrying capacity, the blood increases the number of its red cells and becomes thickened and more concentrated.

In the end, the right side of the heart fails. This is Eisenmenger's complex. Because of the danger of this, early recognition of the presence of the hole in the heart and evaluation of its effects is very important. In cases in which there is risk of proceeding to the Eisenmenger's complex, surgical treatment of heart holes or patent ductus arteriosus become imperative, so as to prevent the secondary lung changes from developing.

Encephalitis

This is inflammation of the brain. Fortunately, this is uncommon. Most cases are caused by infection, especially by viruses such as HERPES SIMPLEX, herpes zoster, polioviruses, echoviruses or coxsackie viruses. Herpes encephalitis usually occurs in children whose immune systems have been interfered with by inborn immune deficiency, by AIDS or by necessary medical treatment. The other forms tend to occur in epidemics and may follow MUMPS, MEASLES, RUBELLA, and CHICKENPOX.

Encephalitis causes:

- severe HEADACHE
- FEVER
- VOMITING
- sickness
- often a stiff neck and back
- epileptic fits
- mental confusion
- coma

A fatal outcome may occur within hours of onset, but even gravely ill patients may make a full recovery. Drugs like acyclovir have changed the outlook in cases of HERPES SIMPLEX encephalitis. Long-term effects are sometimes serious and may include LEARNING DIFFICULTY, EPILEPSY and DEAFNESS.

Enlarged tonsils see TONSILLITIS.

Enuresis see BEDWETTING.

Epicanthus see EYELID ABNORMALITIES.

Epiglottitis

The epiglottis is the leaf-shaped plate of cartilage and mucous membrane at the base of the tongue, that lies like a lid over the entrance to the voice box (larynx). Epiglottitis is inflammation of the epiglottis. The condition, although fortunately rare, is always dangerous because of the risk that swelling of the part may cause obstruction of the airway and suffocation. If this happens, the only hope is to make an emergency opening into the windpipe (TRACHEOSTOMY).

Epiglottitis may be a complication of severe infection of the tissues of the throat with *Haemophilus influenzae* organisms or, rarely, streptococci. It occurs most often in children between the ages of 2 and 5. The symptoms are:

- acute sore throat
- severe difficulty in swallowing, with drooling
- rapid, laboured and very noisy breathing
- restlessness and panic

This is an emergency situation calling for urgent admission to hospital for intensive antibiotic treatment and the passage of a tube to ensure continuity of the airway. Because of the suddenness with which obstruction can occur, it is often thought necessary to perform a tracheostomy, as a precaution.

Happily, *Haemophilus influenzae*, type B (HIB or Hib) vaccination of infants has led to an almost complete disappearance of invasive *Haemophilus* infections in vaccinated children.

Epilepsy

Epilepsy and epileptic seizures are commoner in childhood than in later life, which implies that the condition often disappears as the child gets older. In fact, about 50 per cent of children with epilepsy are fortunate enough to grow out of it. It is hard to give figures for the prevalence of epilepsy because it takes so many different forms and because many seizures, such as fever fits, should not really be classified as epilepsy. In very general terms, the condition affects about seven children in every 1,000, and about seven adults in every 2,000.

Epilepsy is not really a disease. It is a physical sign, an indication that the orderly flow of electrical signals between the different parts of the brain is replaced by abnormal electrical discharges. This is not a pleasant subject, but a full understanding of what happens and why, is greatly to be preferred to ignorance and rejection of the subject. If the subject is faced, the terrors are dispelled.

Generalised epilepsy, or 'grand mal', is the best known manifestation of epilepsy and is what most people think of when they hear the word. In this form, the electrical discharge in the brain is widespread and the effects on the body correspondingly extensive. Many epileptics have a prior warning for up to several hours before the onset of the convulsion, but this is not always recognized. Such a warning can be valuable and it is important to note any unusual states of mind or odd bodily effects which are then followed by a fit.

Such effects, occurring well before the convulsive stage, are called the 'prodrome' and should not be confused with the 'aura', described below. Prodromal indications of an impending fit may include one effect familiar to at least 80 per cent of people: the alarming body jerk commonly felt in a drowsy state or when falling asleep. Sometimes the jerk involves a single limb only. These common effects are called 'myoclonic jerks' and, in the case of an epileptic child, should alert him or her to the possibility that a fit may occur later that day. Probably more significant is a feeling of depression or apathy or, commonly, irritability. Such a feeling may precede a grand mal fit by several hours. Occasionally, the prodrome may consist of a throbbing HEADACHE or some form of intestinal upset, such as DIAR-RHOEA or even constipation.

When the grand mal attack starts there is, in about half the cases, a preliminary stage in which the discharge is beginning to have its effect but has not yet reached full intensity. This spread of discharge causes the 'aura' and during it the child experiences one or more of several possible effects. For each individual, the aura tends to be standardised and it may consist of:

- a feeling of fear or apprehension
- a sense of NAUSEA
- the perception of a powerful smell or taste
- a strong recollection of some event or place, or even a formed image of some scene
- an illusion of having experienced something before which is really being experienced for the first time (déjà vu)
- a conviction that something static is moving

The precise nature of the aura gives an indication of the location, in the brain, of the focus of electrical discharge, or even of the site of the injured area, should this be the cause of the epilepsy.

The aura, if it occurs, is a part of the fit proper. It may be very brief and provide insufficient time for the child to take any precautions to protect him or herself from the coming fit. But in some cases, it lasts long enough for the affected child to have time to loosen tight clothing, get into a safer place, perhaps to lie down on a soft bed. In about 50 per cent of cases, the sufferer is unaware either of a prodromal stage or of an aura and passes straight into the major fit without any warning, and simply falls unconscious to the ground.

This stage of the grand mal attack is caused by massive electrical discharge right across the whole of the surface of the brain on both sides. The most obvious effect of this is on the motor system of the brain, with powerful impulses being sent to almost every muscle in the body, causing them to contract. This is called the 'tonic' stage because the affected muscles go into a state of prolonged, maximal contraction. The effect has to be seen to be appreciated but, fortunately for the person most immediately concerned, consciousness, or at least a later awareness of what has happened, is lost early in the tonic stage. Because opposing groups of muscles are contracted simultaneously, the arms and legs will be rigid. Commonly, the legs are stiffly extended and the arms in the 'hands-up' position. The eyes and mouth tend to open wide at first and then the jaw snaps shut, sometimes biting the tongue.

It is not only the muscles of the arms, legs and jaw that are driven into sudden contraction. The same thing happens to the diaphragm and the respiratory muscles of the chest. The result is a temporary paralysis of breathing. Before this happens, however, it is common for air to be forced out of the lungs and this air, as it passes between the tightened vocal cords in the voice box (larynx), may cause a sound like a high-pitched cry or scream. This is not a real cry indicating distress, but simply an involuntary sound caused by the rush of air through the voice box.

Because the sustained contraction of the respiratory muscles may last for up to half a minute, there is no possibility of breathing and the body is temporarily deprived of oxygen. Soon the skin assumes a dusky bluish-grey colour. At the same time the large veins in the neck, which are meant to carry blood back to the heart from the head, become compressed at the root of the neck, and the blood, which is unable to flow, causes them to be distended. The same applies to all the veins of the face and head. So the face of the child having the grand mal attack turns blue and the veins become very prominent. The pupils of the eyes are widely dilated. The whole effect is very distressing to witness, but the child is quite unaware of what is happening.

After about 20 or 30 seconds the tightly knotted muscles begin to relax and air can, once again, flow into the lungs. As it does, normal colour begins to return to the skin and the distention of the veins subsides. But now starts the third, and perhaps the most upsetting, part of the fit to witness – the clonic stage. In this, all the muscles that were previously tightly contracted pass into a stage of generalised slight trembling which soon becomes a sequence of violent, repetitive, rhythmical jerky contractions. The head and limbs are jerked about, and the contractions of the muscles of the face cause a series of unpleasant grimaces as if the child were suffering great pain or distress. In this stage, also, the tongue may be bitten and the contraction of the muscles in the wall of the abdomen may squeeze the bladder or the rectum so that urine or faeces are involuntarily passed.

During the whole of the fit, normal swallowing is usually impossible and saliva accumulates in the mouth. This may be turned to foam by the forced emptying of the lungs at the onset of the tonic stage.

Gradually, over the course of two or three minutes, the interval between clonic contractions becomes greater and so the fit passes off altogether. The breathing, which has been suppressed during the whole of the clonic stage, now re-starts with a deep inspiration. For about five minutes the child may lie limply in deep coma with all muscles relaxed, and may then open the eyes and look around, obviously wondering what has happened. If undisturbed, he or she may pass into a deep sleep and may not wake for some hours. Alternatively, full consciousness and control may soon be regained. In either case, the child retains no memory for any detail of the event except the aura.

When grand mal epilepsy occurs between the ages of 5 and 15, the outlook is good. Such children are unlikely to have epilepsy in later life. Unfortunately, there is another form of epilepsy that affects children – focal epilepsy.

FOCAL EPILEPSY

In partial seizure, or focal epilepsy, the disturbance is confined to a well localised area of the brain, and the effects usually indicate to the doctor which area is involved. If only one bodily or mental function is affected, the partial seizure is described as 'simple'. If there is a wider spread of effects, it is called a 'complex partial seizure'. Probably the commonest types of simple partial seizure are the focal motor and sensory seizures. Usually, there is little or no warning and the attacks often start and end with a jerk of the arm or leg, or an area of tingling or numbness anywhere on the skin. There is no loss of consciousness and none of the confusion of mind that follows major epilepsy. Often the muscular jerking goes on rhythmically for several seconds, but the child remains normally alert throughout.

Quite commonly, the part of the back of the brain concerned with vision may be the site of a simple partial attack and the affected child will have the illusion of flashing lights or of seeing various patterns. Detailed visual hallucinations do not occur in simple partial seizures, but may occur in complex partial seizures. Another area of the brain commonly involved in simple seizures is the part of the temporal lobe responsible for the perception of sounds. In this case, noises will be heard. Similarly, powerful smells and tastes of all kinds – often quite unpleasant – are features of this kind of disorder. There may also be nausea and severe loss of balance. In all of these cases, it is possible to localise, quite precisely, the area of the brain affected.

Complex partial seizures are usually more distressing than simple partial seizures. Most of them begin in the temporal lobe and there is usually an aura. In this case, however, the aura tends to differ from that preceding an attack of grand mal. Typically, the affected child experiences an elaborate hallucination, perhaps a fully formed visual image or the sounds of voices or music, or he or she may enter a dream-like state in which some former memory comes back with striking clarity and reality. Often there are strong sensations related to the stomach, sensations so remote from normal experience that they cannot be adequately described. The chief emotions felt are anxiety or fear, but occasionally there is intense anger and this may lead to violent behaviour. There may be a feeling of being separated from the body, so that the actions can be watched as if they are those of a stranger.

The attack proper may consist only of a period during which the affected child is inaccessible and unresponsive. But more often the child behaves in an automatic manner, carrying out certain actions in a robot-like way and later having no recollection of having done so. At the time, however, there is a feeling of being forced to do these things: rotating the head in a particular direction, going to the sink and filling a glass with water, continuing to turn the pages of a book, sometimes even urinating or removing clothing in public. The affected child commonly makes chewing, sucking or swallowing movements and may spit repeatedly. Such features are very common in epilepsy and the reason is that, in the motor area of the brain, a disproportionately large area is devoted to the function of eating.

During this period of automatic behaviour, it is dangerous to try to restrain the child too forcibly. Usually he or she may be gently led or directed, but forcible restraint may cause an outburst of blind fury with violent results. Such outbursts are rare unless provoked by interference. In children, temporal lobe epilepsy tends to cause hyperactivity and uncontrollable rage. These effects may be the result, not of the brain defect itself, but of the child's and the parents' reaction to the experience of the epilepsy. If the child has an aura that is frightening, he or she will tend to try to dispel this fear by activity. The child may try, quite literally, to run away from the source of the fear. Again, the very natural anxiety which the diagnosis of epilepsy induces in the parents is bound to be apparent to the child who will, in turn, react by fear and restlessness.

About one child in three with temporal lobe epilepsy shows severe and uncontrollable rage. It is important for parents to understand the true nature of this rage, so that they can try to respond to it in a constructive and understanding manner rather than in the instinctive way. This rage is a release of high emotional pressure arising from an overburdening of the child's brain by excess emotional stimuli. Viewed in this way, and with awareness that the expression of rage is helpful, the unpleasantness can be more readily tolerated.

Educational problems are common in children with temporal lobe epilepsy. The repeated attacks interfere with the normal functioning of the brain and will, cumulatively, add up to significant loss of educational time. Again, children whose emotions are unstable and variable and who are anxious and restless inevitably have a poor level of concentration and attention. In some cases, epilepsy causes a temporary, or permanent, drop in the actual intelligence level. Both the IQ and the ability to learn may fluctuate considerably in epileptic children. The reason for this is not apparent. Although, on the whole, epilepsy tends to interfere with educational progress, many epileptic children have an outstanding scholastic performance and there have been numerous examples of high academic achievement.

Some cases of focal epilepsy can be cured by brain surgery to destroy the area that triggers off the attack. But the basic, and highly effective method of management of epilepsy is by anticonvulsant medication. Treatment of epilepsy with drugs such as phenobarbitone, sodium valproate or carbamazepine, can be highly effective.

See also ABSENCE ATTACKS, FEBRILE CONVULSIONS.

Exercise

The Broadcasting Audience Research Board, in its 1993 report, showed that British children between the ages of 4 and 15 are watching between two and three hours of television each day. This means that about one-third of the time available to children for exercise in each 24-hour period (after sleeping, school and eating are subtracted) is spent in a sedentary occupation. When it is remembered that many children are now driven to school and that the National Curriculum now provides for only an hour of physical education a week, it becomes clear that today's children are exercising considerably less than those of past generations.

It is an established medical fact that a sedentary lifestyle in adult life is one of the small number of factors leading to the top killer, coronary heart disease. Unfortunately, it also seems more than likely that habits of physical activity – or inactivity – are laid down in childhood, and that these habits are hard to break. Once an inactive lifestyle is established in childhood, it is likely to persist. Unfortunately the converse does not follow: highly active children do not necessarily become highly active adults. However, inactive children are much less likely to become active adults. Only about 2 per cent do so. Of active children, some 25 per cent become active adults.

Surprisingly, there is no evidence that highly physically-active children are less fit than their couch potato companions. Numerous studies have failed to show that contemporary children are any less fit than their parents or grandparents were as children. But to assume that this justifies or excuses a sedentary lifestyle is a dangerous generalization. The fact is that the processes that lead to heart disease and the other serious health risks of middle age and later take years to develop and do not show their effects during childhood. They have, however, already started in these idle children. The serious arterial disease ATHERO-SCLEROSIS has already begun to develop. And the earlier this destructive process starts in life, the earlier it will lead to blocked arteries with the attendant risk of heart attacks, strokes, kidney disorders and limb gangrene.

One reason why a sedentary childhood is so important is that it is strongly associated with the consumption of far too much junk food with a high fat content. Over 40 per cent of British children have blood cholesterol levels above the recommended safety limit. Raised blood cholesterol is another of the established risk factors for atherosclerosis, and it has an insidious tendency to rise with increasing age. Paradoxically, people, including children, who exercise regularly eat less food.

Extra chromosomes see TRISOMY.

Eye deviation see SQUINT.

Eye infections see RED EYE.

Eye disorders see AMBLYOPIA, BLEPHARITIS, CATARACT, COLOUR BLINDNESS, RED EYE, CONTACT LENSES, EPICANTHUS, NYSTAGMUS, PTOSIS, REFRACTIVE ERRORS, RETINOBLASTOMA, RETROLENTAL FIBROPLASIA, SPECTACLES, SQUINT, STYES, TOXOCARIASIS, TOXOPLASMOSIS, WATERING EYE.

Eye focusing problems see REFRACTIVE ERRORS.

Eyelid abnormalities

There is a condition of lid inturning that affects fat babies. This is called puppy-fat entropion and, although it looks very uncomfortable, the remarkable thing about it is that the affected babies don't seem to be worried. The fact is that, at that age, the eyelashes are so soft that they are very unlikely to do any harm even if they lie on the cornea. Eye specialists never operate on puppy-fat entropion as the condition can be relied on to clear up on its own.

Epicanthus is a variant on the normal appearance of the upper eyelid. In epicanthus, the margin of the upper lid curves round and downwards so as to cover and conceal the inner corner of the eye. Epicanthus is common in babies and, if marked, may cause an appearance somewhat similar to convergent squint. In most cases, it reverts to normal as the face and nose grow. Persistent epicanthus is easily corrected by a plastic surgery, should it be thought disfiguring.

A potentially much more serious eyelid abnormality is drooping lid, or blepharoptosis (see PTOSIS). The danger here is that the condition will be thought to be of cosmetic significance only. It is nothing of the sort. A drooping lid that covers half the pupil may lead to permanent loss of vision in the affected eye (see AMBLYOPIA).

Other common eyelid problems in children are STYES and BLEPHARITIS.

Eyelid inflammation see
BLEPHARITIS.

Eye pressure see GLAUCOMA.

Eye wobbling

Children with persistent jerky or wobbling movement of the eyes, usually together, have a condition called NYSTAGMUS. The movement is most commonly horizontal, but may be vertical, or even circular. The commonest type of nystagmus, 'sawtooth' nystagmus, involves a repetitive slow movement in one direction followed by a sudden recovery jerk in the other. You can observe this kind, as a normal phenomenon, in underground railway passengers trying to read the station name from a moving train. Permanent sawtooth nystagmus is almost always present from birth (congenital) and seldom implies anything serious. Although the eyes are normal, it is, however, usually associated with a slight reduction in visual acuity. The exception to this is sawtooth nystagmus secondary to the condition of ALBINISM. In this case, the visual deficit may be considerable.

Nystagmus, of a searching type, as if the affected person is constantly looking for something, is a feature of very severe visual defect, such as might occur from dense congenital cataract (see CATARACT) or other serious eye defects present from birth. Nystagmus appearing *for the first time* later in life (acquired nystagmus) indicates a probably serious disorder of the nervous system and requires immediate medical attention.

F

Facial pallor see SKIN PALLOR.

Facial puffiness see
GLOMERULONEPHRITIS.

Facial swelling see MUMPS.

Fainting

Fainting is a temporary loss of consciousness due to a drop in the blood pressure, so that the brain is deprived of an adequate supply of fuel (glucose) and oxygen. The drop in blood pressure may result from a reduction in the rate of pumping of blood by the heart or from a general widening of the arteries of the body.

Common faints usually occur after prolonged standing, especially in hot conditions, when the return of blood to the heart by the veins is impeded. A severe fright or shock may cause sudden slowing of the heart. Fainting is also more likely when the volume of the blood is reduced as in fluid loss from prolonged DIARRHOEA or excessive sweating. Fainting on taking exercise suggests heart disease.

The fainting person falls and this is exactly what is required to restore the flow of blood to the brain. This can be encouraged by raising the legs. Convulsions or even brain damage can result if the fainting person is foolishly kept upright.

Genuine fainting is rare in children and should always be reported.

Fallot's tetralogy

Although relatively uncommon, this is one of the most frequent forms of CONGENITAL HEART DISEASE. Four defects occur. These are:

- narrowing of the main artery to the lungs

- a hole in the wall between the two sides of the heart
- an abnormality in the position of the main artery of the body (the aorta)
- considerable enlargement of the main pumping chamber (the ventricle) on the right side of the heart

Affected children usually show bluish skin colour (see CYANOSIS) and are breathless and easily tired. They often show a characteristic squatting position after exercise. They may have spells in which they are acutely cyanosed and floppy. Excellent results can be obtained by radical surgical correction of the various defects.

Family therapy

Many serious behavioural and emotional problems in children have their roots in defective interaction within the family. Many others are affected by the family relationships. Family therapy, in which the whole family participates, can therefore be more effective than therapy directed only to the child who has been identified as the patient, or who is the person deemed to be most seriously disturbed. Some of the problems dealt with by family therapy are:

- the inability of parents to agree on matters of importance to the children
- marital conflict which affects the children
- severe emotional separation between members
- blockage of communication between members
- lack of congruence between verbal and non-verbal communication

A social unit as well-established as a family is not easy to change because patterns of behaviour are deeply ingrained and largely unconscious. Short periods of therapy – perhaps three to five sessions of less than one hour each – may be sufficient, and therapy does not call for great psychiatric expertise. Much family therapy is now conducted by general practitioners, paediatricians and other experienced counsellors.

Patterns of family structure, illness and behaviour tend to be repeated over many generations. One way in which therapists proceed is to guide the family through the construction of a 'genogram', based on the family tree, in which a picture of how the current family relates to the previous generation is built up. In eliciting the facts on which this is based, much information comes to light, not only from the answers, but also from the way in which the therapist's questions are answered. Problems that are alleged to be entirely intrinsic to ('the fault of') a child may be shown to arise from conflicts essentially between the parents, recurrent patterns of illness or undesirable behaviour, alcoholism, family secrets or other factors relevant to the present family.

Once the therapist has established the nature of the group and has begun to see where the problems lie, it becomes possible to give all members of the family an insight into what is happening. Failure of communication, not only with the child but also between the parents, is one of the commonest problems and it is one of the most important functions of the therapist to ensure that proper communication techniques are applied. As a respected moderator or chairperson, he or she is able to prevent one member from dominating, two people from talking at once, shouting down, and so on. Anger shown by one member against another must be carefully channelled, recognized and analyzed so as to avoid escalation towards worsening relationships or breaking off of the therapy. Scape-goating must be detected and discussed. Constant harping on the supposed faults of the child or other members of the family is discouraged in favour of a consideration of how these faults may possibly be modified.

Family therapy can be found helpful in the management of severe family tension, truancy, defiant antisocial behaviour deliberate soiling, and child neglect and other forms of child abuse.

Febrile convulsions

These are seizures similar in appearance to EPILEPSY but caused solely by a sudden rise in temperature. They are relatively common in young children and may be a horrifying experience for parents, who often fear that the child is going to die. But death, in such cases, is extremely rare. The great majority of children who suffer these episodes are not epileptic and these fits do not occur because of any brain defect. The term 'febrile convulsions' simply means 'fits occurring in the course of a fever'.

Between three and four children in every 100 have one or more febrile convulsions by the time they are 5 years old. In most cases, the fits occur after the age of 6 months. Seizures occurring earlier than that are a matter for more concern.

It appears that the brains of many young children are exceptionally sensitive to a raised body temperature and that this, in itself, is enough to produce an electrical discharge. Febrile convulsions are usually fairly brief.. They seldom last for longer than about 10 minutes, and recovery is complete. But the convulsion will often resemble a full 'grand mal' attack of epilepsy and parents inevitably become seriously alarmed and may be convinced that their child is going to be a life-long epileptic.

But even children who have many fits will not necessarily become epileptic. In 19 cases out of 20, the sensitivity of the brain to fever decreases as the child grows and that is the end of the matter. As a general rule, isolated febrile convulsions may be considered unlikely to cause any permanent harm and need not occasion great anxiety.

It would be wrong, however, to suggest that febrile convulsions are unimportant. Convulsions themselves can cause brain damage – especially in the temporal lobes – which, in turn, can cause severe epilepsy. Most febrile convulsions occur between the ages of 9 months and 2 years and it seems likely that certain individuals have an inherited tendency to be more sensitive to fever than average. Boys are affected more often than girls.

The higher the fever, the more likely is there to be a convulsion. Three quarters of all convulsions occur with a temperature of more than 39.2° C (102.5° F). The younger the child, the more likely are the convulsions to be severe and prolonged, and the more severe the fits the more likely they are to cause permanent brain damage. Also, the probability of recurrence rises with the severity of the attack, and life-long epilepsy is much more likely if there are prolonged and severe febrile convulsions in infancy.

The implication is, of course, that every effort must be made to prevent febrile convulsions. Fever, in this age-group, should be controlled with paracetamol and deliberate cooling, and medical advice sought so that the cause of the fever may be treated as effectively as possible. Many childhood fevers are caused by infections which will respond rapidly to ANTIBIOTICS and these will be prescribed whenever necessary. Conditions commonly causing fevers include middle ear infection (OTITIS MEDIA), TONSILLITIS, kidney or urinary infection, pneumonia and any of the common infectious diseases of childhood, such as MEASLES, MUMPS, CHICKEN-POX and WHOOPING-COUGH. Many paediatricians believe it so important to avoid recurrent febrile convulsions that they view the start of any fever in a child who has already had a fever fit as a signal for the use of an anticonvulsant drug. Many doctors have found that the best drug to use, for this purpose, is the old-fashioned phenobarbitone.

Infantile convulsions have, in the past, been attributed to all sorts of alleged causes, such as TEETHING, THREADWORMS, CONSTIPATION, and so on, but there is no reason to believe that any of these minor conditions can cause fits. Modern methods of investigation will usually bring out the true cause.

As soon as you suspect that a febrile convulsion may be starting, you should try to prevent the fit by cool sponging. This should also be done even if the full fit occurs. Put the child on a large polythene sheet, or other waterproof surface, surround with bath towels and sponge down

thoroughly with lots of tepid water. In some cases it may be quicker simply to strip off the child's clothing and take him or her out into a colder environment. Get someone to phone for an ambulance. If the convulsion is severe, don't try to restrain the child – just gently protect him or her from injury. Remove all hard objects such as toys, and pad the cot sides with a folded towel or blanket, if necessary. Don't try to force open the mouth: to do so may cause the tongue to fall back and obstruct the airway.

If consciousness is lost, see to it that there is no obstruction to the breathing. As soon as the convulsion is over, the child should be turned face-down with the head turned to one side. If the leg on the same side is drawn well up, with the knee bent, this will stabilise the position. Should there be any indication of obstruction to the breathing, clear the mouth with a finger and suck out anything in the back of the throat with some form of tubing. Continue the sponging if the fever remains.

Try to be observant. It may be difficult for you to be detached, but it can be helpful if you note down any unusual features, as this may help the doctor to decide whether or not the fit has serious significance. Note whether the convulsion is generalised or, if local, which parts of the body are affected; how long the attack lasts; whether there is incontinence; note whether consciousness is lost and, if so, for how long. Remember that almost all seizures are self-limiting and will pass. Try to remain calm.

Feeding see introductory section.

Fetal alcohol syndrome

This is the group of effects on the growing fetus caused by repeated high levels of alcohol in the mother's blood. Maternal alcohol abuse during pregnancy is the commonest cause of drug-induced fetal abnormality. Few women can now be unaware that drinking during pregnancy is undesirable. But many are still uncertain about the actual degree of risk to the growing fetus. The syndrome is likely in those who drink heavily throughout pregnancy, and the severity of the effects is proportional to the amount of alcohol consumed. Exposure of the fetus to alcohol can cause any of the following effects:

- an eightfold rise in the death rate in the period immediately after birth
- defective body growth leading to low birthweight
- an abnormally small head (microcephaly)
- LEARNING DIFFICULTY, with IQ below 80 in 50 per cent of cases
- abnormal facial features – small eyelid openings, defective growth of the upper jaw, with receding teeth and protrusion of the lower jaw
- CLEFT PALATE
- limitation of joint movement
- congenital dislocation of the hip
- an increase in the likelihood of CONGENITAL HEART DISEASE

The fetal death rate and the death rate in the period immediately after birth are both markedly higher than in other pregnancies. Nearly one-fifth of affected babies die during the first few weeks of life. Of those who survive, many suffer some degree of physical or mental backwardness. Newborn babies with the syndrome suck poorly, sleep badly and are very irritable. Such babies are actually suffering alcohol withdrawal symptoms.

The trouble with alcohol is that it enters the blood very quickly and is immediately carried to all parts of the body. Alcohol gets everywhere including the brain – yours and the baby's. Women can take a lot more alcohol than a tiny fetus growing in the womb. So, if you feel drunk, what kind of an effect do you suppose the alcohol is having on your baby?

Alcohol, or, more accurately, its breakdown product, acetaldehyde, is a poison and the fetal alcohol syndrome is simply the effect of sustained poisoning of the fetus throughout the pregnancy. The younger the fetus, the more sensitive it is to the effects of alcohol. Unfortunately, the worst time of all is the period from 4 to 10 weeks. As pregnancy is usually diagnosed somewhere between 3 and 8 weeks, women who are liable to get pregnant should obviously avoid heavy drinking. The severity of the effects on the fetus are roughly proportional to the amount of alcohol consumed, but there is no known lower level of safety.

Incidentally, the drug Flagyl (metronidazole), commonly used for vaginal *Trichomonas* infections, causes accumulation of the alcohol breakdown product acetaldehyde. This may make you feel extremely ill and, as it is acetaldehyde that is believed to cause the fetal damage, it is likely to do your baby even more harm.

There has been a lot of medical controversy on how common the fetal alcohol syndrome actually is. It is true that the fully established syndrome, featuring most of the effects shown above, is not very common. It has been reported in about one-third of babies born to mothers with a chronic alcohol problem who go on drinking steadily throughout the pregnancy. But there is now little doubt that lesser, but still serious, effects are very common and that there is no lower limit of safety. Even small amounts of alcohol may produce permanent harm. So it really comes down to how you define the syndrome. If you mean the severe physical and mental effects listed above, then it is rare. But if you mean depriving your baby of the very best possible start in life, then the syndrome is distressingly common.

You do not need to drink much to damage your baby. Visible or measurable effects can occur if you take two shorts or two or three bottles of beer or glasses of wine each day (30 ml of pure alcohol). There is no reason to suppose that an occasional glass of wine or beer is likely to do harm, but there is every reason to go along with the universal medical advice that women should abstain completely from alcohol during pregnancy. Heavy drinking during pregnancy is permanently damaging to the fetus. Total abstinence from alcohol immediately before and throughout the pregnancy is the only positive safe way of avoiding such damage. Women with a drinking problem need advice and treatment before embarking on pregnancy.

Fetal skin coating see VERNIX.

Fetal jaundice see JAUNDICE, RHESUS INCOMPATIBILITY.

Fever

A fever is a rise in body temperature above the normal range of 37° to 37.5° C (98.6° to 99.5° F), taken in the mouth. Rectal temperatures are a little higher.

In childhood, fever is nearly always caused by infections, common examples being conditions such as TONSILLITIS, OTITIS MEDIA, MEASLES, MUMPS and CHICKENPOX. Infecting organisms grow best at normal body temperature and are discouraged by fever. So it is not always desirable to bring down the temperature. But high temperatures in children often cause FEBRILE CONVULSIONS and should always be brought down. Temperatures above about 44.5° C (112° F) usually cause fatal brain damage and, in such cases, urgent cooling, by any available means, is vital.

Fever fits see FEBRILE CONVULSIONS.

Finger and toe inflammation see CHILBLAINS.

First aid for children see introductory section (Safety and First Aid).

Flipper limbs see PHOCOMELIA, THALIDOMIDE EFFECT.

Floppy infant syndrome

When a normal baby is supported, face down, with a hand under the chest, the head is held back, the back is held straight, or almost so, and the arms and legs are partly bent. A floppy infant droops over the hand like an inverted U. This state is called 'hypotonia' and it is not, in itself, a disease, but rather an indication of one of a wide variety of conditions. Investigation is needed to determine whether any of these conditions is present. The possibilities include:

- any major debilitating disease
- malnutrition
- a hormonal disorder such as hypothyroidism
- DOWN'S SYNDROME
- TURNER'S SYNDROME
- a connective tissue disorder, such as MARFAN'S SYNDROME, osteogenesis imperfecta or the 'elastic skin' Ehlers-Danlos syndrome
- a birth brain injury
- progressive spinal muscular atrophy
- a MUSCULAR DYSTROPHY or other muscle disorder
- the muscle weakness disorder myasthenia gravis
- infection with the paralyzing botulinum organism (infant botulism)

Many floppy infants do not have any of these disorders, but this should not discourage investigation, for urgent treatment may be needed.

Flu see INFLUENZA.

Fontanelles

The vault of the growing skull of the baby and young infant is made of separate plates of bone which are close together except at the points where more than two meet. Towards the front of the vertex of the head, the meeting of four large plates – the two forehead (frontal) bones and the two side (parietal) bones – leaves a central gap known as the anterior fontanelle. The rear (posterior) fontanelle also lies centrally between the two parietal bones and the single rear occipital bone. The fontanelles are covered by scalp and skin and can easily be felt, as soft depressions, by gentle pressure with the fingers.

The fontanelles allow moulding of the skull during birth and allow for growth of the bone. The anterior fontanelle normally closes between 10 and 14 months of age, but the limits are wide and may extend from 3 to 18 months. The posterior fontanelle usually closes by 2 months.

Two important changes in the fontanelles may occur. Depression of the fontanelles implies a shortage of body fluid (DEHYDRATION), a state that can be very dangerous in babies. A sustained bulging of the fontanelles implies a rise in the pressure of the cerebrospinal fluid. This may have various causes, all of them potentially serious. Either effect should be reported urgently to your doctor. Transient bulging of the anterior fontanelle during crying or coughing is normal. This fontanelle may also be felt to pulsate. This, too, is normal.

Food poisoning

This is caused either by living organisms present in food, which incubate and reproduce in the body until enough are present to cause illness, or by contamination of food by the toxins of organisms which have grown outside the body. In the former case, there is usually a delay of a day or two before symptoms occur, in the latter, symptoms come on within hours. Bacterial toxins are very powerful and produce severe, but usually short-lived effects. A common cause of toxin contamination of food is the presence of septic spots on the fingers of people preparing food.

Food poisoning causes NAUSEA, VOMITING, loss of appetite, FEVER, abdominal pain and DIARRHOEA. The commonest bacterial contamination of food is by *Salmonella* organisms which are commonly found in meats and eggs. Food handled by people with poor standards of personal hygiene is often contaminated by human faeces. The most dangerous form of food poisoning is botulism, which, fortunately, is rare. The organism is found in meat pastes and other processed animal products, usually prepared in the home and inadequately sterilised. It causes widespread paralysis and death.

Food poisoning can also be caused by poisons such as metal salts or plant or animal poisons. Naturally-occurring poisons include those in mushrooms, such as *Amanita phalloides*.

Foreign body in ear see EAR, FOREIGN BODY IN

Foreskin see CIRCUMCISION.

G

Galactosaemia

This is a rare genetic disorder of babies, inherited as an autosomal recessive trait (see GENETICS – AN OUTLINE), in which a chemical activator (enzyme) necessary for the breakdown of galactose, a sugar present in milk, is absent. As a result, galactose, instead of being converted to glucose, accumulates in the body and may cause LEARNING DIFFICULTY, cataract (see CATARACT IN CHILDREN), liver enlargement, JAUNDICE, DIARRHOEA, VOMITING and malnutrition. There is a great variation in severity.

The gene for the enzyme is located on chromosome number 9 and it is absent in one in 150 of the population. The inheritance is recessive (see GENETICS – AN OUTLINE), so the condition can occur only if both parents carry the gene on at least one of the pair of corresponding chromosomes, and both of them happen to pass this one on to the child. The incidence of galactosaemia in Britain is about one in 80,000 births. Fetal antenatal screening can detect the condition before birth and, if the mother has high galactose levels, amniocentesis can demonstrate whether the fetal brain is likely to have been been damaged.

Affected babies appear normal when born, but within a few days of starting to take milk have diarrhoea and vomiting. Soon wasting becomes apparent and within seven to 10 days JAUNDICE appears. The rapid enlargement of the liver is a notable feature of the condition. The lower edge of the enlarged organ can easily be felt. Because of failure of the breakdown of milk sugar to usable monosaccharides, the baby is being starved of the normal body fuel – glucose – and may suffer hypoglycaemia (see DIABETES). This can cause convulsions. In an untreated baby, cataracts will develop within a few weeks.

If the condition is diagnosed early, the infant can be fed on a galactose free diet and will grow up entirely normal. Even if lens opacities have begun to form, a change to a galactose-free diet may be followed by restoration of lens transparency.

Gamma globulin

Antibodies are also called immunoglobulins. They are protective soluble proteins, produced by B lymphocytes, which attach to invading organisms or foreign substances and neutralise them so that they can be destroyed by the body's scavenging cells (the phagocytes). There are five classes of immunoglobulins, the most prevalent being immunoglobulin G, or gamma globulin. This provides the body's main defence against bacteria, viruses and toxins.

Gamma globulin is so widely effective that it is produced commercially, from pooled human plasma, and used as a means of passive protection against many childhood infections. It is useful for protection, when the need arises, against such infections as HEPATITIS A and B CHICKENPOX, MEASLES and POLIO. It is also very useful for children who have an inherent or acquired immune deficiency, such as the condition of agammaglobulinaemia.

Gargoylism see HURLER'S SYNDROME.

Gastroenteritis see DEHYDRATION.

Gender identity problems

Fortunately, these are uncommon, but for the children concerned, and for their parents, they are of central importance. Uncertainty as to gender identity gives rise to severe distress and is prolific source of emotional and behavioural problems. In many cases parents may be quite unaware of the source of the young person's unhappiness. Suicide or suicidal attempts are common in young people affected in this way. This is often what brings the matter to the attention of the medical and psychiatric professions.

The term 'gender' has extended its meaning in recent years and is no longer limited in its application to grammatical terms. It is now usefully applied to the feeling of belonging to one or other biological sex. In the enormous majority, the gender will correspond to the anatomical structure of the external genitalia. But it need not necessarily do so. In this context, gender is the mental and behavioural component of sex. It is the inherent sense of either masculinity or femininity as the case may be. Gender identity disorders arise when the gender differs from the anatomical sex.

By the age of 2 or 3 almost all children have a perfectly clear perception of their own gender and make frequent references to it. It is important to distinguish a real gender identity disorder from a mere apparent tendency to possess some of the characteristics of the other sex. Thus, the condition is not present simply because a girl has a tendency to boyish interests or conduct – she will be acknowledged as a tomboy. Nor is it present if a boy appears girlish or evinces feminine behaviour or traditional female interests. Gender identity problems are not the same as homosexuality, notwithstanding the facts that some homosexual women seem to favour mannish behaviour and some homosexual men enjoy drag. At the same time, research shows that children with genuine gender identity problems commonly turn out to be homosexual or bisexual rather than heterosexual. Transvestism – the desire to dress as the other sex – is not a common outcome. Very few children with gender identity disorder become transvestites.

According to the *American Diagnostic and Statistical Manual of Mental Disorders-IV* (DSM-IV), children with gender identity problems show at least four of the following:

- repeatedly stated desire to be of the opposite anatomical sex or insistence that he or she is of the opposite sex

- a preference, in boys, for cross-dressing or simulated female attire; an insistence, in girls, on wearing only stereotyped male clothing
- strong and persistent preference for taking the role of the other sex in make-believe play; or persistent fantasies of being of the other sex
- an intense desire to participate in characteristic games and pastimes of the other sex
- strong preference for playmates of the other physical sex
- in adolescents, frequent passing off as belonging to the other physical sex, a desire to live and be treated as a member of the other sex, and the conviction that he or she has the typical feelings and reaction of the other sex.
- persistent discomfort with his or her sex or a sense of inappropriateness in the gender role of that sex

Boys will assert that their external genitalia are disgusting and hope that they will disappear or ought to disappear. Girls feel that they should urinate standing up and resent having to sit down to do so. They insist that they do not want to grow breasts or menstruate, and will sometimes assert that they will grow a penis.

The cause of gender identity disorder remains unclear and most of the more obvious possibilities, such as hormonal irregularities before and after birth, have been dismissed. Some experts believe that gender identity is determined early in life by the effect of the parents' behaviour and attitudes to the child brought about by their wish for a child of the other sex. In some cases, there may have been genital ambiguity at birth and a genuine mistake as to the sex of the child, potentiated, perhaps, by wishful thinking on the part of the parents (see PSEUDOHERMAPHRODITISM). Recent studies, however, have shown that this, alone, is not enough to account for the prevalence of the condition.

It seems probable that a number of conditions, operating early in the life of the child, must co-exist for the problem to arise. These may include:

- boys with unduly close attachment to the mother and an uncaring and distant father
- girls with a depressed mother and an unsupportive father
- a dominant and important attachment to a person other than a parent in early childhood
- the inability to mourn the death of a parent in early childhood
- a family history of gender identity problems

The first step in the management of the problem is to recognize that it exists. This requires skilled and specialized attention by experts in this rare disorder. Recognition and acknowledgement can, in itself, result in considerable relief for the unfortunate victim. Later in life, a proportion of them seek sex-change surgery and, in some cases, this is highly successful. It is never agreed to, however, without the most searching and careful preliminary investigation.

Gene therapy

This contentious subject is still in its infancy but is advancing rapidly. At the time of writing, no single inheritable disease has been cured by gene therapy. But the possibilities – as well as the risks – are enormous and it is only an awareness of the latter that has, quite rightly, delayed progress.

Gene therapy is concerned with the treatment of hereditary disease by introducing normal genes into the body. There are about 4000 known GENETIC DISORDERS and few of them can be effectively treated by conventional means. Some of these diseases are so distressing that pressures to adopt potentially effective genetic treatments have become overwhelming. Ethical committees and other authorities are now progressively giving way in carefully selected areas.

There is a great divide in gene therapy: genes can be introduced into the general body cells (somatic cells) or they can be introduced into the germ cells – sperms, ova or early embryos. The difference is fundamental. In the first case, only the individual is affected; in the second, all that person's future offspring will be af-

fected. For this reason germ cell gene therapy is currently almost universally prohibited. It simply raises too many dangerous possibilities and ethical problems.

Gene therapy involving somatic cells is now going ahead. The condition severe combined immunodeficiency (SCID) is so dangerous that affected children have to be kept in plastic bubbles to insulate them from infection. The condition is caused in many cases by the absence of a gene that codes for the enzyme adenosine deaminase (ADA) necessary for the integrity of the immune system. In September 1990, scientists began to insert the gene for this enzyme into affected children. Bone marrow transplants of genetically engineered cells are being done to treat leukaemia and other blood disorders in which new clones of blood cells can be expected to survive and give rise to healthy populations of blood cells. The gene has to be inserted in the stem cells which clone the cell populations. These are difficult to find.

Genes can be introduced into cells by various methods. Micro-injection using a fine glass pipette, works very well but requires skill and is hardly practicable if many cells are to be processed. Electroporation involves exposure of cells to an electric shock which makes the membrane more permeable and allows material to enter the cell, but is often severely damaging. Perhaps the most efficient method is the use of retroviruses to carry in the new gene. Many viruses have now been engineered to serve as vectors for gene transfer. Retroviruses convert their own RNA to DNA in infected cells and insert the DNA into a chromosome. So if a retrovirus contains the required gene and is otherwise harmless, it makes an ideal delivery system. Unfortunately, retroviruses can cause cancer, especially if they are allowed to multiply in the body. This is a major problem that is being energetically tackled.

Research is in progress to study the possibility of engineering skin cells, such as fibroblasts, to make them produce needed proteins that are normally produced in other cells. If this succeeds, implants of skin cells could correct many disorders in which a protein is absent –

conditions such as HAEMOPHILIA or DWARF-ISM from growth hormone deficiency.

We are only at the beginning of a new and very exciting chapter in the history of medicine.

See also GENETICS – AN OUTLINE

Genetic counselling

In all of the many conditions known to be caused by a defect in a particular single gene, the chances of producing an affected baby can be mathematically determined. Genetic counselling is based on a detailed knowledge of the principles of genetics and of the conditions caused by gene defect. Counsellors must be able to construct a family pedigree, draw inferences from it and convey difficult information to sometimes distressed parents in a form that can be understood. Only then can rational decisions be made about having children.

The subject is so difficult that it is best dealt with in centres specialising in genetic counselling, where a high level of expertise and knowledge of recent developments can be brought to bear effectively on these often tragic human problems.

If you already have a child with a hereditary disease, or if a close relative has a hereditary disease, you will naturally want to know the chances of the disease appearing in your next child. There are several reasons why genetic counselling could be important for you. There may be a family tradition of a particular disease and you may be doubtful whether or not it is hereditary. Like many parents, you may have a horror of bringing a deformed or severely defective child into the world. If you are a woman of 40 plus and pregnant, or think-ing about getting pregnant, you will be concerned about the higher risk of genetic disease in the child. These are all reasonable and realistic concerns and the right way to get answers to your questions is to seek genetic counselling.

Genetic counselling is a service available to people who need information or advice about the chances of bearing children with a disease caused by an inherited abnormal gene. If you think you need counselling, go and see your GP first. He or she may be able to counsel you, but this is a complicated matter and most GPs will prefer to refer you to the experts.

In some cases, hospitals have teams that, in addition to geneticists, include a baby doctor (paediatrician), a childbirth specia-list (obstetrician) a social worker, a nurse and, as required, special consultants who are experts in particular diseases.

After asking what has been worrying you, the counsellor will take a careful fa-mily history, so it will be very helpful if you find out as much as you possibly can about previous cases of the same condition in your family. Contact all your relatives and ask them. Check especially with the older people. Ask particularly about *any* diseases about which there is any doubt.

The counsellor will then perform a full physical examination of anyone known to be suffering from, or suspected of having, the disease in question. In some cases, the physical signs of the disease are so obvious that the condition can immediately be re-cognised and counselling can be given. Laboratory tests will probably also be ar-ranged. The first thing to be found out is whether or not the problem actually is genetic, and if so, how it is passed on. This is called the mode of inheritance. If the condition is hereditary, the counsellor will try to draw a family tree showing all cases in which the condition occurred. Such a tree will show the mode of inheritance. Labora-tory tests are often helpful and may show such things such as:

- microscopically visible abnormalities in chromosomes
- an extra chromosome, as in DOWN'S SYNDROME
- abnormal haemoglobin, as in SICKLE CELL DISEASE
- absence of a particular blood-clotting factor, as in HAEMOPHILIA

If the disease can be identified, the risks of it happening again can usually be stated accurately. For certain chromosome disor-ders the risk may be 100 per cent. In con-ditions caused by a single gene, the risk may be as high as one in four or even one in two. If the gene is known to be on one of the two sex chromosomes, the mode of inheritance and the risks will be clearly explained. If many different factors have to be present the risk will be much smaller, perhaps as low as one in 20.

Even if you are already pregnant, genetic counselling may be valuable, but you must not delay. A genetic defect can be identified by amniocentesis or chorionic villus sampling – procedures performed in hospital. Small samples of fluid surrounding the fetus, or even, in the case of chorionic villus sampling, of the part of the developing placenta of the embryo, can be withdrawn through a fine tube or needle passed into the womb. Amniotic fluid contains fetal cells which can be studied for chromosomal or chemical abnormalities and may indicate the presence of certain birth defects. A great many hereditary diseases can now be identified in this way. The sex of the fetus can also be checked and this may be important as some genetic diseases only occur in one sex, and this can sometimes rule out a suspected condition.

If the worst happens and the embryo is found to have a serious genetic disorder, you will have the option of deciding to have the pregnancy stopped at this early stage.

See also GENETICS – AN OUTLINE.

Genetic disorders

A gene is a short piece of one of the very long strands of DNA which form the chromosomes present in every cell of your body. It is simply a particular sequence of chemical groups called bases, and an abnormal gene is one in which the order of the bases has become mixed up or some of them have been lost. The genes model thousands of different body proteins and these, in turn, determine the functioning of our body chemistry and how our bodies differ from those of other people. Most of the proteins formed in this way are called enzymes. These bring about the chemical reactions in the body necessary for its growth and development. Single gene disorders occur when there is a mistake in the sequence of bases that form the gene so that the necessary enzymes are defective or non-operative.

Chromosomes are arranged in pairs, each pair with the same sequence of genes, so each gene is present twice. If a condition results when only one gene of a pair is abnormal, it is said to be dominant. If a condition occurs only when both genes of the pair are abnormal, it is said to be recessive. Single gene disorders may be dominant or recessive. In recessive disorders, when one gene is normal, the enzyme produced by the normal gene is sufficient to allow normal function. But in dominant disorders, or when both genes are affected in recessive disorders, the enzyme is missing and a biochemical reaction essential to health cannot proceed normally.

Genetic disorders occur when one or more genes have been changed at any time before conception. These changes are called mutations. Mutations can occur in the sex glands of either parent, or they may have occurred perhaps generations before and have been passed down from person to person. Genetic disorders also arise if there is anything wrong with whole chromosomes. Unlike gene defects, whole chromosome defects can be seen under a microscope. They include bits missing from chromosomes, extra bits stuck on to chromosomes, and additional complete chromosomes. DOWN'S SYNDROME, for instance, is caused by an additional chromosome number 21.

About one baby in 200, born alive, has a genetic defect, but gene defects are much commoner than this would suggest. Many of the fetuses that abort spontaneously at an early stage of pregnancy are genetically abnormal.

There are thousands of different genetic disorders and, happily, most of them are rare. They include such conditions as:

- SICKLE CELL DISEASE
- CYSTIC FIBROSIS
- DOWN'S SYNDROME
- MUSCULAR DYSTROPHY
- PYLORIC STENOSIS
- SPINA BIFIDA
- PHENYLKETONURIA
- TAY-SACHS DISEASE
- GALACTOSAEMIA

Other less common single gene disorders are:

- HAEMOPHILIA, affecting males and causing severe bleeding.
- Agammaglobulinaemia, an immune deficiency disorder featuring the absence of certain antibodies. Affected children suffer recurrent infections but can be kept healthy by regular injections of gamma globulin.
- Testicular feminization syndrome, in which males appear like normal females because of an enzyme defect that prevents male sex hormone from working.
- Cystinuria, a recessive disorder causing abnormal excretion of the amino acid cystine in the urine. Stones form in the kidney and bladder but effective treatment exists.
- The Ehlers-Danlos syndrome, characterized by extraordinary elasticity of the skin and excessive laxity and increased mobility of the joints which may dislocate easily. It is due to defective formation of the protein collagen.
- Haemochromatosis, in which abnormal absorption of iron from the intestine results in deposition of iron in the tissues with damage from excessive formation of fibrous tissue. Regular bleeding helps to dispose of excess iron and can prevent tissue damage from iron accumulation.
- Huntington's disease, a dominant disorder causing involuntary jerky movements of the limbs and body so that the affected child may appear to be dancing and grimacing. There is usually progression to dementia. There is no treatment, but diagnosis can be made before birth and the pregnancy terminated.
- Osteogenesis imperfecta, or 'brittle bone' disease, a dominant disorder that leads to repeated bone fractures. The whites of the eyes are exceptionally thin so that the underlying pigment shows through, producing a blue appearance.
- Otosclerosis, a hereditary form of deafness due to a dominant gene. One of the bones in the middle ear becomes fused and immobile, but the condition can be treated with microsurgery.
- Retinitis pigmentosa, a condition of very variable course involving degeneration of the retinas that may lead to blindness. There is poor night vision and a progressive loss of the field of vision. There is no known treatment.
- Nephroblastoma (Wilms' tumour), a dominant condition featuring a malignant tumour in the kidney in about one child in 10,000. It is the commonest form of kidney cancer and, if detected early, can be cured by surgery, radiation and chemotherapy.

See also GENETICS – AN OUTLINE.

Genetics – an outline

It would be inappropriate in a book of this kind to go into great detail about the way children acquire their physical and mental characteristics, but this subject is so important and is of such interest to many parents that a brief outline is included.

Every cell in the body has a length of DNA in it about a metre long. The DNA is normally in a big tangle in the middle of the cell but when cells are dividing to form new cells the DNA gets coiled up tightly to form chromosomes. Genes are just lengths of DNA consisting of variable numbers of four chemical units, called bases, arranged in different orders. Each group of three bases stands for a particular one of 20 protein-building units known as amino acids. So the sequence of groups of three tells the cell which amino acids to select, and in what order, to make proteins. This is the genetic code.

The body is mainly made of proteins but most of the genes are codes for making another class of proteins known as enzymes. And it is these that determine how the body is put together and how it works. Genes that cause disorders or diseases are normal genes with some mistakes in their base sequence. These are called mutations and they result in defective proteins being formed, most of which are enzymes. Other differences occur between gene pairs, differences that do not cause disease but merely different normal characteristics. In this case, one gene has one effect and the other a different effect. For instance, one might cause brown eyes and the other blue eyes. Here, we do not talk of 'normality', although at one stage in human evolution, one state must, have been 'normal' and the other a mutation.

Half of the child's genes come from the mother and half from the father. But, of course, the same applies to their parents, so you can consider that the mother and father contribute a quarter each and all the previous forebears the other half. The mother's genes come in the egg and the father's in the sperm. Eggs, being cells in the female body, contain one X (sex) chromosome. Sperms carry either an X chromosome or a Y chromosome. Only one sperm gets lucky and that one will, by pure chance, carry either an X or a Y. If it carries a Y, the result will be a boy; if an X, a girl. So boys have an X and a Y chromosome in each cell of their bodies (XY), and girls two X chromosomes (XX).

There are 46 chromosomes altogether and they come in 23 pairs, of which one pair is the sex-determining chromosomes just mentioned. The two members of a chromosome pair are called homologous chromosomes. One of each pair comes from the mother and the other from the father. The chromosomes other than the sex chromosomes are called autosomes and in each pair the two chromosomes are very similar to each other but not quite identical. Homologous chromosomes have their genes in corresponding positions (loci) along the chromosomes. So genes, too, come in pairs. Mostly, the members of the pairs are the same and are entirely normal. But in some cases, one gene of the pair is normal and the other has a mutation. Much less often, both genes of the pair have mutations.

Children do not inherit complete unchanged chromosomes from their parents. If they did, they would more closely resemble their parents than they actually do. While the eggs and sperm are being prepared from normal body cells, the two members of each chromosome pair come close together and randomly exchange segments. This mixes up the gene pairs considerably so that the differences between the members of each pair of chromosomes have changed. There is another cause of mixing. Eggs and sperm each have half the full complement of chromosomes – 23 instead of 46. This is so that when the sperm enters the egg the right number is made up. So when sperm and eggs are being formed during cell division, the members of the pairs in each cell have to separate and go to two different eggs in the case of females, or to two sperm in the case of males. When they do so, it is a completely random matter which of the pairs goes to which of the two new egg or sperm cells being formed.

DOMINANCE

Each pair of homologous chromosomes have their corresponding pairs of genes, but, as we have seen, the genes need not be identical. When they are, the characteristic which the gene produces, appears. If one of the genes of the pair has a mutation that can cause a particular effect, it may do so, over-ruling the normal gene. In this case, the gene that causes this effect is said to be the *dominant* gene and the other the recessive. The effect, physically, will be the same as if both genes had been identical to the dominant gene. People with a dominant gene disorder will usually have a long family history of the condition, which can usually be traced through the generations. Because only one of the gene pair is affected, they are said to be heterozygous. And they have a 50–50 chance of passing on the trait to their offspring regardless of whether these are boys or girls. Of course, unaffected children do not carry the gene so they cannot pass on the condition.

Autosomal dominant conditions are not at all common. Among the best known are Marfan's syndrome causing 'spider fingers', dislocated eye lenses and floppy aorta; neurofibromatosis (von Recklinghausen's disease); otosclerosis that causes progressive deafness; ACHONDROPLASIA; brittle bone disease (osteogenesis imperfecta); polycystic kidney; Huntington's disease; and elastic skin disorder (Ehlers-Danlos syndrome).

Often a mutation in one of the gene pairs will not matter a great deal because the other gene is normal and produces enough protein to do the job. In this case, the gene with the mutation is said to be *recessive*. But remember that every cell in the affected person's body, including those producing sperm and eggs, contains the recessive gene. Such a person is said to be heterozygous for that gene and is also known as a 'carrier' of the gene. When a cell divides to form a sperm or an egg, one of this pair of chromosomes goes to each. So for each sperm or egg there is a 50–50 chance that it will be the one with the mutated recessive gene. In the unlikely event of a sperm with the recessive gene fertilizing an egg which also happens to have the recessive gene, the situation is quite different. Every cell in the resulting child's body will contain only the mutated gene and there is bound to be an effect – which may be serious.

From this we see that an autosomal recessive condition appears only if both father and mother carry the recessive gene, and if both the sperm and the egg happen to be carrying it. Most mutations are recessive and do not cause trouble because, although they code for a defective protein, the normal gene of the pair usually produces enough normal protein to keep things going normally. With recessive disorders there is not usually a family history because carriers produce no discernible effect. But if both parents carry the same recessive gene, the chances of a child getting the disorder are one in four. Probably the best known autosomal recessive condition is CYSTIC FIBROSIS. Others are PHENYLKETONURIA, SICKLE CELL ANAEMIA, THALASSAEMIA, Tay-Sachs disease, GALACTOSAEMIA and homocystinuria.

There is an interesting special case of recessive inheritance in which the affected gene is carried, not on an autosomal chromosome, but on a sex chromosome.

SEX-LINKED, RECESSIVE INHERITANCE

This is a mode of inheritance in which the gene for the condition is carried on the male X chromosome. The condition almost always affects males, but is never transmitted directly from father to son. This is easily explained.

Males have X and Y chromosomes, the latter being responsible for maleness and little else. It seems likely that Y chromosomes do not carry genes for any disorder. So X-linked is really the same as sex-linked. Females have two X chromosomes, one inherited from the father by way of an X-carrying, daughter-producing sperm, and the other inherited from the mother in the egg. Because a father transmits his X chromosomes only to his daughters, he can only pass on the gene for the condition to a daughter and never to a son; the son, of course, gets the father's Y chromosome. The daughter will have the mutated gene on one of her X chromosomes, and the chances are that she will have a normal gene on the other X chromosome. Like all her sisters, she will simply be a carrier of the gene. For a recessive condition to appear in a girl, both members of the gene pair must be affected. So, for a girl to develop a sex-linked recessive condition, she would have to inherit an X chromosome, with the gene, from her father, and an X chromosome, with the affected gene, from her carrier mother. This mating of a man, suffering from the condition, with a woman who happens to be a carrier, is very unlikely except in close relatives. This is why inbreeding can cause trouble, but it will only do so if a recessive gene mutation of importance is present in the family.

There are no male carriers of X-linked recessive conditions. Healthy males don't have the gene and can't pass on the condition. A female carrier of the sex-linked recessive condition has the gene on half her X chromosomes and has a 50–50 chance of passing the condition on to her sons. If she does so, all the sons with the gene will develop the condition, because their other sex chromosome is a Y chromosome which cannot 'cancel out' the gene on the X chromosome. The best-known sex-linked recessive condition is HAEMOPHILIA. Others are Duchenne MUSCULAR DYSTRO-PHY; fish-skin disease (ichthyosis); and the fragile X syndrome.

New single-gene conditions are constantly being detected so it is difficult to say how many there are and what are the proportions of the various types. But a recent authoritative work gives a total of nearly 4,500 proven and probable such conditions. Of the 2,208 proven conditions, 1,443 are autosomal dominant, 626 are autosomal recessive and 139 are X-linked.

A great many disorders are known to have a genetic element in their causation but are not caused, like all those mentioned above, by a single defective gene. These conditions, which may prove to be a majority of all diseases, are believed to result from the interaction of the effect of several genes at different locations with the total environment. The total effect is thus known as multifactorial. Much remains to be discovered about multifactorial inheritance.

WHOLE CHROMOSOME DISORDERS

These are conditions caused by major defects in the visible structure, or number, of whole chromosomes. They are different from gene disorders, in which the chromosomes appear normal but have errors somewhere along the length of DNA. One liveborn baby in about 200 has a detectable chromosome defect, but the actual number occurring at the time of fertilization is much higher than this. Many conceptions with chromosomal defects abort spontaneously within a week or two because the defect is incompatible with survival and is of a kind never found in live babies.

Chromosomal abnormalities take various forms. Pieces of a chromosome may be missing (deletion), or parts from one or more chromosomes may be attached to another. This is called translocation. Sometimes a chromosome forms into a ring.

As well as structural differences, there may be more or less than the normal number of chromosomes. If an autosomal chromosome is missing altogether, essential genes are absent and survival is impossible. The presence of an extra chromosome, however, has a less serious effect because all the necessary genetic material is present. But the duplication of genes will always cause trouble of some kind. An extra chromosome means that instead of one of the pairs there are three of one kind. This is known as TRISOMY.

An additional chromosome number 21 is the cause of DOWN'S SYNDROME. The defect is called trisomy 21 because all the cells in the body have three samples of chromosome 21. Like other forms of trisomy, it is more likely if the child is conceived towards the end of the mother's reproductive life. Other forms of trisomy are the Patau syndrome (trisomy 13) and Edward's syndrome (trisomy 18). Both of these are associated with multiple birth defects, learning difficulty and a limited lifespan. A proportion of people with trisomy have an extra chromosome in some of the body cells and the normal number in the others. This is called mosaicism. A child with trisomy 21 mosaicism will have much less obvious Down's syndrome characteristics than a child with three number 21 chromosomes in every cell.

Additional sex chromosomes also occur. Most commonly there are three (trisomy), but sometimes four. One of the commonest sex chromosome abnormalities is Klinefelter's syndrome. This affects males and they usually have an extra X chromosome, so each cell contains two X chromosomes and one Y chromosome (XXY). Occasionally there are four chromosomes, giving an XXYY constitution or sometimes XXXY. Because of the extra female sex chromosome, boys with Klinefelter's syndrome develop a female-like body pattern with underdevelopment of the genitals and enlargement of the breasts. About a quarter of those with the commoner XXY pattern are mentally retarded. Men with the XXXY pattern are always mentally retarded.

Another numerical chromosomal disorder in males is the XYY configuration. Many such men appear to be entirely normal, but surveys in institutions for mentally retarded men with criminal tendencies have shown that up to 5 per cent of the inmates have the XYY pattern. This is a far higher proportion than in the general population.

Only one important chromosomal numerical abnormality affects females. This is TURNER'S SYNDROME in which each cell contains only one X chromosome (XO configuration). At least 90 per cent of Turner's syndrome embryos and 60 per cent of Down's syndrome embryos abort spontaneously in early pregnancy.

Chromosomal disorders are easily diagnosed because the bodily effects are usually so obvious that they can at once be recognized by doctors. It is usual, however, to confirm this by examining the actual chromosome pattern (the karyotype). This simply involves taking a cell sample by gently scraping the inside of the cheek, culturing the cells, prompting them to enter the chromosome stage before division, and then taking a microphotograph of the chromosomes. This is enlarged and the chromosomes cut out of the print and arranged as homologous pairs. Any abnormality in the patterns can then be detected. There is no practicable treatment for conditions as widespread as those caused by whole chromosome abnormalities, but much can be done to encourage the best possible development and outcome in any case.

All human chromosome abnormalities can be detected in the developing fetus by the 14th to 16th week by sampling the cells in the fluid surrounding the fetus (amniocentesis). DNA can be obtained even earlier – as early as the 9th week – by chorionic villus sampling. If a chromosomal abnormality is found, there is the option of agreeing to have the pregnancy terminated.

See also GENETIC DISORDERS.

Genital stimulation see
MASTURBATION.

Gifted children

If unusually gifted or precocious children are to fulfil their potential, they cannot be considered to be adequately served by the same educational and cultural environments as average children. They need special opportunities, special challenges and,

above all, a special appreciation of what they can, and should, attain, such as can be offered by institutions dedicated to that purpose.

Such children attending ordinary schools are nearly always bored mainly because they are forced to spend so much time listening to instruction on matters already completely familiar to them. In addition to being bored, such children are often unhappy for other reasons. Because they are so bright they are, *ipso facto*, different from their contemporaries and, because of this, often disliked. Their companions frequently tease and bully them and they commonly feel – and are – misunderstood and alienated.

It is not enough to provide these children with supplementary instruction or to move them up to higher forms.

Studies show that exceptionally gifted children usually overcome the inadequacies of their educational opportunities, and do very well as adults. A Stanford University Press report by LM Terman and MH Oden, called *The Gifted Group at Mid-life*, recounts how 1,528 unusually gifted children were followed and up from the age of 12 to middle age. These authors found that 'the superior child, with few exceptions, becomes the able adult, superior in nearly every aspect to the generality. The superiority is greatest in intellectual ability, in scholastic accomplishments, and in vocational achievements'.

Gilles de la Tourette syndrome

This extraordinary, but rare, disorder begins in childhood with simple, involuntary, uncontrollable body movements such as shrugs, twitches, jerks or blinks (TICS), but, instead of disappearing spontaneously as these childhood tics normally do, progresses to a repertoire of ever more extensive and grotesque manifestations. Initially, these are complex bodily movements only, but eventually the sufferer begins to emit noises, at first minor barks, grunts or coughs, but later compulsive utterances, usually of an obscene nature. Coprolalia – involuntary scatological remarks – occurs in about half the cases and so the condition becomes a severe social disability.

Gilles de la Tourette syndrome requires skilled treatment with antipsychotic drugs (neuroleptics) which cause emotional quieting, promote indifference and slow down bodily and mental overactivity. Haloperidol (Serenace) is often used.

Glandular fever

In childhood, this disease is usually mild and inapparent, and most children acquire the infection without knowing it. One attack confers permanent immunity. During the acute phase and convalescence the virus is present in large numbers in the saliva. This is why the condition is sometimes called the 'kissing disease'.

In an obvious case, there is misery, FEVER, HEADACHE, sore throat and a general enlargement of lymph nodes which may be felt, as rubbery swellings, in the neck, armpits, elbows, groins and behind the knees. The spleen is also enlarged. In about 10 per cent of cases, there is a rash of small, slightly raised, red spots. If this does not occur spontaneously, mistaken treatment with the antibiotic ampicillin will bring it on. The lungs may be involved, with chest pain, difficulty in breathing and cough.

Usually there is complete recovery in less than a month, but one person in 10 complains for months, or even years, of fatigue with occasional recurrences of fever and lymph node enlargement. There is no specific treatment, but bed rest is desirable during the acute stage and strenuous exercise should be avoided as long as the spleen is enlarged.

Glaucoma

Glaucoma is an eye disorder in which the pressure of the fluids within the eye is abnormally raised. The effect of this is to compress and occlude tiny internal blood vessels supplying blood to the nerves running from the retina. As a result more and more of these nerves are destroyed and vision is progressively lost. Glaucoma present at birth (congenital glaucoma) causes enlargement of the eyeballs, a condition known as buphthalmos. This form of glaucoma is rare and is caused by a developmental defect of the eye that results in failure of adequate drainage from the eye of the internal fluid (aqueous humour) that maintains its shape. Because the fluid continues to be secreted within the eye but cannot escape normally, the pressure rises.

Up to about 3 years of age the elastic coats of the eye are still capable of stretching and the affected eye enlarges, sometimes markedly. This is readily apparent from an increase in the diameter of the cornea. Examination of the cornea with the slit-lamp microscope – the basic diagnostic tool of the ophthalmologist – shows ridge-like cracks or breaks in one of the inner membranes of the tissue. There is constant watering, acute sensitivity to light and a strong tendency to keep the eyes shut.

Congenital glaucoma requires urgent treatment. The pressure in the affected eye or eyes must be measured, usually under anaesthesia, and an operation performed to open up the drainage channels of the eye at the root of the iris. Careful follow-up is essential to ensure that the eye pressure is kept within safe limits so that vision is preserved.

Glomerulonephritis

This is inflammation of the kidneys caused by an immunological disorder. When bacteria, such as streptococci, invade the body, they prompt an antibody response from the immune system which is usually sufficient to destroy them. Sometimes, however, the quantity of antibody produced is insufficient to do this and the battle becomes a kind of stalemate, with millions of little groups of bacteria, tightly linked to small quantities of antibody, circulating in the blood. These groups are called 'immune complexes' and they are increasingly recognized as an important cause of disease.

Glomerulonephritis is one of the major disorders caused by circulating immune complexes. These complexes settle in the kidneys and are deposited on the walls of the filtering units (glomeruli) where they cause severe inflammation which may be very damaging to the tissue.

The initial streptococcal infection usually involves the throat and may be quite mild – sometimes passing unnoticed. One to three weeks later, the effects of kidney damage appear. The disease commonly affects children, causing generalised swelling of the tissues of the body (oedema) especially of the face, fever, loss of appetite, vague backache, vomiting and headache. The eyelids may be so puffy that the eyes are difficult to open. The blood pressure is usually raised and examination of the urine shows that this is scanty and contains blood and protein – both abnormal constituents. Sometimes 'coke-coloured' urine, from blood, is the only sign. In severe cases, the urine may stop altogether, for a time. After two or three days the signs and symptoms lessen, the output of urine increases and apparently full recovery occurs. There may, however, be abnormalities in the urine for weeks or months afterwards and, in about 10 per cent of cases, the episode of glomerulonephritis is later seen to have been the start of a prolonged course of progressive disease that may end in kidney failure.

There are several varieties of glomerulonephritis, some with a more serious outlook than others, and these are best distinguished by taking a small sample of kidney tissue (renal biopsy) for microscopic examination. Because of the dangers of streptococcal throat infections, many doctors take throat swabs and treat throat infections routinely with ANTIBIOTICS.

Glue ear

'Glue ear' is an insidious condition of the middle ear, mainly affecting children. The medical term is secretory OTITIS MEDIA. In this condition the free movement of the eardrum and the three small linking bones, which transmit sound vibrations from the air to the cochlea in the inner ear, is impeded by a 'glue' of sticky mucus produced by the inflammation. Glue ear is not primarily caused by infection, as are the other common forms of otitis media. It may occur without any definite cause being apparent. Some causes and contributory factors are, however, known. These include:

- enlarged adenoids that block the opening of the tube (Eustachian tube) draining the middle ear
- inadequately treated acute middle ear infection
- the injudicious use of antibiotics for childhood respiratory infections
- travelling in an aircraft while suffering from a cold
- hay fever (allergic rhinitis)

Parental smoking is thought by some doctors to predispose to secretory otitis media.

Unfortunately, the symptoms of this disorder are often not readily noticed. Pain in the ear may be absent or there may only be mild discomfort. Sometimes there is a complaint of a hissing or singing noise in the ear (tinnitus) and occasionally a child may suffer unsteadiness. Often the only symptom is DEAFNESS. If the condition is suspected, however, examination by an expert will soon confirm the diagnosis. The characteristic appearance and state of indrawing (retraction) of the ear-drum, a visible level of fluid in the middle ear, and the results of a simple tuning-fork test of the hearing all indicate the nature of the problem.

If mild, secretory otitis media will often clear up without treatment, and in such cases the specialist will usually be content with a period of observation. Antihistamine and mucus-dispersing drugs are sometimes helpful. Persistent glue ear causing deafness can fairly easily be treated, and normal function restored, by a simple operation in which a tiny cut is made in the ear-drum and a small plastic drainage tube – a 'grommet' – is inserted. This allows immediate equalization of pressure on the two sides of the drum and free drainage of middle ear secretions.

It is important for parents to remember that glue ear is usually symptomless, the only effect being deafness. This, too, may be unsuspected as the affected child is often unaware that anything is wrong and will seldom complain. Such children are often accused of inattentiveness. A high proportion of young children who fail to meet their parents' educational expectations suffer from glue ear and are found, on audiometric testing, to be incapacitated by deafness.

Undetected severe glue ear is particularly disastrous if it occurs in the first two years of life, for normal hearing is essential for the development of speech and learning. Sensory deprivation during this period may have a life-long effect, not only on comprehension and speech, but on actual intellectual development. Language problems starting in this way persist and cause irremediable later difficulties in acquiring a vocabulary. Audiometry under the age of 5 is very difficult, but simpler tests can demonstrate hearing defect and draw attention to the condition of the ears and the state of the throat.

Glue sniffing see SOLVENT ABUSE.

Green stools see MECONIUM.

Grommet treatment see GLUE EAR.

Growing pains

This idea is a medical fiction, probably invented by doctors at a loss to account for some of the many aches and discomforts complained of by children. All pains have a cause, most of which are trivial, but not all of which can be explained. So long as the child is well, active, free from fever, eating and sleeping normally and gaining size, there is little likelihood that these pains are of significance. Possible causes of vague aches and pains include overuse of muscles, tendon and ligament strain, partial dislocation of joints and hair-line fractures of bone.

Growth disorders

Body growth is influenced by many factors. Heredity is one of the most important. Tall parents tend to have tall children. Certain genetic disorders feature very short stature.

These include ACHONDROPLASIA. Hormones, especially the growth hormone from the pituitary gland, can have a major effect. Deficiency of growth hormone in childhood, which is very uncommon, causes DWARFISM and this can be treated with growth hormone. Too much causes gigantism. Deficiency of thyroid hormones in childhood and sex hormones at puberty also leads to impaired growth.

The state of early nutrition and of general health are also important. Severe, long-term illnesses can limit growth as can the use of STEROIDS. General social and parental deprivation often leads to short stature.

See also SHORT CHILDREN.

Grunting see GILLES DE LA TOURETTE SYNDROME.

Gynaecomastia

This is abnormal enlargement of one or both breasts in boys, so that they resemble the female breast. In most cases, gynaecomastia is temporary and is due to a transient lack of hormonal balance. Such cases, fairly common at puberty, nearly always settle without treatment. Rarely, the condition may be due to:

• liver disease, such as cirrhosis, which prevents the normal liver destruction of female sex hormones
• drug therapy with steroids or oestrogens, or the diuretic spironolactone
• a tumour of the testis or pituitary gland
• a hormone-secreting tumour of the lung, breast or other organ

In such cases, treatment is directed to the cause. Persistent gynaecomastia, that causes embarrassment or annoyance, can easily be corrected by plastic surgery.

Habit formation

It may seem old-fashioned to suggest that parents have a duty to form 'good' habits in their children, but there is more in this than immediately meets the eye. A habit is a sequence of learned behaviour occurring in a particular context or as a response to particular events. Life without habit is inconceivable, and much of our behaviour consists in the working out of sequences of habit. Habits organize life, and if habits are constructive and useful, their formation can be of the greatest value and importance, making for efficiency and social and occupational usefulness. The obvious advantages of possessing a complex of 'good' habits make nonsense of the unthinking reaction against the idea that parents should try to inculcate good habits in the upbringing of their children. Critics are apt to suggest that this is a form of programming – an idea hateful to many.

Habits are often conditioned, are performed automatically and unconsciously, and spare us much decision-making. They start in an observation of the effect produced by behaviour. If the effect seems desirable, the behaviour is repeated. The strength and stability of a habit depends on repetition of rewards, or repeated avoidance of unpleasantness, such as punishment. These lead to reinforcement and eventual strong establishment of the habit. Once a habit is well established, it may be maintained even if the factors that began it no longer operate. We become creatures of habit in more than one sense.

It may be argued that when parents are concerned with the upbringing of their children it is not obvious which habits are 'good'. Much has been written about the supposed damage to children of imposed patterns of behaviour; and much of this is trendy nonsense. It is probable that more harm is done by leaving children to develop their own habits than to encourage them to adopt those that parents have found by hard experience to be useful. There can be little argument that habits such as those of truthfulness, courtesy and reliability are to be encouraged. Many others might be cited, but that would be to go beyond the scope of this book.

The practical importance of recognizing that habit is a matter of programming lies in the corollary that what has been programmed can always be re-programmed. This process is often painful – as when attempts are made to change damaging but self-gratifying habits – but the result can be useful. Behavioural psychology and behaviour therapy are based on the acceptance of this premise.

Haemolytic disease see RHESUS INCOMPATIBILITY, SICKLE CELL DISEASE.

Haemophilia

This is a rare condition, affecting boys and men, and very rarely girls, that causes a life-long tendency to excessive bleeding with very slow clotting of the blood. Haemophilia is due to a gene mutation that leads to the absence of Factor VIII, one of the many elements necessary for normal blood clotting. In rare cases, the disease may be due to absence of Factor IX and is called haemophilia B or Christmas factor deficiency. In both cases, the condition is a recessive genetic disorder, the gene being on the X (sex) chromosome (see GENETICS – AN OUTLINE). The sons of a haemophilic man do not suffer the disease and do not pass it on to their descendants. All the daughters carry the gene on one X chromosome but, because the gene is recessive, do not suffer the disease. They are, however, carriers, and there is a 50 per cent chance that the X chromosome they transmit to their sons will be the one with the mutated gene. Because the other sex chromosome in males is a small Y chromosome that carries few if any operative genes, it does not cancel out the inherited X chromosome. So, on average, half the sons of a female carrier will have haemophilia. Female haemophiliacs are very rare and occur only if haemophiliacs marry carrier females and transmit two affected X chromosomes to the daughter.

In haemophilia, bleeding occurs either spontaneously or after minor trauma, most commonly into the joints, causing severe pain, swelling and spasm of the associated muscles. The blood absorbs within a few days and the symptoms settle. Repeated episodes, however, lead to damage and chronic joint disability. Bleeding may also occur into the bowel, causing symptoms which mimic other acute abdominal emergencies and problems from excessive blood loss. External bleeding, from injury, whether accidental or surgical, continues indefinitely unless special measures are taken to stop it. Dental extraction is followed by very prolonged bleeding. The severity of haemophilia varies with the level of Factor VIII activity in the individual, and in severe cases this may be less than 2 per cent of normal.

All of these troubles can be prevented by giving Factor VIII whenever bleeding occurs. The concentrate is derived from donated blood and, unfortunately, is active only for a short period so repeated injections are necessary. Haemophiliacs are advised to try to avoid trauma, but to lead as normal lives as possible.

Before the dangers of AIDS were fully recognised, pooled blood containing HIV the virus, was used to produce Factor VIII concentrates and many haemophiliacs acquired the disease. All concentrate is now heat treated to kill the virus. HEPATITIS, type B which causes AIDS, is also a problem, and many haemophiliacs contract the disease.

Hair loss see ALOPECIA.

Hair pulling see ALOPECIA.

Hamster face see MUMPS.

Handedness

By this is meant the preferential use of one hand, rather than the other, in voluntary actions. Ambidexterity – the ability to use either hand, indifferently, with equal skill – is very rare. About 90 per cent of children are right-handed. The two brain hemispheres are not identical. In right-handed people, the neurological connections for understanding and performing speech are nearly always in the left hemisphere. This is also true for 40 per cent of left-handed people. But in 60 per cent of left-handers, the nervous tissue relating to the speech functions are in the right hemisphere.

Hare lip

This is the appearance caused by a badly repaired cleft lip. With advances in understanding of the principles of plastic surgery and a recognition that these principles, and the appropriate skills, should always be available when congenital cleft lip is to be repaired, the condition, at least in an obvious form, has become quite rare. See also CLEFT PALATE.

Headache

Only a tiny proportion of headaches indicate serious disorder. True headaches are uncommon in children, although they will often complain of them, especially if there is a headache martyr in the family.

In adults, tension headaches are caused by sustained contraction of muscles of the face, scalp and neck, and account for half or more of all headaches, but the situation is quite different in children. In those aged between 5 and 15, tension headaches account for only about 10 per cent of all severe, recurrent headaches. Surprisingly, migraine is the commonest cause of severe headaches in children and is an important cause of loss of time at school. In a major study of 2,165 children selected at random from 67 primary and secondary schools, it was found that the prevalence of migraine was 10.6 per cent and that of tension headache only 0.9 per cent.

Migraine headaches occur at intervals of days, weeks or months. The term comes from the words 'hemi-cranial', meaning 'half-head', and it is a feature of classic migraine that the pain occurs only on one side. The condition is one-sided in a wider sense, however, as it is caused by a temporary shut-down of the blood supply to a part of one side of the brain, followed by a wide and painful dilatation of the affected arteries.

The preliminary spasm of these vessels often interferes seriously, but temporarily, with the function of the brain. As it is often the arteries supplying the back of one side of the brain that are affected, the commonest result is a disturbance of vision. This usually takes the form of a small blind area with sparkling edges (a scintillating scotoma), which expands until a large part of the field of vision is blind, lasts for about 20 to 30 minutes and then reverts fairly quickly to normal. Some children may, at first, be seriously disturbed by this phenomenon, but it can be relied on to fade away and, after experiencing it once or twice, the child will know what it is.

Other parts of the brain can be similarly involved and there may be weakness or loss of sensation on the face or down one side of the body, disturbance of speech or comprehension, or other alarming effects. These are much less common than the visual disturbances. All these preliminary effects are included in the stage known as the aura. 'Classic' migraine of this kind is then followed by a severe headache on the opposite side of the head, with nausea, vomiting, extreme sensitivity to bright light and a strong inclination to go and lie down in a darkened room. The headache may last for up to a day or two, but eventually resolves. Some people suffer a prolonged headache which is followed by paralysis of one half of the body, gradually recovering over the course of several days.

In many cases, the preliminary stage of brain malfunction is absent and the attack starts with the headache and NAUSEA. This type is sometimes called 'common migraine' and is less easy to distinguish from other forms of headache. It is also very common for the initial stage of visual disturbance to constitute the entire attack. This kind of 'migraine without headache' is much commoner than is generally thought. It may occur frequently or only at very long intervals, and the precipitating factors are often unknown.

Migraine runs in families, but so does any form of headache, not because of a hereditary influence, but because children are often deeply impressed by the sufferings of parents who are constantly having headaches.

International Headache Society
Criteria for the diagnosis of migraine
Migraine without aura
At least five attacks lasting for 2 to 48 hours and featuring at least two of the following:
- one-sided headache
- pulsating quality
- severe enough to prevent or interfere with daily activity
- aggravated by climbing stairs or other similar physical activity
- NAUSEA or VOMITING or both or strong dislike of light

Migraine with aura
At least two attacks with at least three of the following:
- one or more aura symptom that fully reverses
- one or more aura symptom developing gradually over more than four minutes or two or more of them occurring in succession
- no aura symptom to last more than 60 minutes
- headache following aura within less than 60 minutes

Migraine can be precipitated by many factors, including fatigue, anxiety, stress, weather changes, fasting, cheese and chocolate, and in adolescents, menstruation, contraceptive pills and alcohol. Triggering foodstuffs and drinks contain the amino acid tyramine and administration of this will provoke an attack. The agent which causes the effect on the blood vessels is probably the highly active neurotransmitter serotonin.

The medical control of migraine calls for expert prescribing and several drugs are useful, among them ergotamine tartrate which acts to prevent or control the secondary dilatation of the blood vessels which is what causes the pain. Ergotamine tartrate is not without danger and should not be given to young children. Other drugs used in migraine include beta-blockers, such as propranolol, and antidepressants, such as amitriptyline. The serotonin antagonist methysergide, widely used to treat migraine in adults, is not recommended for children.

DANGEROUS CAUSES OF HEADACHE

In children, dangerous causes of headache include MENINGITIS, which is accompanied by severe neck stiffness, fever and general upset; BRAIN TUMOUR and other causes of raised pressure within the skull, such as benign intracranial hypertension, both of which are rare; and ENCEPHALITIS.

In trying to decide whether or not a headache is dangerous, consider whether it started recently or has been happening for years. If the latter, it is unlikely to be dangerous. Are there any other symptoms or signs of brain disorder such as loss of vision to the sides, double vision, sudden projectile VOMITING, hormonal changes, weakness, paralysis, vertigo or one-sided deafness? A new and persistent headache, accompanied by any such changes should be urgently investigated.

Head enlargement see
HYDROCEPHALUS.

Head tilt see TORTICOLLIS.

Hearing problems see
DEAFNESS.

Heart disease see BLUE BABY,
CONGENITAL HEART DISEASE, EISENMENGER'S COMPLEX, HOLE IN THE HEART, KAWASAKI DISEASE, RHEUMATIC FEVER.

Heart rate in childhood

Heart rate in babies and children at rest

Age	Average heart rate beats per minute	Normal range
Birth	140	90–190
0–6 months	130	80–180
6–12 months	115	75–155
1–2 years	110	70–150
2–6 years	105	68–138
6–10 years	95	65–125
10–14 years	85	55–115

You can most easily feel the pulse on the front of the wrist, on the thumb side, near the outer border. Use a finger-tip and light pressure.

Heat stroke

Fortunately, this is rare in children but, when it occurs, is very serious. Heat stroke happens when the body's temperature regulating mechanism is unable to cope with excessive heat, or when, as a result of disease or other causes, it fails altogether. Newborn babies, children with CYSTIC FIBROSIS, and those who undertake strenuous exertion in very hot conditions are especially liable. The temperature rises rapidly and the situation is highly dangerous. Initially, there may be warning indications in the form of faintness, dizziness, HEADACHE, dry skin, absence of sweating, thirst and NAUSEA. Later there may be lethargy and confusion or agitation progressing to epileptic-like seizures (see EPILEPSY), coma and death. This is a medical emergency. The rising temperature causes brain damage which worsens the longer the high temperature continues. It can also cause multiple organ damage.

The treatment, which must never be delayed, is to bring the temperature down by any available means. Call for an ambulance but start treatment at once. The child's whole body should be immersed in cool water and ice-packs, and fans used to supplement the cooling. The temperature must be monitored continuously and not allowed to drop below 38° C (101° F) as excess cooling may convert hyperthermia to hypothermia.

Hepatitis

This is inflammation of the liver. Of the two main types, hepatitis A is much commoner in children than hepatitis B and, fortunately, is much less serious. Hepatitis A is due to infection with a virus usually acquired by food contaminated with human faeces. Children are the main cause of spread. In a healthy, well-nourished child, the illness is very mild. Eighty per cent of those affected are not aware that it has occurred. In severe infections there is fever, severe loss of appetite, loss of energy, slight enlargement of the liver with tenderness, yellowing of the skin (JAUNDICE) and darkening of the urine. The stools look very pale and clay-like. The appearance of jaundice usually brings improvement and complications are few.

Hepatitis B is spread by blood or other body fluids, such as saliva, semen, vaginal secretions and urine and is rare in children. The disease can, however, be spread from mother to baby at, or soon after, birth. Vaccination against hepatitis B is effective and should be considered by all those at special risk, including babies born to women carriers.

Hereditary disease see GENETIC COUNSELLING, GENETIC DISORDERS, CHROMOSOMAL DISORDERS.

Hereditary spherocytosis

This disorder of the envelope of the red blood cells is inherited as an autosomal dominant condition (see GENETICS – AN OUTLINE). As a result of the changes in the red cells they are more fragile than normal ones and can rupture easily. This breaking of the cell membrane and release of haemoglobin is called haemolysis and it causes a haemolytic anaemia. Affected children develop mild to severe anaemia and yellowing of the skin (see JAUNDICE).

Many cases can be treated with folic acid supplements, but severe cases may require more energetic measures. Because much of the red cell destruction occurs in the spleen, the condition can be treated by removal of this organ (splenectomy). This is not without dangers and is usually deferred until the early teens. Loss of the spleen increases the danger of certain infections and children who have had the operation are given long-term penicillin and anti-pneumococcal vaccination.

Hermaphroditism

This is a rare condition in which both male and female reproductive organs are present. True human hermaphroditism is rare and most of those affected have external genitalia of ambiguous character. There may be one ovary and one testis, or gonads with a combination of ovarian and testicular features. The external genitalia may be female or male, or a combination of both, and some hermaphrodites are said to be capable of sexual intercourse with either sex.

There are several possible causes for ambiguous genitalia. These include abnormalities of the sex chromosomes (normally XX for a girl and XY for a boy) such as the XXY or the Y only (YO) karyotypes. Other cases are associated with multiple congenital abnormalities of the urinary tract. Hormonal anomalies cause PSEUDO-HERMAPHRODITISM.

Most of the affected children are raised as males, but at the time of puberty about half of them menstruate and 80 per cent develop breasts of the female type. Often there is difficulty in deciding which sex to elect, but, in general, surgery to achieve feminisation is easier and more satisfactory and should, ideally, be performed in infancy. If left until puberty or later, surgical correction must be determined by the gender identity accepted by the individual.

Heroin babies

Heroin converts to morphine soon after entering the body and morphine in the mother's blood passes through the placenta into the blood of the fetus. Seventy-five per cent of babies born to addicted mothers show withdrawal signs and most require treatment. The signs include:

- tremor
- hyperactivity

- FEVER
- VOMITING
- DIARRHOEA
- sweating
- sneezing
- respiratory distress
- convulsions

These effects last for an average of about a week, but sometimes persist for three weeks.

Reports of the long-term effect on babies differ and it is difficult to separate the purely medical effects of morphine from the high level of socially disadvantageous factors common in heroin addicts. In one series, for instance, only one-quarter of the mothers were living in a stable relationship. Another study, from the United States, showed a baby mortality rate, within a few weeks of birth, of nearly 7 per cent. But this may well have been because of social rather than drug effects, and there is no very convincing evidence that morphine, by itself, has a major influence on the health of these babies.

Herpes simplex

There are two strains of herpes simplex viruses: herpes simplex virus, type 1 (HSV-1), which causes 'cold sores' around the mouth and nose; and herpes simplex virus, type 2 (HSV-2), which causes venereal herpes. Herpes viruses are highly contagious and few people are free from them. Children usually acquire the infection by kissing infected people. Most of us carry herpes simplex viruses lying dormant in the nerves at the junction of skin and mucous membranes of the mouth and nose.

Every now and then, as immunity varies, dormant viruses become active, reproducing rapidly, moving to the skin and causing the well-known itching, tingling discomfort and spreading clusters of painful little crusting blisters we call 'cold sores'. Flare-up often occurs during a feverish illness, or at times of stress or emotional upset, or after exposure to bright sunlight. The virus can cause sight-threatening ulcers on the cornea.

One of the most serious forms of herpes in children is that which can affect children with ECZEMA. This is called Kaposi's varicelliform eruption or eczema herpeticum. It is one that should be familiar to every person with eczema old enough to understand, and especially to the parents of children with eczema. Kaposi's varicelliform eruption is a secondary infection of eczema patches with the herpes simplex virus, or, occasionally another virus called the coxsackie virus. Before the eradication of smallpox, the condition was commonly caused by the vaccinia virus deliberately given to protect against smallpox. There is now no reason to vaccinate anyone against smallpox and this should never be done. Previously, eczema was one of the main reasons for avoiding smallpox vaccination.

Kaposi's varicelliform eruption is so called because of its resemblance to CHICKENPOX (varicella), but the condition is very much more serious than any attack of chickenpox. It features high fever, severe illness, and an extensive rash with small skin blisters filled with blood. The rash can readily cover almost the whole of the body surface. Worst of all, herpes virus infection can involve the brain and the spinal cord.

Fortunately, since the development of the drug acyclovir (Zovirax), which can be taken by mouth, doctors have had an effective weapon against this most serious complication of eczema. Even so, the death rate from severe cases is by no means negligible. The importance of knowing about Kaposi's varicelliform eruption lies in the fact that anyone with a cold sore or other manifest herpes simplex infection must stay well away from anyone with eczema. If you have a cold sore on the mouth, don't kiss a child with atopic eczema under any circumstances. Don't kiss anyone.

Acyclovir is also the safest and most effective treatment for all other forms of herpes and is usually applied as a cream or taken in tablet form. It must be used at the earliest possible stage in the attack.

High fever see HYPERPYREXIA.

Hiccup

This is very common in children and is rarely of any significance. Hiccup is a succession of involuntary spasms of the diaphragm, each followed by sudden closure of the vocal cords, which checks the inrush of air and causes the characteristic sound. Hiccup can be caused by irritation of the nerves to the diaphragm (phrenic nerves) or by abnormal stimulation of the input nerves to the brain which supply the respiratory centres there. In most cases, as already implied, the cause is unknown and harmless. Very rarely, hiccup is so persistent as to be seriously exhausting.

The tendency to hiccup is reduced if the level of carbon dioxide in the blood is raised. This is most easily achieved by holding the breath for as long as possible or by re-breathing air in a paper bag or *small* plastic bag. A child should, of course, never be allowed to do this unsupervised. Other tricks include drinking water out of the 'wrong' side of a glass, pulling on the tongue or pressing, but not too firmly, on the eyeballs.

In extreme cases, sedative drugs may be prescribed, but if all else fails, a phrenic nerve can be temporarily prevented from transmitting impulses by injecting a small dose of local anaesthetic around it.

Hip, congenital dislocation of

Now usually known as developmental dysplasia of the hip, this is the condition, present at birth or starting in the early months, in which the sphere-like head of the thigh bone does not fit normally into its socket in the side of the pelvis. Congenital dislocation is commoner in girl babies, and one or both joints may be affected. The condition appears to be due to lax ligaments around the hip joint. In most cases it recovers without treatment, but if it does not, or if it is not detected, treatment is necessary to prevent severe defects of walking and subsequent arthritis. The earlier the condition is spotted, the easier it is to treat. Because the condition can appear after birth, repeated screening at designated intervals is essential if late cases are not to be missed. This is incorporated into the child health surveillance programme in the UK.

If the head of the thigh bone is held in its socket by light splinting for a few weeks,

normal growth and development can occur. The splints hold the thighs apart and are rotated outwards. If congenital dislocation is not diagnosed until the child begins to walk, the problem then becomes apparent. If one joint is affected there will be a limp and a lurch to the affected side. If both joints are dislocated, the gait is waddling. Delayed treatment means greater difficulty in management and usually a less satisfactory result.

There is a routine test for congenital dislocation of the hip which all babies should have in a baby clinic. The baby is put on his or her back on a table. The knee and hip joints are held bent and an attempt is then made to swing the thighs gently outwards until the knees touch the table. Normally this is easily accomplished, but in congenital dislocation it will be found that this movement is resisted by spasm of the muscles which pull the thighs inward, so that the thighs cannot reach the surface of the table. This test should be left to the doctor and is best not tried at home. Inexpert manipulation of the hip joints could cause damage. Any suspicion of hip defect, however, should be reported without delay.

Hole in the heart

The presence of this condition does not mean that the blood can leak through the outer wall of the heart. The heart is divided into two sides by a central wall. The right side pumps blood that has returned from the body to the lungs; the left side pumps blood that has returned from the lungs to the rest of the body. So blood in the right side of the heart is short of oxygen and blood in the left side has plenty of oxygen.

A hole in the heart is an opening in the wall between the two sides. This may be in the upper part of the wall between the upper chambers (atrial septal defect), or in the lower part between the lower chambers (ventricular septal defect). Hole in the heart may cause little trouble, but may be serious if it results in excessive shunting of blood from one side to the other. This can interfere with the normal action of the heart and can sometimes lead to heart failure in infancy. If the pressure on the right side exceeds that on the left, deoxygenated blood will pass straight to the main output chamber of the heart – the left ventricle – without first going through the lungs. Oxygenated blood is bright red and confers a healthy pink colour to the skin; blood that has lost its oxygen is a dark purplish colour and causes a blueness in the skin known as CYANOSIS. Babies with a hole in the heart may show this worrying sign, as may those with other CONGENITAL HEART DEFECTS. They are often known as 'blue babies'.

In severe cases, septal defects require surgical correction in which the hole is closed with stitches or with a small plastic patch sewn into place over the hole.

Hookworm infection

Although this is almost unknown in developed countries, world-wide, many millions of children suffer infestation with one or both of the parasitic roundworms *Ancylostoma duodenale* and *Necator americanus*. These occur in rural areas almost everywhere, but present a major problem only in regions where much of the population go bare-foot and the standards of hygiene and sanitation are low. The condition is also known as ancylostomiasis, the term referring to a mouth equipped with hooks.

The life-cycle of these parasites is extraordinary. Worm eggs are deposited in the soil in human excreta and hatch to release larvae which are able to penetrate the skin of the feet, causing the condition of 'ground itch'. These tiny worms migrate inwards and enter small blood vessels and are then carried to the lungs in the bloodstream. In the lungs they are trapped in the small capillaries, causing a form of lung inflammation (pneumonitis) and a cough, sometimes with blood in the sputum. They then break through into the air sacs (alveoli), migrate up the air passages (bronchial tubes) and windpipe (trachea) to the mouth, and are swallowed. In this way the larvae reach the intestine, where they grow to adult worms in about five weeks. The worms hook themselves into the bowel wall and derive their nourishment from blood and mucus, often causing severe ANAEMIA, debility, abdominal pain and DIARRHOEA in the process. Individual worms can live for as long as 10 years and the pregnant females may release several million eggs a day into the stools.

The control of ancylostomiasis is an administrative rather than a medical problem and is entirely a matter of the economic level of the community. Proper sanitation and hygiene, or even just the wearing of shoes, soon eliminate the threat. For children infested, there are effective anthelmintic drugs, but such treatment is of limited value in a situation where re-infestation is inevitable.

Hurler's syndrome

Once known as 'gargoylism', this is one of the group of very rare inherited disorders called the mucopolysaccharidoses. Hurler's syndrome is due to the absence of an important chemical activator (enzyme) necessary for the normal growth and development of most parts of the body. Certain carbohydrate-protein-linked substances called mucopolysaccharides accumulate abnormally, causing defects that appear in the first few months of life. The condition features:

- DWARFISM
- widespread skeletal deformity
- LEARNING DIFFICULTY
- heart abnormalities
- opacities of the cornea
- early death

X-ray of the spine shows a characteristic bony deformity, and large quantities of the chemical dermatan sulphate are found in the urine. Unfortunately, there is no treatment. In the future, conditions such as this may well be treated or prevented by GENE THERAPY.

Hydrocephalus

Usually known as 'water on the brain', this uncommon condition is an abnormal accumulation of the water fluid (cerebrospinal fluid) that normally bathes the brain and occupies spaces within it known as the ventricles. Hydrocephalus results when this fluid cannot be properly reabsorbed, usually because its flow is blocked, either by a congenital abnormality or by later acquired disease.

In babies or young children the pressure from accumulated fluid readily expands the skull, sometimes greatly, because the bones of the vault have not yet fused together and are still separate. There may be VOMITING and lethargy and the child will often show a downward deviation of the eyes, known as the 'setting sun' sign. If the cause of the raised pressure cannot be removed, it is necessary to shunt, or bypass, the normal channels by means of a tube passed into one of the spaces in the brain (ventricle) and carried down under the skin of the neck to be inserted, by way of a jugular vein, into the heart. Alternatively, the shunt tube can be carried right down to open into the abdominal cavity. In either case, the tube contains a one-way valve so that fluid can pass out of the brain but not back in. Unfortunately, blockage of the tube is common and replacements may be required.

Unrelieved hydrocephalus causes compression of the brain, especially after the skull bones have fused together, and this leads to HEADACHE, vomiting, and damage to function, including visual disturbance.

Hyperactivity

This is the description usually applied to children who are excessively restless and inattentive and who have a low threshold of frustration. An alternative term is the 'hyperkinetic syndrome'. Hyperactive children are unable to concentrate, throw tantrums, are aggressive, restless, fidgety and generally infuriating to adults. They are often intelligent, but their low attention span sometimes results in poor academic performance. Many normal children are labelled in this way. But a child who can concentrate on TV for more than five minutes is unlikely to be hyperactive. The condition starts before the age of 5 years.

Widespread doubt has been expressed among the experts as to whether hyperactivity is a real medical or psychological condition and most think of it as a variety of conduct disorder or temperament. Parents of hyperkinetic children, however, are in no possible doubt as to the existence of the condition, and pressure from parental groups has drawn professional attention more closely to the condition. Furthermore, there is clear evidence that children who display these characteristics do not necessarily 'grow out of it' and that almost one-third of them may continue to show them in early adult life. There is also evidence that these children are much more prone than others to subsequent conduct disorder, including DRUG ABUSE, stealing and violence.

These findings are not really surprising. Those who, by reason of defective attention, have been unable to obtain the data input necessary for good social and mental functioning, might be expected to suffer behavioural disorder. The quality of this 'programming' is likely also to have been affected by the inevitable deterioration in relationships with older people, including parents and teachers, caused by these children's inability to conform to expected norms of behaviour. As a result they tend to have low self-esteem and to withdraw from normal social contacts.

No one knows for certain what causes hyperactivity, and the view that it is always caused by food additives, such as tartrazine, salicylates or the antioxidant preservatives butylated hydroxyanisole (BHA) and butylated hydroxytoluene (BHT), is almost certainly untrue. Diets designed to eliminate all such additives have been used experimentally with inconclusive results, although some children appear to have improved. If this approach is to succeed, meticulous identification of the exact substance to which the child shows intolerance is necessary. It has also been suggested that child diets high in sugar or the sweetening agent aspartame are responsible. But the report of a carefully-conducted double-blind trial of this, published in 1994, showed that even when intakes exceed normal dietary levels, neither of these substances affects the behaviour of children.

Much has been discovered about methods of controlling the disorder. Paradoxically, *stimulant* drugs, such as amphetamine, have been found very helpful in some cases. Monoamine oxidase inhibitor drugs have also been found useful.

The drug methylphenidate hydrochloride (Ritalin), which is a stimulant, is now freely available for prescription in Britain, although it must be used under the supervision of a specialist in behavioural disorders. This drug has been shown to be very effective in some cases. A four-week trial will show whether it is going to be useful. Drug treatment is not necessarily required. In many cases, behaviour therapy can produce a better response. Often both are needed.

These methods are, of course, only a means to the end of ensuring that such children are not deprived of the vitally important elements of proper behaviour training. There is plenty of evidence that children who learn early to conform to reasonable patterns of behaviour, and who have a clear idea of the rules, are not only happier, but are much more likely to become effective, productive and contented adults.

See also HABIT FORMATION.

Hyperlexia

A very small proportion of children show an extraordinary ability to read at a remarkably early age, without really understanding what they are reading. Such children use reading as a substitute for other activities and even human relationships. Analysis of their skills may show that although they have unusual powers of translating printed or written words into the correctly pronounced sounds, the words, in fact, have little or no meaning for them. These children actually have serious problems with language and may be very slow in other respects. Sadly, they may turn out not to be exceptionally gifted but, in fact, autistic.

For them, reading – at least in the sense of what they actually do – is a compulsive activity that displaces most other normal childhood action, especially normal play. And, of course, it serves little or no useful purpose.

The majority of children who show gratifying early reading skills are, in fact, genuinely gifted. But if you suspect that your child is reading in an abnormally compulsive manner and is deriving no real sense from what he or she reads, you should waste no time in seeking professional advice and help. This is the one minor exception to the excellent general rule that children should be given every encouragement to read as early as possible.

Hyperpyrexia

This simply means an abnormally high, and dangerous, level of body temperature. Hyperpyrexia exists if the temperature rises above 41.1° C (106° F) At this level, urgent treatment to cool the body is required to lower the temperature, if permanent brain damage is to be avoided. See also HEAT STROKE.

Hypospadias

This is a rare congenital abnormality of the penis in which the tube for the urine (the urethra), instead of running the full length and opening at the tip, terminates and opens on the underside of the organ. The opening may be at the junction of the bulb (glans) and the shaft, or further back on the shaft. It may be associated with other abnormalities of the urinary system.

Hypospadias causes inconvenience in urination and subsequent difficulty in achieving conception, but plastic surgical correction is possible. Recent developments have shown that a perfectly normal lining for the newly constructed passage-way can be grown artificially in a tissue culture of the person's own cells and then applied to the inside of the new urethra.

I

Idiot savant

In technical terminology, an idiot is a person with a mental age of not more than 2 years or an IQ of 25 or below. A very small proportion of people in this category have an extraordinary talent of some kind – often for music or for the ability to memorize certain categories of fact, or to perform certain kinds of mental arithmetic. Some are able to play chess to a high standard or to produce drawings or sculpture with great skill. The idiot savant, however, has little appreciation of his or her capabilities or their uses.

Such people are often physically handicapped and manifest clear signs of brain damage or AUTISM. Sometimes, when their talents are encouraged and promoted, however, they may show some improvement in their general abilities.

The observation of the creative ability of some idiot savants has prompted the idea that the phenomenon might be explained on the basis of left-sided, but not right-sided, brain damage. The left half of the brain is concerned with verbal and general intellectual activity; the right half with artistic and creative activity. The suggestion is that following partial loss of left-side brain function, the right side of the brain becomes over-developed in compensation.

Immunization

The terms immunization and vaccination mean exactly the same thing. Immunization against infectious disease has been highly successful and, in areas where there has been a good acceptance rate, has led to a large reduction in the incidence of diseases such as DIPHTHERIA, MEASLES, RUBELLA (German measles), POLIO and WHOOPING COUGH (pertussis). Smallpox has been eradicated, largely due to immunization.

The effect of these successes has been a substantial reduction in the human tragedy of early death and of congenital and acquired defects. But Public Health authorities are anxious that generations of parents, who have never known the horrors of diphtheria, or seen their children crippled by polio, may not have the necessary motivation to see that their children are immunized. Moreover, after a generation of freedom from such diseases as diphtheria, there is little or no natural immunity in the population and the re-introduction of the disease could lead to major epidemics.

Some children are at special risk from infectious disease and should be immunized as a matter of urgency. These include children with:

- ASTHMA
- CONGENITAL HEART DISEASE
- chronic lung disease
- DOWN'S SYNDROME
- those who were premature babies and remain small for their ages
- children who are HIV positive

Active immunization with vaccines containing live, but modified organisms, which is, in general, very safe in normal children, can offer dangers to certain groups. These include:

- those who have shown a previous severe reaction to vaccines
- anyone suffering from any acute illness
- anyone on high dosages of steroids or on immunosuppressive treatment

Immunization is readily available against diphtheria, whooping cough, tetanus, poliomyelitis, measles, rubella, *Haemophilus* influenza type B (HIB), tuberculosis (see BCG), mumps, hepatitis A and B, rabies, cholera, typhoid, anthrax, and yellow fever. Every child should be protected against the first seven of these as a matter of routine policy. In addition, all girls must be vaccinated against rubella between their 10th and 14th birthdays. The tragedy of a baby with major congenital abnormalities from rubella infection in the mother in early pregnancy is compounded by the fact that such a disaster is so easily avoided. Although rubella is generally a trivial infection in males, rubella vaccination should not, however, be limited to girls. If the disaster of congenital rubella infection is to be reduced to the lowest possible level, or ever to be eliminated, immunization must also be provided for all boys.

Immunodeficiency disorders

This is an important class of diseases in which the body's immunological system of defence against infection, foreign material generally and some forms of cancer, is in some way defective. The best known example of this group of disorders is, of course, the acquired immune deficiency syndrome, AIDS, but immunodeficiency disorders were well known in medical circles long before AIDS appeared. Immunodeficiency disorders may be present at birth (congenital) and may be of genetic origin, or may be acquired later. The immunological mechanisms are so important for survival that major defects are seldom seen.

Some deficiency in the production of immunoglobulins is normal in the early years of life and it is not until adult life that full production occurs. This is why children are so susceptible to infections. Children depend on antibodies supplied by the mother before birth and provided in the early breast milk (colostrum) after birth. Premature babies may not, because of early birth, have received the full quota from the mother.

Antibodies, which are produced by the B lymphocyte system, are proteins known as immunoglobulins. Immunoglobulin deficiency is the most important of these congenital disorders and occurs as a sex-linked recessive trait (see GENETICS – AN OUTLINE). Although the name, agammaglobulinae-

mia, implies complete absence of the important antibody type, gamma globulin, total deficiency does not, in fact, occur. Such children have a variable degree of B cell deficiency (hypogammaglobulinaemia) and may survive for many years, although very susceptible to bacterial and other infection, and requiring constant treatment.

Another form of immunodeficiency disorder is a selective deficiency of the T cell group of lymphocytes. When this is present from birth, the outlook is poor, but in some cases treatment by human fetal thymus gland transplantation has been effective. The most serious form of congenital immunodeficiency is the severe combined immune deficiency (SCID) whose victims have to become 'bubble babies' enclosed in plastic from birth to keep out infecting organisms.

Children with immunodeficiency disorders suffer recurrent infection, not only from the common organisms, but also by those which do not normally cause disease. These infections are known as opportunistic and include such conditions as *Pneumocystis carinii* pneumonia, cytomegalovirus infections and extensive HERPES SIMPLEX and THRUSH infections, involving not only the skin, but also the intestinal and respiratory systems – all the features that have become so familiar in the AIDS era.

See AIDS.

Impetigo

Impetigo appears as characteristic small blisters, often ring-like, which soon crust and form scabs. If neglected, the condition may quickly become widespread, suggesting poor standards of baby or child skin-care. Both staphylococci and streptococci can cause impetigo. ANTIBIOTICS, such as erythromycin, in ointment form, are usually effective, but recurrence is likely unless the child is carefully washed all over, every day.

Inattentiveness see ABSENCE ATTACKS.

Incubation period

This is the time interval between the entry of germs into the body and the first appearance of symptoms of the resulting disease.

In spite of considerable variation in the number of organisms and in the resistance of the person concerned, the incubation period is remarkably constant. This is because it is a characteristic of the organism itself rather than of these other factors. It reflects the germ's rate of reproduction, its mode of infection and the route it takes to reach its objective. The incubation periods of different organisms vary widely. Cholera, for instance, may strike a child down within a very few hours of drinking contaminated water; rabies may start several months after a bite on the foot. In the former, the organisms reach the point of attack – the bowel – almost at once; in the latter, the viruses have to make the immensely long journey by way of the nerve fibres, to reach the brain. The incubation period of rabies depends on how close the bite was to the brain.

Some typical averaged incubation periods	
Virus diseases	*Incubation period*
Common cold	4 days
Influenza	5 days
Measles	10 days
Chickenpox	14 days
Poliomyelitis	17 days
Rubella	18 days
Mumps	28 days
Hepatitis A	32 days
Rabies	30 days to several months
Bacterial diseases	
Food poisoning	Hours to a few days
Cholera	Hours to a few days
Gonorrhoea	4 days
Scarlet fever	5 days
Meningitis	6 days
Diphtheria	6 days
Whooping cough	9 days
Tetanus	10 days
Typhoid	14 days

Incubator

Premature babies require, for a time, a controlled environment which provides them with optimal conditions for survival. The baby incubator offers such an environment. It is a closed, insulated and transparent box, with ports for access, in which temperature, humidity and oxygen concentration can be suitably adjusted and the relative absence of infecting organisms can be achieved. Tiny babies can be tube-fed while remaining in incubator.

Very small babies are often nursed naked in the incubator for purposes of observation. Small babies can lose heat very rapidly because they have a large surface area in relation to their weight. They are also short of brown fat, normally used by full-term babies to produce heat rapidly. So internal incubator temperatures have to be carefully maintained at a level depending on the baby's weight. A 1 kg infant, for instance, will require a temperature of 35° C to keep the baby's core temperature at the normal 37° C. A 3 kg baby will require an incubator temperature of 33° C. Incubator temperature is normally reduced at a rate of about 1° C each week.

Humidification of the incubator air is used less often nowadays because this increases the risk of infection. But very small babies still require humidified air.

Infant blindness see TAY-SACHS DISEASE, CATARACT, RETROLENTAL FIBROPLASIA.

Infant feeding SEE introductory section (Baby Care).

Infant mortality

The infant mortality rate is the number of infants under the age of 1 year who die, for every 1,000 live births. This is a sensitive index of the level of social and medical advance in a society and of the standards of public health. In 1900, in Britain, the infant mortality rate was around 150 – about one baby in seven died before reaching its first birthday. By 1950, the figure had dropped to 35 and by 1984 it was down to about 11. Some regions, such as Oxford, had a mortality rate of as low as eight per thousand.

As the common former causes of infant mortality – respiratory and gastrointestinal infection and malnutrition – are brought under control, the emphasis, in reducing the figures still further, swings across to the more specialised services – obstetric and neonatal care, the early identification of severe congenital disorders by prenatal diagnosis and the surgical and other treatment of congenital defects. In underdeveloped parts of the world, babies continue to die from the causes which are now largely eliminated in the industrialized countries.

Infectious diseases see

DIPHTHERIA, FOOD POISONING, GASTROENTERITIS, GLANDULAR FEVER, HEPATITIS, INFLUENZA, MEASLES, MENINGITIS, MUMPS, POLIOMYELITIS, RUBELLA.

Influenza

Popularly described as 'flu', influenza is caused by a virus and is spread mainly by virus-contaminated droplets coughed and sneezed by sufferers. It is highly infectious to the susceptible, and this group includes young children many of whom have not yet had time to acquire resistance. Influenza spreads rapidly through closed communities and in the general population, and tends to occur in epidemics, in the winter time. Each year many people die from influenza. A first attack of influenza in children under 5 years of age can be very severe and may be complicated by pneumonia.

Influenza is an infection of the upper air passages and features:

- FEVER
- sore throat
- running nose
- a dry, unproductive cough
- HEADACHE
- backache
- general muscle pains
- loss of appetite
- insomnia and prostration

In most cases the acute symptoms settle after about four days and then gradually disappear. DIARRHOEA and VOMITING are common in infants. Complications include OTITIS MEDIA, high fever (see HEAT STROKE),

sinusitis acute bronchitis, pneumonia and REYE'S SYNDROME. ANTIBIOTICS have no effect on the viruses, but may be necessary to control secondary respiratory infection, especially pneumonia.

The Department of Health recommends that children over the age of 4 years who are asthmatic be vaccinated against flu.

Insect bites see BITES AND STINGS.

Inhalers

These have become increasingly important as a means of delivering medication, especially in the treatment of diseases of the bronchial tubes and lungs. ASTHMA is the principal disease treated in this way. Inhalers can produce aerosols of liquid solution or may deliver measured doses in powder form, and the contents may be propelled by gas under pressure or may be breath-activated. Drugs commonly taken in this way include corticosteroids and bronchodilators.

The use of inhalers has the notable advantage over treatment by mouth or injection that the drug is delivered directly to the point of action and that, in consequence, a much smaller dose is needed. There is then less likelihood of side-effects. Unfortunately, studies have shown that many patients using inhalers have never been shown how to do so. More seriously, many asthmatics do not appreciate that failure to obtain relief from a bronchodilator inhaler means that the asthma has entered a dangerous refractory state and that more powerful treatment, such as with steroids, is urgently needed.

Intelligence and intelligence tests

Many parents are preoccupied with the question of their children's intelligence, and most of them, if questioned, would claim to be fairly sure that they know what intelligence is. But what this claim really means is that they can recognize intelligence when they come across it – usually by comparing it with their own. This is not a trivial academic point. Parents who insist they know what intelligence is may make decisions about the lack of it in some of their children – decisions based on misapprehension and which can have serious long-term effects.

The truth is that there is still no general consensus among psychologists as to the definition of intelligence. We know that intelligence manifests itself in various abilities, such as a general effectiveness in putting two and two together and coming up with four, or in grasping the essence of difficult ideas, or accumulating mental data. But to describe the manifestations of something is not to define it. When people first began seriously to consider the nature of intelligence it seemed obvious that it was a matter of inherent brain power. Different people inherited brains of different quality and that was that. Intelligence obviously ran in families. Every now and then an exceptionally powerful brain turned up and the possessor became a genius. Sometimes people were born with very low-grade brains and these unfortunates were mentally deficient.

Further consideration, however, showed that this schema was inadequate. The idea of innate brain power, independent of educational and environmental factors, did not fit the facts. A mass of evidence showed that the development of intelligence depended largely on the input to the brain after birth. Children of highly intelligent parents only became intelligent if their environment was conducive to the development of intelligence. And the kind of intelligence that developed was very much determined by the environment, in particular by the way they were educated. It seems clear that two factors are necessary for the development of intelligence – the inheritance of good 'hardware', and the subsequent provision of good 'operating software' and data.

DOES INHERENT BRAIN POWER EXIST?

The early idea that intelligence was a simple power of the mind independently of its separate abilities, has also had to yield to scrutiny. Numerous attempts to find this inherent power have failed. It seems that intelligence, on close inspection, *resolves into a large complex of different abilities or skills present to different degrees*. None of these – not even reasoning power (which, on examination resolves itself into the ability to perform one or other special skills) – can be definitely selected as a central, innate entity we could call intelligence.

The list of mental skills is a long one and includes such things as:

- verbal comprehension
- word fluency
- numerical ability
- the ability to detect significant associations
- the power of spacial visualization
- speed of perception
- the ability to acquire and memorize information
- the power of recall
- the ability to adjust to change
- planning ability
- the ability to chose between alternative courses of action

The disparity in the degree to which these different skills may be present in any one child is remarkable. Two people can be generally acknowledged to be intelligent yet may have few abilities in common. One psychologist claimed that human intelligence comprises 120 distinguishable elementary abilities, each one involving an operation on something to produce a product.

Psychologists have been deeply divided on the question of how many distinguishable mental skills constitute intelligence, and whether there is anything more than the totality of these skills. Some claim that there is no general factor in human intelligence. Most, however, seem to believe that there is such a factor but are a little vague as to its nature. Psychologists are also at variance in their definitions of intelligence. Fourteen notable experts, when asked for a definition, produced 14 entirely different answers. These included such ideas as the ability to learn by experience, to adapt to changing environments, to think in abstractions, to perceive truth, to acquire skills, and so on. One expert defined intelligence as the ability to do well in intelligence tests.

A definition still fairly widely accepted is that of Charles Spearman, who was Professor of Mind and Logic at University College, London. Spearman taught that there is a general ability, which he called 'g', and that this general ability is necessary for the performance of all mental tasks. Surrounding this general ability are several separate specific abilities, present to different degrees and capable of being separately measured. Spearman's concept has been widely discussed and many modifications suggested, but has not been seriously challenged, even by modern cognitive psychologists, who try to understand intelligence in terms of information processing. The nature of the basic quality 'g' has been a source of much argument, although a strong case has been made that it is the capacity to detect new and non-chance associations.

The practical significance of all this is clear. It is a great mistake for parents to categorize a child as lacking in intelligence when what they really mean is that the child appears to perform poorly in a particular sphere of activity arbitrarily selected by the parent as a criterion of intelligence. Such a sphere will, of course, generally be one in which the parent himself, or herself, excels. There are numerous examples of children who have been decreed to be 'slow' or 'stupid' who have turned out to be achievers in the first rank. The list of Nobel Prizewinners in science contains some of these. Many exceptionally gifted children perform very poorly at school simply because their interests lie elsewhere. So long as the opportunities for such children are not prejudiced by their parents' decisions about their 'intelligence', many of them will, in due course, show their full capabilities.

INTELLIGENCE TESTS

Although, as we have seen, intelligence is indefinable, the term is needed and, whether understood or not, is universally used. The intelligence quotient (IQ) is the ratio of the mental age to the chronological age. When these are equal, the IQ is given as 100. The problem in assessing intelligence is to find fair, realistic and reliable ways of measuring the mental age. The difficulty relates closely to the difficulty of defining intelligence and of trying to find abilities to test that are independent of educational and cultural influence, and of the special interests of the children being tested. Intelligence tests compiled without due regard to these factors have, rightly, been condemned as being unfair to those candidates who do not share the educational and cultural background of the people setting the test. Such criticisms have tended to bring all intelligence testing into disrepute.

The first formal tests of intelligence were devised, at the request of the French government, by the French psychologist Alfred Binet, working with Théodore Simon. The purpose was to determine which children were worthy to receive education. Binet originated the idea of IQ. These tests were subsequently repeatedly modified at Stanford University in California by Louis Terman and others, and the original Binet-Simon test became the Stanford-Binet tests. The current Stanford-Binet tests provide tasks for various ages from 2 to adulthood. Very young children are asked to draw copies of objects, to string beads, build with blocks and answer questions on familiar activities. Tests for older children involve such things as detecting absurdities, finding what various pairs of words have in common, completing sentences with omitted words, explaining proverbs, and so on. Such tests are, of course, strongly educationally oriented and really test scholastic ability.

The most widely used intelligence tests today are the Wechsler tests, compiled by the New York psychologist David Wechsler. These are of two basic kinds – the Wechsler Adult Intelligence Scale (WAIS) and the Wechsler Intelligence Scale for Children (WICS). The tests involve progressively increasing difficulty. Each test has verbal and performance parts, and these can be applied independently for people with language difficulties, or combined to give an overall score. The verbal parts test vocabulary, verbal reasoning, verbal memory, arithmetical skill, and general knowledge. The performance sections involve completing pictures, arranging pictures in a logical order, reproducing designs with coloured blocks, assembling puzzles, tracing mazes, and so on. Again, these tests cannot be said to assess much more than the general educational level.

The level of intelligence, whatever it is, cannot be reliably assessed in infancy, and until about the age of 5 years there are usually only the most general indications of whether adult capability is going to be high or low. An occasional child will show evidence of exceptional intelligence or of retardation, but until that age there is little indication in the average child. In most cases, however, from the age of about 12 onwards the results of intelligence tests are consistent with the level of subsequent adult performance.

Intelligence tests are not, except in the most general way, accurate predictors of achievement. Scholastic achievement depends on a number of factors other than intelligence, especially the quality of instruction, parental expectations, and a rich early educational environment. Achievement later in life is even less accurately predictable on the basis of intelligence tests, and is determined by many other factors including quality of personality, physical appearance, opportunity, luck, and the possession of special skills. Good motivation can compensate for restricted intelligence, while low motivation can result in little effective use being made of high intelligence. Nevertheless, there is a general positive correlation between intelligence, as measured by tests, and material and professional success in life. Although intelligence tests purport to measure innate mental ability, they actually tell us little or nothing about the relative importance of heredity and environment in determining intelligence.

The IQ increases with age up to about 18 and remains fairly static during most of adult life. Intelligence is distributed, in the population, in accordance with the standard Gaussian distribution curve. This means that there are as many very stupid people as there are very bright people. About 68 per cent of the population have an IQ of between 85 and 110, and 95 per cent have an IQ between 70 and 130. People of IQ over 130 are exceptionally intelligent, and people below 70 are mentally retarded.

Intussusception

Bowel (intestinal) contents are moved along by a process known as peristalsis in which the muscles in the walls of the intestine contract and relax so as to push the material in one direction. This process, however, sometimes leads to an internal infolding of the bowel wall so that it slides into itself somewhat in the manner of a naval telescope. Intussusception is not particularly common but most cases occur in young children. Occasionally it will happen as a result of polyps in the adult. Once started, intussusception rapidly progresses until the associated blood vessels are also dragged in and become progressively compressed until they are completely closed off. At the same time the bowel itself is becoming obstructed, but this is much less immediately serious than the interference with the blood supply. When this is cut off, the area of bowel affected will die (become gangrenous).

Intussusception causes colicky pain, vomiting and the passage of blood and mucous. It is a surgical emergency calling for prompt surgical intervention. Sometimes the invaginated portion of the bowel can be pulled out and normality restored. But if there is any doubt as to the viability of the affected segment of intestine, it must be removed and the healthy parts joined end-to-end.

IQ tests see INTELLIGENCE AND INTELLIGENCE TESTS.

Iris inflammation see UVEITIS.

Isolation

This is the deliberate separation of a person suffering from an infectious disease, or carrying potentially dangerous organisms, from those uninfected and possibly susceptible. Isolation, once the fate of numerous children and others in infectious disease hospitals, is now much less commonly used. Today, the resources for dealing with infections – especially the use of antibiotics – are greatly improved and isolation tends to be limited to especially dangerous viral infections for which there is no specific treatment. It is still important, however, used in the reverse direction (reverse barrier nursing), for children and others who are immunocompromised and who are very susceptible to infection by organisms present on, but unlikely to affect, healthy individuals.

Itching

This usually trivial symptom is an awareness of a tickling irritation in the skin which prompts one, almost irresistibly, to rub or scratch. In certain conditions, such as ECZEMA, itching is by no means trivial and yielding to the impulse to scratch, although well aware that the relief so obtained is only temporary, may lead to complications. Itching is caused by the stimulation of certain nerve-endings in the skin, but the reason for this is unclear. The substances responsible may include various enzymes called endopeptidases, which occur naturally in the skin and in the bloodstream, and which may be released by some local skin disturbance.

Severe itching is called pruritus and this often occurs in and around the anus or the female genitalia and is commonly associated with THRUSH (candidiasis). This is common in children. Other fungus infections, such as the various forms of tinea, also feature severe itching, and many fungi contain endopeptidases.

In childhood, the outstanding itching condition is ECZEMA. Many sufferers from eczema would be willing to tolerate it were they relieved of the dreadful itching that is such a constant feature of the condition. Itching is the principal symptom of the condition. The itching is not necessarily confined to the areas of the rash but may be generalized. It is, however, mainly localized to the fronts of the arms and the backs of the legs. The severity of the itching varies with the seasons and is often worse in winter. It also varies with the time of day, being worst in the evenings and least around midday.

Itching is a strange symptom, closely tied up with the state of mind of the person concerned and capable of influencing it. The evening increase in itching may be more apparent than real, and is occasioned by the relative lack of concentration on important matters connected with daytime work. There is, however, an increased skin blood flow during the evenings and a slight rise in body temperature, and this may be a factor. It is a common observation and experience that itching can be provoked, or aggravated, by emotional upset or stress. This idea has also been supported by formal research.

In eczema, because of the torturing itch, constant rubbing and scratching is inevitable. The skin responds to this trauma by producing a thicker protective layer of dense, hard protein called keratin. This, in turn, becomes furrowed by scratching, producing the appearance known as lichenification. The thickening of the skin makes the normal skin grooves more prominent. Wherever there is scratching, lichenification is liable to occur; and if the scratching becomes widespread, so will the lichenification.

It is easy to set up a vicious cycle by getting into the habit of scratching a particular area of the skin. Any child who does this persistently will damage the skin in such a way as to produce an itch reaction. Thus, the scratch-itch-scratch-itch cycle is set up. If the cause of the original scratching was some kind of psychological upset, the cycle may be very difficult to break. Skin damage caused in this way is called lichen simplex. The solution to this problem is somehow to avoid the scratching. Often the best way to do this is to cover up the affected area completely with some kind of bandage or dressing. The resulting difficulty in scratching will help to remind the child that scratching is not allowed.

Another important cause of itching, especially in the region of the wrists, is SCABIES.

Itching is usually remediable if the cause can be established and treated. Scratching invariably makes things worse. The use of simple lotions, such as calamine and phenol, is often to be preferred to scratching.

J

Jaundice

Sometimes called icterus, this is a yellowing of the skin and of the whites of the eyes from deposition of a natural colouring substance, bilirubin. This pigment is released from the haemoglobin in red blood cells at the end of their working lives of 120 days. In health, bilirubin is taken up by the liver and passed into the intestine in the bile. But if the liver is diseased, as by HEPATITIS, so that it cannot secrete the bilirubin, or if the bile ducts are blocked, so that the bilirubin cannot get out, it gradually accumulates in the blood and stains the tissues. Jaundice can also be caused if the red blood cells are broken down more rapidly than normal (haemolytic disease) so that more bilirubin is produced than the liver can cope with.

In itself, skin staining with bilirubin is fairly harmless and, assuming the condition causing it is reversed, will soon disappear. But the skin is not the only tissue to be stained with bilirubin. The brain is particularly susceptible to deposition of bilirubin – a condition known as KERNICTERUS – and can be seriously damaged by it. This is one of the main reasons why RHESUS INCOMPATIBILITY in babies is so dangerous. Severe kernicterus may cause death before, or within a week or two after, birth. Surviving infants feed poorly, suffer varying degrees of paralysis, epilepsy, spasticity of the muscles, LEARNING DIFFICULTY, DEAFNESS and blindness. Kernicterus is preventable by prenatal diagnosis and treatment. Exposure of the baby to intense blue light containing a high ultraviolet component soon after birth assists in converting the bilirubin in the skin to a form which is harmless to the brain. The eyes must be protected.

Other much less common causes of jaundice in babies and young children include:

- CYSTIC FIBROSIS
- infection before birth
- blood poisoning (septicaemia)
- CONGENITAL BILIARY ATRESIA
- unduly thick blood (polycythaemia)
- HEPATITIS
- thyroid gland underactivity
- bruising
- bleeding into the skin
- HEREDITARY SPHEROCYTOSIS

Jaundice must never be ignored, and it is essential that the cause should always be discovered and appropriate treatment given.

Jealousy see introductory section (3 to 5 years).

Jerky eyes see NYSTAGMUS.

Joint pains see ARTHRITIS.

Junk food

A popular term for highly refined, processed and ready-prepared food, usually containing a fairly high level of sweeteners and a low level of roughage. Junk food has the same calorific value as any other comparative food and indulgence in it is, in itself, no more harmful than any other comparable kind of food. A diet exclusively of this kind of food may, however, be relatively deficient in vitamins and minerals and especially in the high cellulose content (roughage) of fresh fruit and vegetables. It will also be high in saturated fats and, if the diet contains a high proportion of junk food, it will be liable, long-term, to encourage the development of the serious arterial disease ATHEROSCLEROSIS. On such a diet, weight gain occurs readily. A diet of junk food, or any other diet in which the emphasis is on dairy fats and protein, should certainly be regarded as much less satisfactory than a well-balanced intake, high in roughage and complex carbohydrates and low in animal fats.

Juvenile delinquency see DELINQUENCY.

K

Kaposi's varicelliform eruption

This is a life-threatening complication occurring in children with ECZEMA and which can be caused by kissing by an adult with oral cold sores. See HERPES SIMPLEX.

Kawasaki disease

This disease, relatively common in Japan, but rare elsewhere, was first recognised in 1967 by Tokyo paediatrician Dr Tomisaku Kawasaki, but is now known to occur world-wide. It affects chiefly infants and young children and causes FEVER, a measles-like rash, red eyes, red palms and soles, puffiness of the hands, dry cracking lips, swollen lymph nodes and, in about 40 per cent of cases, changes in the coronary arteries. These are local enlargements (aneurysms) and are transient in most cases; only about 10 per cent of children have long-term involvement of the coronaries. The cause remains obscure and, although the features of the disease suggest an infection, no organism has been isolated and there is no response to ANTIBIOTICS.

Recently, it has been found that children with the disease have an enzyme, reverse transcriptase, which is a feature of a particular class of viruses, the retroviruses. It is also known that viruses can affect the smooth muscle of artery walls. There is some evidence that the disease may be spread by house-dust mites, or cat fleas.

There is no known laboratory test for Kawasaki's disease but the clinical features are now clear and diagnosis is not difficult. Aspirin has been found useful in the treatment and appears to reduce the incidence of heart complications. The death rate is less than 1 per cent and most children make a complete recovery.

Keratomalacia

Literally, 'softening of the cornea', this is a common cause of blindness in severely malnourished children whose body stocks of vitamin A have become exhausted. Vitamin A deficiency causes dryness of the eyes with typical foamy patches (Bitot's spots) in the corners of the whites. So long as some vitamin A remains in the serum, the condition progresses no further, but when none of the vitamin is left, there is 'corneal melt', perforation, a gushing out of the internal fluid and loss of vision. Internal infection follows and the eyes are soon full of pus and irremediably blinded.

This is the fate of millions of children every year. There is a bitter irony in the situation, in that many of these children are going blind within easy reach of green leaves containing more than enough vitamin A to keep their corneas healthy. Happily, keratomalacia is virtually unknown in Western countries.

Kernicterus

This is JAUNDICE of the brain resulting from RHESUS INCOMPATIBILITY in babies. Skin jaundice in newborn babies is very common and is usually completely harmless. Most cases are not due to rhesus problems. All jaundiced babies must, however, be carefully checked because of the possible risk. Rhesus antibodies destroy fetal red blood cells (haemolysis), releasing from them a substance called bilirubin which causes jaundice, but which is also highly toxic to nerve cells, if sufficient is able to pass from the blood into the brain. This happens in severe, untreated cases, especially those in which there has previously been a rhesus problem and the mother has built up a high level of antibodies.

Kernicterus causes irritability, an increase in muscle responsiveness to stretch (spasticity), leading to a severe backwards arching of the back and neck, uncontrollable writhing movements (athetosis), reluctance to feed and often death within a week or two of birth. Surviving infants show varying degrees of paralysis, a tendency to EPILEPSY, spasticity of the muscles, athetosis, LEARNING DIFFICULTY, DEAFNESS and blindness.

Such an outcome is especially tragic as kernicterus is always preventable by early diagnosis and treatment of the underlying cause. The diagnosis is suggested by high levels of antibodies in the mother and subsequent amniocentesis. Treatment is by exchange transfusion, if necessary while the baby is still in the womb.

Kidney disorders in children

Congenital abnormalities of the kidney are quite common. One kidney may be absent or the two kidneys may be joined ('horseshoe kidney'). Neither need affect life or health. Polycystic kidney, in which the kidneys become filled with large cysts, usually becomes apparent later in life, but can show itself in childhood. In this case the condition is of autosomal recessive inheritance (see GENETICS – AN OUTLINE).

Tumours of the kidney (Wilms' tumours) are rare in children. Wilms' tumour is believed to originate at the embryonic stage of development and is associated with various other congenital abnormalities. It should be specially looked for if a child has ambiguous genitalia, HYPOSPADIAS, undescended testicle (see CRYPTORCHIDISM) and absence of the irises of the eyes.

Inflammation of the kidneys is called nephritis, the commonest forms being acute GLOMERULONEPHRITIS and pyelonephritis. These can cause severe illness in children. Obstruction to the outflow of urine can lead to back-pressure which can rapidly damage the kidneys. Obstruction can occur in several ways, including severe narrowing of the foreskin outlet (PHIMOSIS) in boy babies, which may call for CIRCUMCISION. Outflow obstruction can also cause stone formation in the kidneys.

Kidney failure is a serious possible complication of various kidney diseases including glomerulonephritis, severe kidney infections, kidney poisons and severe general infections. It may also be caused by severe dehydration, massive blood loss and uncontrolled DIABETES. It is the state in which the kidneys are unable to excrete enough urine to maintain the normal composition of the body fluids. Usually, there is little or no output of urine or the passage of urine containing only a very small quantity of its usual constituents. Unless treated by dialysis or a kidney graft, total kidney failure is invariably fatal.

Kidney inflammation see GLOMERULONEPHRITIS.

'Kissing disease' see GLANDULAR FEVER.

Knee pain in boys see OSGOOD-SCHLATTER DISEASE.

Knock-knee

Genu valgum, or 'knock-knee' is a minor deformity that features an abnormal increase in the distance between the ankles when the knees are touching. It may result from growth disturbance in RICKETS and is not uncommon in rheumatoid arthritis, in which the inner ligament of the knee joint may weaken. The commonest cause, however, is a natural variation of the normal in children, occurring because the line of weight-bearing falls to the outer side of the centre of the knee joint. Over 20 per cent of all 3 year olds have at least a 5 cm gap between their ankles with the knees touching, while only about 1 per cent of 7 year-olds show an equivalent degree of knock-knee.

For this reason, moderate degrees of genu valgum in healthy children below 7 years may safely be ignored. In some cases it is considered worth raising the inner edge of the heel of the shoes slightly. In severe cases, walking braces or night splints may be used or even operative correction.

Koplik's spots

These are small white specks, about the size of grains of salt, surrounded by a red base, and appearing on the inside of the cheeks and the inner surface of the lower lip. If these are seen in a child who has been exposed to a case of measles, the disease can be confidently expected. Koplik's spots occur during the incubation period of the disease.

Kwashiorkor

Kwashiorkor is a serious nutritional deficiency disease of young children which results from a diet containing grossly inadequate quantities of protein. It is a disease of developing countries and is virtually unknown in Britain and other Western countries. In conditions of extreme poverty, the only resource, for many small children, is for them to eat anything that can be obtained. The result is the consumption of cereals containing very little digestible carbohydrate. To try to meet their energy needs, these children have to have a large volume intake, most of which is roughage of no nutritional value. Kwashiorkor is probably the commonest of all dietary diseases. It occurs when children are weaned and thus deprived of the high nutritional value of breast milk, or when the appetite is affected by infections.

The disease causes:

- delayed growth and development
- fluid retention (oedema)
- reddish discolouration of the skin and hair
- irritability or apathy
- enlargement of the liver
- wasting of the muscles

Characteristically the abdomen protrudes markedly, and the child with kwashiorkor may, superficially, appear to be well nourished. This is an illusion, however, and these children actually have severe loss of muscle bulk and great weakness. Low levels of protein reduce the power of the blood to withdraw fluid from the tissues and these become water-logged (oedematous). This, together with enlargement of the liver, is the cause of the protuberant abdomen. The face, too, is swollen and puffy. Antibodies are protein molecules and these, too, may be deficient, so that resistance to infection is lowered. Such children are highly susceptible to severe infectious diseases, which often prove fatal.

Affected children are always extremely miserable and, if they can summon up the energy, will have a constant, weak, cry. Because of muscle wasting they are capable of hardly any exertion and are seldom able to feed themselves. If help becomes available, kwashiorkor is treated initially by giving feeds of milk with vitamin and mineral supplements and then, if possible, a normal balanced diet with adequate protein content.

Children under 2 years of age who develop kwashiorkor are likely to suffer lifelong severe retardation of both physical and mental development. Thus, the conditions which caused their problem in the first place – poor social development and the provision of the means of health and nutrition – tend to be perpetuated. Protein starvation is a world-wide problem. Attempts have been made to encourage such enterprises as the stocking of fish ponds. These are capable of providing an adequate supply of high-grade protein. Tragically, the immediate need to assuage hunger has often led to these stock fish being caught and eaten.

Kyphosis

This is an abnormal degree of backward curvature of part of the spine. Backward curvature is normal in the upper back region of the spine and in the lowest part (the sacrum). The term kyphosis, which comes from the Greek 'kyphos' meaning 'bowed or bent', is applied to a degree of backward curvature of the spine sufficient to cause deformity.

Kyphosis is due to downward loading on the spine so that the normal curves are exaggerated. This will not happen unless there is inadequate support from poor muscles or faulty posture. It therefore tends to affect adolescents, as a result of slouching or slumping.

Kyphosis

Adolescent kyphosis responds readily to a determined attempt to assume an upright posture, together with regular exercises to strengthen the abdominal muscles and those which extend the spine. Later in life kyphosis becomes increasingly difficult to correct, but, at any age, the same approach can help.

L

Lactose intolerance

This may be a GENETIC DISORDER or may result from damage to the intestinal lining from gastroenteritis or other disease. In the former condition, in which the chemical activator (enzyme) responsible for splitting milk sugar (lactose) is absent from the intestine, there is DIARRHOEA from birth and failure to thrive. Lactose is a double sugar (disaccharide) which is normally broken down by the digestive enzymes to readily absorbable monosaccharides. When the enzyme is missing the lactose remains in the intestine and passes to the colon where it is fermented by bacteria to cause gas production, colic, distension and diarrhoea.

Lactose intolerance is commoner in black, Asian and South American children than in Europeans. It is treated by giving a diet free from milk sugar.

Lazy eye see AMBLYOPIA, SQUINT, PTOSIS.

Lazy vision see AMBLYOPIA.

Lead poisoning

Lead and lead compounds are highly toxic when eaten or inhaled. Small amounts of lead taken in over long periods have a cumulative effect and can be disastrous. Continued exposure to the fumes of leaded petrol, lead paints, pottery glazes, solder or water from lead pipes, causes lead to accumulate gradually in the body especially in the liver, kidneys and brain.

There has been particular concern over the risks from tetraethyl lead used as an anti-knocking agent in petrol. Children exposed to the exhaust fumes from such petrol may suffer chronic lead poisoning and this can cause damage to brain function, with headache, loss of physical coordination, loss of intellectual ability and memory, and abnormal behaviour. Large numbers of children have, in the past, suffered varying degrees of loss of intellectual function – even measurable loss of IQ – as a result of prolonged exposure to atmospheric lead. Public awareness of the problem has, however, led to reduced levels of environmental lead and unleaded petrol has become much more popular.

Learning difficulty

Children vary greatly in intellectual ability and it is impossible to draw a definite line between normality and retardation. There are, however, those whose mental ability is so much below average that, as they grow up, they are unable consistently to perform even simple, work or other social functions and require constant supervision and guidance if they are not to fall into distress or danger. Such people are said to suffer from learning difficulty – formerly described as mental handicap. This is the result of brain defect or malfunction and is often present from birth.

The mentally retarded are usually classified by intelligence quotient (IQ). Mildly defective people have IQs from 70 down to about 55; moderately defective people have IQs from 54 to 40; and severely defective people have IQs below 40. It should be noted, however, that intelligence quotients are very difficult to measure in the lower ranges and often have to be assessed or even guessed. This is likely to lead to inaccuracy and sometimes to unfair assessments.

People of low mental capacity should be strongly encouraged to try to master some form of useful or other work under supervision. Work can be a source of pride and satisfaction to the retarded, and training in work activities often reveals a higher capacity than had been expected.

Learning difficulty is nearly always present in childhood and usually becomes apparent then by a reduced level of performance in the various social and educational skills compared to that of other children. Severely retarded children occur in roughly equal proportions in all socio-economic classes, but mild retardation seems to be commoner in the most deprived groups. Males are more commonly retarded than females.

Learning difficulty is commonly associated with a range of organic problems. These include:

- DOWN'S SYNDROME
- CEREBRAL PALSY
- PHENYLKETONURIA
- brain damage from asphyxia around the time of birth
- RUBELLA affecting the fetus in early pregnancy
- TOXOPLASMOSIS infection of the fetus
- SPINA BIFIDA
- poorly controlled maternal diabetes during pregnancy
- premature separation of the placenta
- FETAL ALCOHOL SYNDROME
- heavy smoking during pregnancy
- MENINGITIS after birth
- head injury after birth

There is no specific treatment for learning difficulty but often, especially in the case of the mildly retarded, the potential for performance is greater than is suspected. Retarded children may usefully be classified as educable, trainable or multi-handicapped. The first group may, by special intensive education, be expected to achieve at least some degree of independence and a fairly normal quality of life. The second can often, by special training, achieve a variable level of ability to attend to their own needs and to participate in social activity in a relatively protected environment. Unhappily, there is little to be done for the multi-handicapped, who require constant supervision and attention.

Mentally retarded children suffer frustration, poor self-esteem and repeated disappointment. This can lead to emotional and behavioural difficulties that may require psychiatric help, such as FAMILY THERAPY and sometimes drug therapy. This may, for instance be needed to help in the management of anxiety, depression, impulsive behaviour or HYPERACTIVITY. Parents, too, often need support and counselling and occasionally family therapy.

See also INTELLIGENCE AND INTELLIGENCE TESTS.

Leukaemia

Leukaemia is a kind of blood cancer, affecting the blood-forming cells in the bone marrow, in which certain groups of white blood cells reproduce in a disorganized and uncontrolled way, so that they progressively replace, and interfere with, the normal constituents of the blood. About 2 per cent of all cancers are leukaemias and there are many different types of leukaemia with different outlooks. Unless effectively treated, however, leukaemia usually ends fatally either from a shortage of red blood cells (ANAEMIA), or from severe bleeding or infection. Leukaemia is not one disease but a group of disorders of different degrees of severity, but with broadly similar features. Leukaemia is one of the few major forms of cancer for which a complete cure has been found. Unfortunately, this applies only to certain forms of the disease, but with these, affected children have an 80 to 90 per cent chance of being completely cured.

The cause of the leukaemias is unknown but there are definite associations with radiation; with some drugs used in the treatment of other cancers; with certain industrial chemicals such as benzene; and with certain viruses. The different types of leukaemia arise from different white cell types and have different outlooks.

Leukaemia often features:

- INFLUENZA-like symptoms
- a feeling of great tiredness
- sore throat
- bleeding from the gums and pinpoint bleeding into the skin
- loss of appetite and weight
- enlargement of the lymph nodes in the neck, armpits and groins
- enlargement of the spleen

A blood check shows a severe ANAEMIA and usually large numbers of primitive white cells.

Characteristics of anti-leukaemia drugs

Methotrexate – interferes with formation of DNA. Can affect the formation of normal and important white cells in the bone marrow.

Vincristine – prevents chromosomes from dividing. Can cause weakness of the legs and constipation. There may be some loss of hair if given in weekly doses.

6-mercaptopurine – interferes with formation of DNA. Can affect other white cell formation.

Adriamycin – affects all cells but damages rapidly-reproducing cells more than normal cells. Causes severe NAUSEA and VOMITING. Can cause temporary loss of hair. May damage the heart.

Daunorubicin – as for adriamycin.

Cyclophosphamide – affects all cells. Causes nausea, vomiting, hair loss, bladder inflammation and blood in the urine (haematuria).

Cytarabine – interferes with DNA formation. Some nausea. Can affect bone marrow formation of blood cells.

Etoposide – can damage all cells. Causes nausea and hair loss in large dosage.

The commonest kind of childhood leukaemia, with a peak incidence around the age of 3 years, is known as acute lymphoblastic leukaemia. About 80 per cent of leukaemias in childhood affect the white cell group called lymphocytes. 'Lymphoblastic' just means that these cells are being reproduced far too quickly. There are two kinds of lymphocyte – T cells and B cells – and either kind can be the basis of the leukaemia. In fact, there are five forms of acute lymphoblastic leukaemia and these respond to treatment in different ways. B cell acute lymphocytic leukaemia is very malignant and dangerous. Fortunately, it

is also very rare and accounts for only about 1 per cent of all cases.

Leukaemia can be cured by chemotherapy but, as will be seen, the treatment is very unpleasant. The basis of treatment is to give drugs that interfere with the excessive production of lymphocytes, usually by preventing cells from dividing. These drugs, known generally as cytotoxic drugs, include methotrexate, vincristine, 6-mercaptopurine, Adriamycin (Doxorubicin), daunorubicin, cyclophosphamide, cytarabine and etoposide. It is impossible to stop abnormal cells dividing without, to some extent, damaging normal cells, so all these drugs have unpleasant side-effects.

Other non-cytotoxic drugs used include 1-asparaginase and the steroids prednisolone and dexamethasone. L-asparaginase is an enzyme that acts directly on leukaemic cells preventing them from dividing. It may cause allergic effects such as asthma. The steroids can be remarkably effective in producing a brief recovery but cannot cure leukaemia on their own.

Many different schemes of treatment have been devised and, as experience is gained, these are gradually producing better results. The general principle of all, however, is to induce remission of the disease, to consolidate it and then to maintain it. A typical scheme of treatment might involve starting with a drug called allopurinol. This is commonly used in the treatment of gout because of its value in preventing the accumulation of the products of cell breakdown, especially uric acid. If these products are kept soluble, they will be safely disposed of in the urine. Here its function is to protect the kidneys from possible crystallization out of these products which will be produced as a result of the definitive treatment. To assist in this, plenty of fluids are given by drip so as to maintain a good urinary output. The allopurinol and the intravenous fluids are continued for two or three days.

Steroids are then given by mouth and vincristine by four weekly injections. A single dose of methotrexate is given by lumbar puncture into the spinal fluid and 6 to 12 injections of asparaginase are given over the course of the first four weeks. At the end of that time a sample of bone marrow is examined to confirm that the disease is completely under control and that the bone marrow now appears normal. This result is expected in at least 95 per cent of children.

It is now time for the consolidation treatment and this may consist of an intensive five-day course of toxic drugs such as cytarabine, daunorubicin or etoposide. These drugs are best given through a tube passed through the chest wall into one of the main veins of the body and left in place for the duration of the treatment. The drugs are so damaging that they will knock out the bone marrow completely for two or three weeks. They are also very likely to cause hair loss. The otherwise inevitable nausea and vomiting can be controlled by highly effective drugs.

In the third month of treatment, steps are taken to ensure that the central nervous system is free of the disease. This is done by giving methotrexate into the spinal fluid or by radiotherapy. The nervous system is remarkably resistant to radiation. The fourth month sees the start of the maintenance stage and this might consist of steroids by mouth, daily doses of 6-mercaptopurine by mouth, weekly tablets of methotrexate and monthly injections of vincristine. Maintenance treatment goes on for over two years and during that time there have to be regular checks to ensure that the treatment is not causing too much damage. At the end of that time all treatment is stopped and the child is seen perhaps monthly for checks. As confidence is gained the intervals between checks are lengthened.

A high percentage of children with leukaemia and other cancers are treated in clinical trials involving different combinations and dosage of the anticancer drugs. It is only in this way that improvements in the effectiveness of treatment can be found. These schemes of treatment are all based on previous studies that have shown what methods are, up to that time, known to be most effective and least distressing. But, inevitably, they impose a dreadful burden on both child and parents. It is very distressing for parents to see their children

suffering sickness and other side-effects, and often to be unable to make them understand what it is all about. Behavioural problems are very common. Parents often need counselling and strong support. One encouraging recent advance brought about by such trials is the introduction of new and highly effective drugs to combat sickness.

There are few consolations – other than the prospect of cure – for parents of children who have to undergo this kind of ordeal, but one positive consideration is that participation in these trials is making a major contribution to knowledge in this very important field.

Lice

Lice are small wingless insects, common parasites of human and other animals. There are three kinds of human lice: head lice, body lice and pubic lice, and these differ in their habits. The head louse, *Pediculus humanus capitis*, lives on the scalp and feeds by sucking blood. This causes intense itching and scratching with secondary DERMATITIS and infection of the skin. The females lay eggs (nits) which they glue to the shaft of hairs near the scalp. These hatch in about a week. Spread is by direct contact.

The body louse, *Pediculus humanus corporis*, lives in the seams of clothing close to the skin, and moves on to the body only to feed. The eggs are laid in the clothing. Body lice are easily disposed of by proper cleaning of the clothes. They are, in general, only a problem for those who do not regularly change their clothes.

The crab louse, *Phthirus pubis*, so called because of its squat, crab-like appearance, in uncommon in children. It infests the pubic hair and, occasionally, when the infestation is very heavy, the chest hair, armpit hair or even the eyebrows. In adolescents, *Phthirus pubis* is usually transmitted by sexual contact, and once established, likes to stick in one place, causing constant irritation. Heavy infestation is called 'pediculosis'. Because of their sedentary habits, crab lice soon become surrounded by louse faeces. The scratching of the infested person disperses both these and the lice bodies into the skin, leading to a severe dermatitis.

Lice can be eliminated by the use of suitable lotions, such as benzyl benzoate, or insecticide powders, and by shaving off the hair or removing eggs with fine-tooth nit combs.

Limb shortness see
ACHONDROPLASIA.

Listeriosis

This once very rare disease is becoming more common but is still seldom seen. It is caused by an organism which can resist low temperatures and has been recovered from lamb meat kept at 0° C for 24 days. The organism is present in most domestic and farm animals and many birds and fish. It has been found in soft cheeses and various precooked foods. Over half the chickens in Britain carry the organism, either internally or externally, but proper cooking will kill it. It is common in sewage and in the stools of up to 30 per cent of healthy people.

Babies can be infected before birth but this is rare – only about one baby in 18,000 is affected. Those who are, however, may suffer widespread damage to most of the systems of the body, and about a quarter of the babies severely infected in this way are born dead.

Human listeriosis is commonest in babies and old people, affecting the throat, the eyes, the skin and the nervous system. The great majority of cases are mild and pass unremarked. Some have an upset similar to GLANDULAR FEVER. There is fever, RED EYE, MUMPS-like swelling of the salivary glands and sometimes pustules on the skin.

Listeriosis responds well to ANTIBIOTICS, which greatly reduce the mortality from this condition in infants.

Liver inflammation see
HEPATITIS.

Lockjaw

A lay term for tight spasm of the powerful chewing muscles which is a feature of the serious infection TETANUS. The muscle spasm clamps the teeth together so that they can barely be separated. The medical term is 'trismus'.

Long sight see REFRACTIVE
ERRORS.

Lordosis

This is an abnormal degree of forward curvature of the lower part of the spine, often associated with abnormal backward curvature of the upper part (KYPHOSIS). Lordosis and kyphosis exaggerate the normal 'S' shape of the spine and commonly lead to backache. Young children often have an apparent lordosis as a result of spinal flexibility. So long as the lordosis is not fixed this is normal and harmless. An abnormal lordosis will respond to treatment of kyphosis.

Lyme disease

This disease was first recognized in Old Lyme, Connecticut, in 1975. It is caused by a spirochaete transmitted by the bite of a tick. It occurs throughout the temperate regions of the world and can affect people of any age. The natural hosts are deer and dogs. It is now occurring increasingly in Britain.

The first sign is a slightly itchy red spot at the site of the mite bite. This expands steadily and forms a slowly growing ring. In about half the cases other similar rings appear and there may be as many as 100, scattered all over the skin. These are not due to multiple bites. There is fatigue, malaise, HEADACHES, FEVER, stiff neck, aches in the muscles and joints and enlarged lymph nodes. In some cases, there is sore throat, COUGH, conjunctivitis, other more severe eye complications and abdominal pain with enlargement and tenderness of the liver.

Weeks or months later, one in six affected people will develop MENINGITIS, ENCEPHALITIS, paralysis of various nerves, muscle weakness or shingles-like pain in the skin. Mental illness or deep fatigue and weakness, lasting for months or years, may occur. Half of those who contract Lyme disease suffer joint problems, usually mild, but sometimes severe, with damage similar to that caused by rheumatoid arthritis. Heart damage may also occur.

Lyme disease can be passed from a mother to her unborn baby, and the spirochaetes have been found in children with severe congenital defects. It is a pity that the features of the disease are not better known. If the early skin pattern is recognised, treatment with ANTIBIOTICS can prevent any further trouble.

Malnutrition

This is the effect of an inadequate diet or failure to absorb a normal diet or to assimilate absorbed food elements. The term is now sometimes used to describe gross overeating.

Malnutrition from insufficient food intake is a world-wide problem for which there is no medical solution. This is essentially a matter of economics, education and social development, likely to be solved only by industrialization for the creation of the necessary wealth. Ironically, in many under developed areas, the natural resources would be more than adequate to support local populations if simple food-production methods could be applied, but attempts to do so have repeatedly been frustrated by social factors.

In babies, infants and young children, malnutrition causes failure to thrive and to grow to the height otherwise genetically determined. It can interfere with the production of immunoglobulins and hence reduce the efficiency of the body's defence against infection. Vitamin deficiencies, which are a common feature of malnutrition, cause a wide spectrum of specific disorders including beriberi, pellagra, ANAEMIA, pernicious anaemia, scurvy, dry eye (xerophthalmia), KERATOMALACIA, RICKETS and bleeding tendencies. Protein deficiency causes marasmus and KWASHIORKOR.

Malocclusion

This is a failure of the upper and lower teeth to come together in an acceptable manner. ORTHODONTICS can do much to correct moderate degrees of malocclusion.

Manipulative behaviour

This is conduct calculated to force another person to act in a manner desired by the manipulator. In the case of babies and young children, the commonest forms of manipulative behaviour are breath-holding attacks and temper tantrums (see introductory section). Older children may resort to flattery, subtle pressures, nagging, even moral blackmail. At worst, manipulative behaviour involves seemingly ruthless, cold, manoeuvring and heartless dealing by which the manipulator hopes to gain an advantage over parents and others.

Such behaviour brings so much unpopularity and unhappiness that every attempt must be made to ensure that children guilty of manipulative behaviour understand what they are doing. It should be made clear to them that this pattern of conduct is severely damaging to any relationship and that they risk incurring strong dislike or even hatred. They must somehow be persuaded to respect other people's rights to personal freedom.

See also HABIT FORMATION.

Marfan's syndrome

This is a rare genetic disease in which all the collagen connective tissue of the body is abnormally weak. Affected people grow tall and thin and characteristically have very long spidery fingers (arachnodactyly) and unusually mobile joints. The thumb can be folded right across the palm of the hand so that the tip can protrude beyond the base of the little finger. The joints dislocate easily, the suspensory ligaments of the lenses of the eyes readily break so that the lenses become displaced, and the main artery of the body, the aorta, is unusually elastic and floppy. There is a strong tendency to develop heart disease. There is commonly a sideways bend to the spine (scoliosis).

Marfan's syndrome is an autosomal dominant condition (see GENETICS – AN

OUTLINE) which often does not cause serious trouble until middle age. So unless the nature of the condition is known, children with the condition may have been produced before its significance is appreciated. It is for consideration whether young people with Marfan's syndrome should be made aware of the desirability of genetic counselling before marrying.

Masturbation

All infants, young children, and most other healthy young animals, soon find that they can derive pleasure from handling or otherwise stimulating their genitalia. You should be quite clear that this is normal, otherwise you may produce an emotional reaction that greatly intrigues the child and concentrates his or her attention even more closely on that part of the body. This normal interest can hardly be described as masturbation.

Genital itchiness or irritation is common in children and the natural reaction to this may be interpreted by parents as masturbation. Regular genital rubbing by young girls, especially if it starts suddenly, should prompt close examination for a local inflammation from a cause such as thrush. Boys occasionally develop an irritation of the glans of the penis (see BALANITIS).

Actual masturbation sometimes occurs in infants and is fairly common in older children. It is usually achieved by making repetitive rocking movements with the thighs pressed together. Sometimes the child seems to go into a trance and may appear to be quite out of contact with the environment. The face may turn red and breathing may become heavier. The pupils may be enlarged and sweating may occur. Childhood masturbation has been confused with an epileptic seizure. This is, in fact, entirely normal behaviour and the secret is to ignore it. The last thing needed is to make a fuss and start up all kinds of wrong associations in the child's mind.

In pubertal children, masturbation is also normal and is accompanied by sexual fantasies, usually until orgasm is achieved. Over 90 per cent of males and 75 per cent of females masturbate at one time or another. Repetitive movement of the skin of the penis or gentle massage of the clitoris is the usual method and once the practice is established it occurs, on average, four times a week. The privacy of young people should be scrupulously respected. Masturbation is, of course, a substitute for sexual intercourse with another person and is usually found unnecessary when such intercourse becomes accessible. Even after many years of regular masturbation, the practice will be abandoned in favour of the more satisfying and significant alternative.

There is no reason to suppose that masturbation is harmful. But many young people have suffered mentally as a result of ridiculous statements about it by pious and ill-informed people.

Measles

This is a highly infectious, often epidemic, disease of childhood that is caused by a virus usually acquired by inhaling infected droplet material. Every two or three years a sufficient number of susceptible children accumulate and an epidemic occurs. About 14 days after infection, and shortly before the rash appears, tiny 'salt-grain' spots (KOPLIK'S SPOTS) may be seen inside the cheeks. There is fever, cough, sneezing, general misery, redness of the eyes, and an irregular, red, mottled, slightly raised rash which lasts for about a week and then fades.

Complications include OTITIS MEDIA, bronchitis and pneumonia, all of which will usually respond to ANTIBIOTIC treatment. Much less commonly, there may be ENCEPHALITIS. Measles cannot cause SQUINT but may precipitate it in children with severe 'long sight' (see REFRACTIVE ERRORS).

Most people have measles during childhood and a second attack is rare. The disease can be prevented by a vaccine which should be given to all children, aged 1 to 2 years, for whom there is no valid medical objection. In 1995, a major national anti-measles campaign was mounted. This has succeeded in interrupting the previously inevitable transmission of measles in school children and represents a substantial public health breakthrough.

Meconium

This is the name given to the stools passed by a baby during the first day or two of life, or before birth if there is 'fetal distress'. Meconium is thick, greenish-black and of a sticky consistency. It consists of cells cast off by the lining of the bowel during uterine life, mixed with bowel mucus and stained with bile from the liver. Once feeding is established the meconium is replaced by normal stools.

Medication dosage

Babies and children differ from adults in many ways and several factors determine the correct dosage. It is unsafe to estimate dosage for a child, from the adult dose, on the proportion of the weight. Children's preparations are packaged in appropriate dosage and these should not be exceeded. In the case of important drugs, the doctor will clearly indicate the dosage and this should be scrupulously followed. Over-the-counter remedies are, however, usually safe even if the spoon size varies. Fortunately, most paediatric mixtures have a considerable margin of safety. But it should be remembered that the claimed safety of much modern medication containing pharmacologically active ingredients, is based on the assumption that the recommended dose will not be exceeded.

The standard 'teaspoon' dose is 5 ml and children's plastic medicine spoons, calibrated so as to deliver accurate dosage, can easily be obtained. Although it is possible to make rough adjustments to dosage on the basis of the child's size (rather than age), for over-the-counter medications, you should be very careful not to modify dosage in the case of prescribed drugs. Children are not just little adults. There are many other factors that determine the appropriate dosage. The doctor's instructions should be carefully followed.

Children hate swallowing tablets or capsules and should be given mixtures if possible. Medication spat out or vomited should be replaced. If the medicine tastes too pleasant, however, there is always a risk of overdosage and this should be guarded against.

Melanomas

Malignant melanomas are dangerous tumours of the cells that colour the skin – the melanocytes. Fortunately, these are very rare. Only about 2 per cent of all malignant melanomas occur in people under 20 and only 0.3 to 0.4 per cent of them occur in children below puberty. As malignant melanoma is still comparatively rare in adults five to ten per 100,000 per year) this is a very small number indeed.

Melanoma may be congenital or may develop in infancy. In older children, it is more likely to occur in skin that has been damaged by the sun. Certain other conditions make melanoma more likely in children. These include heavily pigmented giant congenital naevi, the dysplastic naevus syndrome, xeroderma pigmentosum and immunodeficiency states. Dysplastic naevi are multiple pigmented areas, of diameter greater than 5 mm with irregular edges and irregular pigmentation. Xeroderma pigmentosum is a rare genetic skin disease featuring excessive sensitivity to sunlight, premature ageing of the skin and the development of skin cancers. The unfortunate victims are almost confined to an indoor existence and have to rely on protective covering and skin sunscreen creams.

Danger signs of malignant melanoma

Obvious changes in pigmented moles, especially:

- swelling
- increasing size
- change in shape
- irregularity of, and alteration in, borders
- irregularity and changes in the distribution of pigment
- bleeding on minor trauma
- inflammation
- surface ulceration
- itching and pain

Particular risk factors for children are fair skin and inappropriate exposure to the sun with burning. White infant skin may be especially susceptible. Every precaution must be taken to protect the skin against the dangers of ultraviolet radiation. T-shirts or other protective clothing should be worn during swimming, effective sunscreen creams should be used, and children (and adults) should wear hats. Remember that during the midday period, the ambient rays of the sun pass through the thinnest atmospheric distance and are thus most intense.

It is very unusual for a child to develop malignant melanoma, but, for this very reason, and because of the nature of the condition, doctors are hesitant to make the diagnosis. This may result in unacceptable delay in starting treatment. Any genuinely suspicious lesion should be entirely removed (excisional biopsy) and sent for expert examination.

Meningitis

This serious disease is inflammation of the membranes covering the brain and spinal cord (the meninges). The commonest cause of meningitis today is infection with viruses such as HERPES SIMPLEX CHICKENPOX, POLIO, echo viruses, coxsackie viruses and MUMPS.

Viral meningitis is often a minor disorder but may be acute, with headache, fever and drowsiness which may progress rapidly to deep coma. In severe cases, there may be weakness of the muscles, paralysis, speech disturbances, double vision or partial loss of the field of vision, and epileptic fits. Most children make a complete recovery, but some may have residual effects. There is no specific treatment for most virus infections, but in the case of herpes meningitis, the drug acyclovir can be valuable.

Meningococcal meningitis is an epidemic form of the disease which tends to occur in institutions and overcrowded dwellings, such as orphanages or boarding schools, but may affect any community of children. It is usually much more serious than viral meningitis. All parents should be aware of the characteristic signs and symptoms (see box).

Signs and symptoms of meningitis
- sore throat
- rising temperature
- severe HEADACHE
- marked stiffness of the neck
- VOMITING
- rash of red spots appearing on the trunk
- confusion
- drowsiness
- coma

Babies and infants show fever, vomiting, convulsions and have a characteristic high-pitched cry. In babies, the soft areas on the head between the skull bones (the fontanelles) often bulge outwards and feel much tenser than normal. Because of the typical rash, the condition is sometimes called 'spotted fever'.

The affected child may become gravely ill within a day of onset and may pass quickly into coma. Without treatment, death may occur within days or even hours. So treatment is urgent and should never be delayed. Fortunately, bacterial meningitis nearly always responds well to antibiotics and full recovery is usual.

Metabolic disorders

There are about 180 of these rare conditions, and all are caused by genetic errors which result in the absence, or abnormal functioning, of a particular enzyme – a substance needed for the normal chemical processes of the body. The more important conditions include PHENYLKETONURIA, GALACTOSAEMIA, TAY-SACH'S DISEASE, porphyria, HURLER'S SYNDROME and glycogen storage disease. These conditions cause various effects including failure to thrive, floppiness, developmental delay, vomiting, a mousy body odour, CATARACT, JAUNDICE or rashes.

Some of the metabolic disorders are mild and require no treatment, some can be effectively treated. Some of the more severe can be detected early by amniocentesis and termination of pregnancy can then be considered.

Mewing baby cry see CRI DU CHAT SYNDROME.

Microcephaly

Abnormal smallness of the skull. This often reflects poor brain growth and is usually associated with some degree of LEARNING DIFFICULTY.

Milk see introductory section (Baby Care).

Milk intolerance see LACTOSE INTOLERANCE.

Misbehaviour

Around 10 per cent of children behave, consistently, in a manner unacceptable to their parents, but many of these children are merely 'difficult' and will turn out well in the end. Less than 2 per cent of children consistently behave in such a way as to interfere with normal educational progress or to damage social relationships. Most commonly, these children show aggressive non-co-operation, a pattern of automatic opposition to suggestion, unwillingness to adapt to changing circumstances, outbursts of anger and periods of sulkiness.

Sometimes the problem lies with the parent rather than the child. Many parents have an unrealistic idea of normal behaviour and of what may be expected of a child at various stages. Many are overprotective to the point of interfering with the child's need to explore and seek information and stimulation. This induces boredom and frustration in the child. At the same time, parents of problem children often feel guilty and helpless. Most are unaware that tensions of this kind are, to a greater or lesser degree, almost universal.

You should not tolerate seemingly severe problems of this kind for long, because the longer they persist, the more difficult they are to deal with. A little professional advice from a child psychologist or psychiatrist, at an early stage, can completely alter the outlook. If you do seek such help, you will be advised to make reasonable but firm rules and stick to them, to avoid obvious expression of annoyance or anger, and to spend more time actively engaged in play and other activities with the child. Children respond well to positive and consistent programming and are always happier if there is no doubt in anyone's mind about the rules. They will, of course, always try to break or bend the rules and to extend the limits of what they can get away with. Such attempts must be blocked with firmness, but, if possible, with good humour.

Physical punishment may be useful as an ultimate sanction, but should be a rare and noteworthy event. If and when applied, it should be unequivocally clear to the child that the punishment actually does hurt the inflictor more than the victim. Useful, for general disciplinary purposes, is positive reinforcement. The object of punishments, such as brief, timed periods of banishment to a boring place, must be carefully and unemotionally explained to the child prior to the sentence, and at the end of the punishment, the child should be asked to state the reason for it. Soon after, if possible, the child should be praised for some action. Such methods can be highly effective.

You must, at all costs, avoid the all too common emotional outburst – shouting, scolding, striking – in response to the child's stubborn aggressiveness and indiscipline. This induces a vicious cycle in which the child will seek for, and find, all sorts of ways to hit back – sullenness, refusal to eat, temper tantrums, breathholding attacks (see introductory section), the eating of soil or dirt (PICA), deliberate defaecation into the clothes, refusal to go to bed, BEDWETTING, night waking, and so on. This cycle must be broken, but to do so may call for unusual control on the part of the parents. Tantrums and refusal of food must be ignored. Food should be cleared away at the normal time and should not be available until the next meal. There need be no concern about the effect on the child's health. Appetite will assert itself. However difficult, the parent must at all times bear in mind the critical importance of maintaining the child's sense of security and of being loved.

See also BEHAVIOUR DISORDER, DELINQUENCY, SMACKING.

Mongolian spot

A kind of pigmented birthmark (naevus) found on the buttocks or lower part of the back. Mongolian spots have a bluish-black appearance and are caused by a local accumulation of the normal skin pigment. They are commonest in non-white children and have usually disappeared by the age of about 4 years.

Mongolism

The outdated name for DOWN'S SYNDROME.

Mongoloid appearance see
DOWN'S SYNDROME.

Mosaicism

This is the existence of two or more genetically different types of cell in the same individual. Normal human body cells contain 23 pairs of chromosomes. In mosaicism, the cells do not all possess the same number of chromosomes, although they are all derived from the same fertilized egg. In some cases of mosaicism, some cells have an additional chromosome while the other cells are normal.

Mosaicism may, for instance, occur in DOWN'S SYNDROME. This is caused by an additional chromosome 21 (trisomy 21). But in about 1 per cent of cases of Down's syndrome, there are two different cell lines, one of which is normal and the other of which has the additional chromosome 21. Mosaicism may considerably modify the effect of the chromosome abnormality, sometimes reducing it almost to insignificance.

Motion sickness

This is the general term applied to nausea or vomiting induced by any form of passive motion of the body, whether by boat, car, aircraft, swing, space-rocket or simulator.

The word 'nausea' derives from the Greek word 'naus', meaning a 'ship'.

The features of motion sickness are well known to many children. After a variable period of exposure to unaccustomed motion, there is abdominal discomfort, progressive nausea, pallor, sweating of the face and hands, increased salivation, a sense of depression, and vomiting. If the motion continues, the symptoms persist for several days, with variable severity. There is apathy, depression, total loss of appetite and sometimes a loss of the will to live, so that action to maintain personal safety may be abandoned.

The cause of motion sickness is unknown, but it is not experienced by people whose inner ear balancing mechanisms are destroyed. The condition seems to be related to a sustained loss of any fixed base by which to judge bodily position, and it is relieved if the eyes can be focused on some unmoving point or line, such as the horizon.

Motion sickness is best treated with small doses of one of the drugs found, by experience, to be effective. Useful drugs include atropine (Belladonna) and its derivative hyoscine (Kwells), and atropine-like antihistamine drugs such as cyclizine (Valoid), promethazine (Phenergan or Avomine), or dimenhydrinate (Dramamine). Sometimes the phenothiazine tranquillizers and the barbiturates may be used. Any drugs must be taken at least an hour before the motion starts and great care should be taken to avoid overdosage, especially in children, by repeating the dose too frequently.

Mousy-smelling infant see
PHENYLKETONURIA.

Mumps

Mumps is a virus infection, most commonly affecting children, which causes fever and swelling of the main pair of salivary glands (the parotids), so that the face assumes a hamster-like appearance. An attack of mumps confers permanent immunity.

The disease is spread by aerosol droplet transfer during coughing and sneezing and the first symptoms appear after an incubation period of about three weeks. The period of fever is brief – two or three days – and the illness is often very mild, perhaps no more than a slight discomfort in front of the ears and on chewing. If more severe, there may be headache. The swelling of the parotid glands resolves in about 10 days. Occasionally a mild form of meningitis may occur, but this is seldom serious.

The complication most commonly causing concern is inflammation of the testicle (orchitis). This affects about a quarter of the adolescent boys who contract mumps and it may cause much distress. As a rule, only one testicle is affected, but this may become considerably swollen, exquisitely tender and painful and may remain so for several days, before returning to its normal state. Occasionally mumps orchitis leads to sterility of the affected testicle, but this seldom affects fertility. Total sterility from this cause is rare.

Münchausen's by proxy

This extraordinary phenomenon is included simply to make the point that the medical profession is now thoroughly alive to it and will quickly suspect it in any case in which a parent is guilty of such an atrocity.

Münchausen's syndrome is a sustained course of deliberate and calculated deception of the medical profession for the purposes of obtaining attention, personal status and free accommodation and food. People with this condition make a career of simulating disease. They read medical books with close attention and then report to a doctor complaining of the symptoms of a specific disease, preferably a serious one. Such people are usually very plausible and sometimes subtle, and if previously unknown to the doctor or hospital concerned, are likely to carry conviction and succeed in their desire to be admitted for investigation and treatment. They have a preference for surgical conditions and often have an unusual number of surgical scars. On being detected, as they invariably eventually are, these people immediately discharge themselves from hospital.

In recent years, a new variant of this strange disorder has appeared. In Münchausen's by proxy, a parent uses a child as a subject and actually inflicts on the child purported diseases or injuries so that the child will be treated in hospital. Often, the parent continues to inflict damage to the child while it is in hospital. In some cases it has been thought justified to use hidden closed-circuit TV cameras to observe what is happening. Needless to say, parents found to be behaving in this way are liable to criminal proceedings.

Muscle weakness see MUSCULAR DYSTROPHY.

Muscular dystrophy

This is a rare disorder in which slow, progressive degeneration of muscle occurs, leading to increasing weakness and disability. There are three main types of muscular dystrophy. Duchenne dystrophy is almost confined to males as it is nearly always an X-linked recessive condition (see GENETICS – AN OUTLINE). The gene that is affected is one of the largest in the whole genome and this may account for its high mutation rate. The mutation often involves deletion of part of the gene. About 30 per cent of cases arise as a new mutation and in these cases there is, of course, no family history.

The first signs usually appear before the age of 3 years and in most cases the muscles appear bulkier than normal. This is called pseudohypertrophy. The bulk of actual muscle tissue is not, however, increased and there is progressive weakening. The disorder initially affects the buttocks and leg muscles, causing a characteristic waddle in walking. The weakness causes the child to get up from lying in a typical way – by rolling onto his or her face and using the arms to push himself or herself up by 'hand-walking' up the legs. Unfortunately, nothing can arrest the progress of the disease. By the age of about 10 the child is usually unable to walk, and it is common for the heart muscle to become affected as part of the general process. Unfortunately, the disease usually proves fatal by the mid-teens. The affected children commonly die peacefully from pneumonia.

There are two other main forms of muscular dystrophy – the limb girdle type, affecting the shoulders, pelvic and uppermost limb muscles, which usually causes severe disablement within 20 years; and the facio-scapulohumeral type, affecting the muscles of the face, upper back and upper arm, which progresses very slowly and does not necessarily shorten life. Most people with this form of muscular dystrophy remain active throughout a life of normal duration.

Myopia see REFRACTIVE ERRORS.

Myringotomy

This is a surgical incision made in the eardrum. It may be done to allow the insertion of a grommet in cases of GLUE EAR (secretory OTITIS MEDIA) so as to drain the middle ear and relieve deafness. Rarely, the operation may be needed to release pus and relieve pressure in the middle ear in cases of acute otitis media, so as to prevent dangerous internal spread of infection. This is seldom required, nowadays, but was a common operation in the pre-antibiotic era.

Myringotomy is usually performed under general anaesthesia, using an operating microscope and a fine scalpel, with a very small blade, which is introduced through a conical 'speculum' pushed into the ear canal.

Nail biting

This common habit is symbolic of anxiety, but, in reality, is no more than a mild habit disorder, or an indication of boredom. Nail biting may start as early as 1 year of age and becomes increasingly common up to about 12. There is no reason to suppose that nail biting is an indication of any emotional disorder.

Some nail biters, however, carry the habit to the extremity of causing actual damage to the finger-tips by nibbling at the cuticles and causing secondary infection of the fingers and nail beds. The effect is markedly unsightly and, with growing consciousness of the importance of personal appearance, the adolescent nail biter will often find the discipline to desist. Bitter-tasting applications may help to remind the biter of his or her resolution.

Nappy rash

Babies with a nappy rash show obvious discomfort and cry a lot. An extensive rash is usually caused by prolonged skin contact with a wet nappy in which the urine has been acted on by bacteria, so that some of the urea in it has been converted to ammonia. You can smell the ammonia in these cases, and this strong alkali is, of course, highly irritating.

The remedy is to change the nappies frequently and to try to keep the nappy area of the skin as clean and free from contamination as possible. Disposable nappies are better than towelling. Disposable liners are available from most chemists. As the problem is primarily due to bacteria, a mild antiseptic cream containing cetrimide (Savlon) is helpful.

If the rash is confined to the area immediately around the baby's anus, it is probably due to irritants in the faeces. These irritants also irritate the bowel, so there is likely to be DIARRHOEA also. Don't neglect baby diarrhoea. When the diarrhoea settles, the rash should settle also. The affected skin should be kept as clean as possible. A bland protective barrier cream, such as dimethicone cream, can be helpful. The most widely available over-the-counter preparation for the prevention of nappy rash is Sudocrem. Waterproof pants should be used only when strictly necessary and nappies should be left off as much as is reasonably possible.

Narrowed penile outlet see
PHIMOSIS.

Nasal congestion

COLDS and other upper respiratory infections lead to swelling (oedema) of the mucous membranes lining the nose and this causes partial or total blockage of the airway. This is a very common problem in childhood. There is distress, mouth breathing and, in babies, difficulty in both breast- and bottle-feeding. Nasal catarrh, with mucus accumulation, will cause similar problems and these can be relieved by the sparing use of decongestants containing volatile oils such as menthol (eg. Vick's) or Olbus oil. Decongestants containing ephedrine or ephedrine-like substances should not be used in young children. They may be dangerous and the 're-bound' effect leads to increased congestion.

Nasal obstruction

The commonest cause of obstruction to the nasal airway is NASAL CONGESTION, but this may also result from greatly enlarged ADE-NOIDS, nasal polyps, or, very rarely, a tumour in the nose. One-sided blockage is very common and this is usually due to deflection to one side of the central partition of the nose (the nasal septum). This may be natural or the result of injury.

Nasal speech see ADENOIDS.

Nausea see VOMITING.

Navel protrusion see UMBILICAL HERNIA.

Neck rigidity

Stiffness and pain on movement, caused by spasm of the neck and spinal muscles, is a cardinal sign of MENINGITIS.

Neck webbing see TURNER'S SYNDROME.

Neonatologist

This is the term for a doctor who specialises in the care of newborn babies. This important branch of paediatrics covers the special problems of premature or low-birth weight babies and those born with congenital abnormalities. The neonatologist takes charge during the first four weeks of life, after which the child comes under the care of a general paediatrician.

Nervous habit see TICS.

Nightmares

These are intensely vivid and unpleasant dreams, suffered more by children than by adults. Nightmares are often connected with some prior event of a highly traumatic nature such as an assault, a serious accident or injury, severe frights or fears. They may be caused by the withdrawal of sleeping medicine.

Nightmares are anxiety dreams and occur during the periods of rapid eye movement (REM) sleep. They are distinguished from NIGHT TERRORS which occur in the early part of the night during the period of deep, non-REM sleep.

Night terrors

Night terrors produce much more powerful physiological effects than the nightmare –

the heart rate accelerations have been among the highest recorded, the respiratory rate is very high and there is marked sweating. There is often loud screaming. The deeper the non-REM sleep, the more severe the night terror tends to be. The content of the night terror is usually a conviction of suffocation, choking, entrapment in a small space or impending death. Night terrors are commonest around the age of 5 or 6 and tend to stop in adolescence.

Night waking see SLEEP PROBLEMS.

Nose bleed

This very common event usually results from minor injury, such as nose-picking or a blow to the nose, but may also result from infection of the mucous membrane, local drying and crusting. Nose bleed can almost always be controlled by pinching the nostrils firmly together for five minutes and breathing through the mouth. Pressure maintained for this length of time will allow the blood to clot and the bleeding is unlikely to recur unless the site is disturbed. Failure to control bleeding by this method may call for medical attention.

Bleeding in children, arising from persistent crusting of the insides of the nostrils, is best treated by the use of a softening ointment such as petroleum jelly.

Nystagmus

This is persistent jerky or wobbling movement of the eyes, usually together. The movement is most commonly horizontal, but may be vertical, or even circular. The commonest type of nystagmus, 'sawtooth' nystagmus, involves a repetitive slow movement in one direction followed by a sudden recovery jerk in the other. This kind of eye movement can be observed at any time, as a normal phenomenon, in underground railway passengers trying to determine the station name from a moving train.

Permanent sawtooth nystagmus is almost always present from birth (congenital) and seldom implies anything serious. Although the eyes are normal, it is, however, usually associated with a slight reduction in visual acuity. It is an almost constant feature of the condition of ALBINISM. Nystagmus, of a searching type, as if the affected child is constantly looking for something, is a feature of very severe visual defect, such as might occur from dense congenital CATARACT or other serious eye defects present from birth. Nystagmus appearing for the first time later in life indicates a probably serious disorder of the nervous system and should prompt immediate medical attention.

Obesity see WEIGHT PROBLEMS.

Obstruction of intestine see INTUSSUSCEPTION.

Oedipus complex

This is the Freudian notion that all sorts of evils, including all the neuroses, spring from the young male child's unconscious wish to kill his father and have sexual intercourse with his mother. Freud got the idea from his own experience and the name from the swollen-footed, mythical hero of Sophocles' tragedies. Much of the edifice of Freudian psychoanalysis was built up on this remarkable concept, but it is now progressively being relegated to mythology – where, in the opinion of many, it belongs.

Orchidopexy

The testicles are formed inside the abdomen and normally descend into the scrotum before birth, by passing down a tube called the inguinal canal. Sometimes one or both testicles fail to descend, remaining in the abdomen or in the inguinal canal. Orchidopexy is an operation to bring an undescended testicle down into the scrotum and to fix it in place. A testicle which remains in the abdomen will become sterile because the lower temperature of the scrotum is necessary if normal sperm are to be produced. It is also considerably more liable to subsequent cancer than a normally descended testicle.

Ten per cent of undescended testicles remain in the abdomen and in such cases, orchidopexy is difficult and has to be done in stages, but most lie in the canal and can usually be brought down in a single-stage operation. This should ideally be done before the age of 3 years.

Orthodontics

This is the dental specialty concerned with the cosmetic and functional state of the position of the teeth, and the relationship of the upper teeth to the lower (occlusion). Orthodontics takes advantage of the remarkable degree to which tooth positioning can be influenced by sustained pressure, and several different kinds of appliances are used to apply this. These include various types of braces, springs, wires and harnesses. Sometimes small metal attachments are cemented to the teeth so that force may be applied, and sometimes teeth are deliberately extracted to make room.

Pressure applied to a tooth causes absorption of socket bone on the side opposite to the pressure, and new bone production on the same side. The process is slow, but the effect on the position of the tooth is permanent. Orthodontic treatment may also involve the removal of teeth to overcome crowding. Once this is done, displaced teeth may be moved to their proper position.

Orthoptics

Orthoptics is a specialty, ancillary to ophthalmology, concerned mainly with the management of SQUINT in childhood and the avoidance of the visual loss (AMBYLOPIA) which readily results from squint. Orthoptists are experts in the diagnosis of inapparent squint and in obtaining information about the state of the visual acuity, in both eyes, in children. They are also able to determine the degree to which the child is able to perceive simultaneously with the two eyes (binocular vision).

Orthoptists use a variety of ingenious instruments in their work. The central instrument is the major amblyoscope, better known as the synoptophore. This is a device which children will enjoy using once they have got over their initial anxiety. The instrument is adjusted to the child's eye separation and the child is invited to look in. By placing pairs of coloured slides in the synoptophore, one or each side, the orthoptist presents a different coloured image to each of the child's eyes. Thus, one eye might see a goldfish and the other a glass bowl full of water; one may see a lion and the other a cage; and so on.

The child is asked to say what he or she sees. A child with normal binocular vision will see the goldfish in the bowl and the lion in the cage. The arms of the synoptophore can be swung out or in at an angle and a normal child will be able to retain the dual image over a range of convergence and even slight divergence. A child with suppressed vision (amblyopia) will see only the goldfish or the bowl, depending on which eye is affected and on which way round the slides are inserted.

A normal child will also be able to fuse the images from pairs of slides, each being incomplete, into one image. Thus, one slide may show a rabbit and the other an appropriately placed pair of ears. The child is asked to describe the rabbit. 'Does he have ears? Are they in the right place'? In this way the presence or absence of the visual fusional capacity is demonstrated. The range of convergence and divergence over which fusion can be maintained is also measurable.

Once a diagnosis of amblyopia has been made, it is treated largely by the judicious covering, for variable periods, of the better-seeing eye (occlusion). The younger the child, the more quickly will occlusion restore vision.

Osgood-Schlatter disease

This fairly common knee disorder affects mostly boys, usually around puberty. The bulky group of muscles on the front of the thigh run down together into a heavy tendon which contains the knee-cap, and which is inserted into a bony lump on the front of the main bone of the lower leg (the tibia). The repetitive strong pulls on this tendon, as the knee is straightened against resistance – an inevitable occurrence in normal boyhood activity – sometimes cause damage at the point of insertion of the tendon. Some authorities believe this to be due to interference with the blood supply of the region. There is swelling of the upper end of the tibia and sometimes acute tenderness on pressure.

Fortunately, the problem resolves rapidly with no more treatment than a period of avoidance of activities such as climbing, cycling and rugby-playing. If these are persisted in, an unsightly protuberance may develop below the knee. In severe cases, a plaster cast to prevent bending may be required.

Osteomyelitis

This is a serious infection of bone and bone marrow. Osteomyelitis usually results from spread of germs from a boil or other skin infection, or from an open (compound) fracture. The disease is commonest in children and starts abruptly with fever and severe pain at the affected bone site. An adjacent joint may swell and stiffen and confuse the diagnosis. X-ray changes do not occur for several days or weeks, but isotope scanning can establish the cause of the trouble.

Intensive ANTIBIOTIC treatment is necessary if the condition is not to become long-term (chronic), with abscess formation and death of an isolated piece of bone (sequestrum formation). In pre-antibiotic days osteomyelitis was almost always permanent and was curable only by amputation.

Otitis externa

Otitis means inflammation of the ear. Otitis externa is inflammation of the skin of the external ear canal. This is a common problem in children. The skin of the visible part of the ear may or may not be involved. Otitis externa may be a local disorder or part of any general inflammatory disorder of the skin. These include a wide variety of infections. Staphylococci may cause a painful boil in the canal; herpes viruses, both simplex (cold sores) and zoster (shingles), may cause the characteristic blisters and crusting; and fungi of various kinds, including thrush, may cause persistent and sometimes intractable inflammation. Fungal infection of the ear is called otomycosis. ECZEMA and seborrhoeic DERMATITIS are common causes of otitis externa. Most forms of the disorder cause pain, sometimes severe, and there is usually a discharge from the ear. Unless the canal becomes blocked, hearing is not usually affected.

Otitis externa may be persistent (chronic) and difficult to treat, and the management varies with the cause. Thorough cleaning of the canal and specific antibiotic or antifungal treatment are often necessary, and solutions of such drugs may be applied locally soaked into gauze 'wicks' that are gently pushed into the ear canal.

Otitis media

This disorder, which is particularly common in children, is an inflammation in the middle ear cavity, between the ear-drum and the inner ear. Otitis media usually results from spread of infection from the nose or throat by way of the eustachian tube. Although this is the route of access, outward drainage through the eustachian tube is also important in maintaining the health of the middle ear, and blockage commonly leads to infection. Eustachian tube obstruction may be caused by ADE-NOIDS or by inflammation in the tube itself as a result of repeated infection.

Acute suppurative otitis media is a form in which the onset is sudden with a rapid production of pus in the middle ear so that the pressure rises and the ear-drum bulges outwards. There is severe pain and fever with general upset and a risk of perforation of the drum. Urgent pain relief with paracetamol is needed and treatment with ANTIBIOTICS should be given as soon as possible. In chronic suppurative otitis media, the infection has caused a hole (perforation) in the drum, through which the pus persistently drains. DEAFNESS and OTITIS EXTERNA are common complications.

Chronic otitis media requires thorough aural cleansing by a specialist and effective antibiotic treatment. Swabs are taken to determine the infecting organisms and an appropriate antibiotic prescribed. Cleansing is done by dry mopping and sometimes suction. Once the ear is dry the perforation will usually heal. If it does not, an operation may sometimes be done to close it with a tiny tissue graft.

See also GLUE EAR.

Otoplasty

A plastic surgery operation to correct prominent, bat-like ears, usually performed on children.

See BAT EARS.

P

Paediatrics

Paediatrics is the medical specialty concerned with the care of children. But it deals with more than simply children's diseases. It covers all aspects of child health and development in the context of the family and the whole environment. The specialty is very wide and calls for a knowledge of:

- genetics and the whole range of GENETIC DISORDERS
- normal and abnormal physical and mental development
- the special bodily functions (physiology) of the child
- child psychiatry
- behaviour and learning problems
- the nutritional requirements and problems of childhood
- immunization
- the infectious fevers and other disorders common to childhood
- the whole range of diseases that affect people of all ages, but have special features or dangers in childhood

With the growth of medical knowledge, paediatrics, like other medical and surgical disciplines, has become too large to be mastered by only one specialist and is rapidly becoming fragmented into sub-specialties.

Pain

Pain is a sensation, usually unpleasant, and often localised, caused by strong stimulation of sensory nerve endings by an event or process damaging to, or liable to damage, tissue. Pain causes distress and anxiety and sometimes fear, and the psychological and physiological changes associated with it may be similar to those experienced during anger and aggression. This is particularly so in children as it may be impossible to explain to them why they are suffering and why they should have to suffer. Fortunately, there have been great advances in pain control in children.

Experts on pain control emphasize that it should be treated by the simplest and safest available means, but that attempts should always be made to relieve it at the earliest stage, once the cause is clearly known. Prolonged pain is inhumane, demoralizing and debilitating, and should be controlled as early as possible. Neglected pain becomes more difficult to control. Pain-controlling drugs work best if they are used as soon as the pain reappears, and they should not be withheld until pain becomes unbearable.

Severe pain in children presents particular problems and its control requires special paediatric expertise. Recurrent abdominal pain and HEADACHE are very common in children, affecting 10–20 per cent at one time or another. Only a small proportion of these have organic disease, but complaints should never be ignored. Persistent complaint of pain without obvious cause often arises from psychological causes and these, unless checked early, tend to persist into adult life. Stressed children who continue to complain of pain after full investigation should never be told that they are imagining the symptom. The pain must be acknowledged but strong reassurance given that it does not mean anything serious.

There have also been great developments in recent years in the understanding of pain control in infants and children who require surgery. Formerly small children were often denied effective pain control. This was partly because there was no way of knowing how much they were suffering and partly through fear of causing harm by using powerful drugs. Some doctors rationalized that babies either did not feel severe pain or that it caused them no harm. It is now recognized that, quite apart from immediate humanitarian reasons, adequate pain control is essential because the lack of it can have serious long-term effects and can even be fatal.

Doctors now have a wide range of safe and effective ways of controlling pain even in newborn babies. It has been shown, by monitoring various physiological responses, that mild pain can be safely controlled in young infants and children by means of a range of well-known drugs. In the case of more severe pain, carefully measured infusions of morphine have been used safely and effectively. Nerve block or epidural anaesthesia have also been found to be highly effective and safe ways of controlling pain in small children after surgery. These methods have also permitted smaller doses of general anaesthetic agents and lighter planes of anaesthesia. Recovery from surgery is much improved by such methods, especially in children with respiratory problems such as cystic fibrosis.

Painful cough see TRACHEITIS.

Pale skin see SKIN PALLOR.

Passive smoking

The rate of lung cancer in non-smokers rises significantly if they are regularly exposed to other people's cigarette smoke, as, for instance, by children living with parents who smoke. There is no safe threshold for the effects of carcinogens, and non-smokers who breathe environmental cigarette smoke are exposed to known carcinogenic substances. Such non-smokers are found to have nicotine and other tobacco products in their urine.

Although nicotine is not a carcinogen, some of the other 3,000 or so chemical substances in cigarette smoke are, and these are being inhaled also. Ten separate studies have shown an increase of up to 30 per cent in the risk of lung cancer among non-smokers living with smokers, compared with non-smokers living with non-smokers.

Cancer is not the only hazard of passive smoking. Although tobacco tars can affect the lungs directly, many of the other ingredients are absorbed from the lungs into the general circulation and those of them that are damaging can have their effect anywhere in the body. Smoking is one of the principal risk factors for coronary heart disease and this is the major cause of death in the developed world. A considerable range of other conditions can also be caused by substances acquired by active or passive smoking.

Parents who smoke cigarettes compromise the future health of their children. And no amount of exhortation for their children not to smoke, by parents who are regular smokers, is likely to be either convincing or effective.

Patchy baldness see ALOPECIA.

Patent ductus arteriosus

The fetus in the womb is floating in fluid and cannot breathe. So the blood supply to the lungs, which is considerable after birth, has to be bypassed. This is done by a short connection between the main artery to the lungs and the main artery to the body. This connection, the ductus arteriosus, remains open during fetal life but normally closes automatically soon after birth. If it does not, the condition of patent ductus arteriosus exists. This condition causes a loud murmur and may sometimes lead to heart failure and lung disease. Fortunately, the operation to tie off or clip the connection is comparatively simple and safe and the results are excellent.

Patients' rights

The rights of the parents of young patients, especially those in hospital, include considerate and respectful care, an entitlement to information about what is being done to their children, or what is proposed, and the right to knowledge of the diagnosis and probable outlook (prognosis). Parents are especially entitled to all information necessary to enable them to give informed consent to any surgical operation or other form of treatment, especially if associated with risk.

Parents of young patients have a right to refuse treatment and to be informed of the probable consequences of such refusal. They should, however, have extremely cogent reasons for refusing treatment. They are entitled to privacy and confidentiality over their children's medical details, and their children may not be included in any form of medical trial or experiment without full knowledge and consent. Parents may discharge their children from hospital at any time, but may be required to sign a document to the effect that they understand the possible consequences.

There is also a good deal of government legislation protecting the general rights of children. This includes the Children and Young Persons Act of 1933, which covers a wide range of safeguards against physical and mental cruelty and unsuitable employment, and deals with court procedures for children; the Children Act of 1948, detailing provisions for the care and welfare of children without normal parental or guardian care; the Children and Young Persons Act of 1963, dealing with the extent to which, and the conditions under which, children can be employed in the theatre, TV and film industries; and the Children and Young Persons Act of 1969 governing fostering of children and the provision of care.

Penile abnormality see
HYPOSPADIAS.

Penis disorders

Disorders of the penis are uncommon in babies. There is one, however, which may cause concern. Normally, the opening of the urine passage, the urethra, is at the tip of the glans. In rare cases, the urethra may open on the underside of the penis, sometimes as far back as the root. Later, this can, of course, cause both urinary and reproductive problems. Fortunately, HYPOSPADIAS, as it is called, can be corrected by a plastic surgery procedure and the results are usually good.

Occasionally, the opening of the urethra at the tip of the penis is so narrow that the urine is hardly able to get out. This uncom-mon condition, of urethral stenosis, is very easily remedied by a simple operation. It should not be confused with tightness in the opening of the foreskin (see PHIMOSIS).

See also CIRCUMCISION.

Percentile

This is a useful general scientific concept much used by doctors concerned with child development. Any variable quantity, such as height, weight or IQ, can be expressed as a percentile if it is desired to compare it with the rest of a comparable population. A percentile, or centile, is one of 99 values that divides the range of the variable quantity into 100 groups with equal frequencies. Thus, in the context of children's weight, a child on the 75th centile would be heavier than 74 per cent of the children of that age and lighter than 25 per cent of the children of that age. The average is the 50th percentile.

The normal distribution pattern for several variables, such as height, weight and head circumference, has been determined for every month of age from birth to 2 years, and for every two months from 2 to 12 years. These data were obtained by carefully measuring hundreds of normal children in each of these 84 age groups.

A child developing normally will often remain on the same centile for variables such as height and weight. Movement to higher or lower centiles would be noteworthy. See also introductory section (Child Development).

Perforated ear-drum see OTITIS
MEDIA.

Pertussis

This is the medical term for WHOOPING COUGH.

Petit mal see ABSENCE ATTACKS.

Phenylketonuria

This is a rare genetic metabolic disease in which a normal constituent of dietary protein, phenylalanine, cannot be broken down normally but is converted to substances which are very toxic and cause LEARNING

DIFFICULTY. This happens because a body enzyme, which normally converts phenylalanine to a simpler and safe compound, is missing. About one baby in 16,000 has phenylketonuria and because some of the phenylalanine and its breakdown products are excreted in the urine, a simple urine test with a special paper test strip on a wet nappy will detect the abnormality. This test becomes positive at the age of 4 to 6 weeks, but a more sensitive test is available for babies at birth. This is called the Guthrie test and requires a drop of blood from an almost painless heel prick.

Newborn babies with phenylketonuria are often strikingly blond with blue eyes and have a 'mousy' smell. They appear normal at birth but mental deterioration occurs after a few weeks. Vomiting and convulsions follow. Any affected baby taking milk will receive enough phenylalanine to cause damage to the brain. It is thus essential to ensure that the baby has a special diet, very low in phenylalanine. Such a diet must be substituted for milk from the first few days of life until about the age of 10 when brain growth is complete.

Phimosis

This is a very narrow outlet in the foreskin (prepuce) so that the skin cannot be pulled back over the glans of the penis. Phimosis is commonly congenital, but may result from swelling (oedema), infection or scarring. Some degree of phimosis is normal in infancy, but an extreme degree leads to ballooning of the foreskin on urination. Inability to pass urine freely can lead to back-pressure all the way up to the kidneys, which may then become damaged.

Phimosis later in life is liable to cause trouble. If full retraction of the foreskin is eventually achieved, the tight prepuce may become fixed around the neck of the glans (paraphimosis) and this may have serious consequences.

Phimosis also interferes with the important hygienic necessity to wash away accumulated smegma and this becomes offensive and irritating. Phimosis persisting after the age of 4 or 5 years is an indication for CIRCUMCISION.

Phocomelia

This is the major congenital abnormality in which the limbs are replaced by short, flipper-like stumps. This is a very rare disorder, but was a common feature of children born to mothers who took the drug thalidomide in early pregnancy.

Pica

Pica is a persistent tendency to eat non-nutritional substances, such as earth, ice, match-heads, coal, chalk or wood. Pica is common in children under 18 months, and, in these, although undesirable, is not considered abnormal. Pica is a feature of nutritional deficiency and iron-deficiency anaemia and sometimes succeeds in providing a needed supply of minerals. It will often stop if anaemia is effectively treated. It occurs in mentally retarded people and in people with severe psychiatric disorders. Pica in pregnancy has been known throughout the ages and the bizarre catalogue of substances eaten include mothballs, soap, insects, clay, baking soda and excrement.

In most cases, pica does little harm, but there have been many medical reports of obstruction or perforation of the bowel, lead poisoning, parasite infestation and other misfortunes from this cause. No satisfactory explanation of many of the types of pica has been produced.

Pimple

A pimple is a small area of localised inflammation in the skin, often caused by accumulation of sebaceous material in the dermis, in a person with ACNE. The irritation causes a red papule and this may progress to an accumulation of sterile pus, when it is known as a 'yellow head' or pustule. A pimple may also result from infection of a hair follicle in the skin to produce a small boil or furuncle.

Plantar wart

This is a wart (verruca) on the sole of the foot. Like other common warts, the plantar wart is caused by a papillomavirus. The infection is commonly acquired in young people from contaminated wet floors, changing room showers or duck-boards in swimming pools.

Were it not for their situation, plantar warts would appear identical to other warts. But because of pressure from the weight of the body, plantar warts are flattened and forced into the thickened skin of the sole. They may occur as single warts or as a 'mosaic' of many tiny warts closely packed together.

Plantar warts are always a nuisance and may be disabling from extreme tenderness, so that a plastic foam or felt ring or pad may have to be used to avoid pressure and permit comfortable walking. Sometimes they are confused with corns, but the distinction becomes clear on attempts at paring, when the wart will bleed.

Treatment includes freezing with liquid nitrogen, the use of salicylic acid plasters or trichloroacetic acid applications, electrodesiccation or cutting out with a sharp-edged spoon (curettage) under local anaesthesia. In many cases, treatment is unnecessary as the wart may disappear spontaneously. If they are treated, it is important that the treatment should not cause permanently sensitive scars. Treated warts may recur.

Children should be made aware of the danger of contracting plantar warts in public swimming pools and should, if possible, avoid situations likely to lead to infection. Light flip-flops should be worn when walking around changing rooms and showers.

Plaque stain see DISCLOSING AGENTS.

Play for sick children

Children need to play. This is not a luxury for them, but a necessity. Play is one of the processes of development and one of the important ways of releasing tension and anxiety. So sick children need to play within the limits imposed by their illness. Forcing them to keep quiet and lie still is counterproductive and unwise. Play can be a major factor in recovery and in rehabilitation. Making a game of necessary activities, including the taking of medicines, the checking of temperature, making up the child's bed, and so on, can work wonders for the child's morale and can often ease otherwise difficult tasks.

Remember, however, that a sick child will often regress a little and may prefer play activities that have already been outgrown. He or she will also have a shorter interest span than normal and greater effort will be needed to provide sustained distraction. Even a manifestly sick child will nearly always want to have stories read or told. He or she will usually prefer TV or favourite tapes or records to being left alone with nothing to do. Peace and quiet may seem an obviously good thing to the parents, but they are not usually what a sick child wants. Most very sick children, unable to play themselves, much prefer to watch other children playing rather than to be left to their own thoughts and company.

Toys and other play material should be practical and usable, if possible. Writing and painting books, crayons, felt-tip pens and large sheets of paper, cutting-out materials, paste, play-dough and shape cutters, Lego and other construction toys, jigsaw puzzles and puzzle books are always very popular. All of these can be therapeutic. If the child is able to get about, a play house is a great asset.

Polio

Poliomyelitis is an infectious disease caused by viruses which inhabit the intestine and are passed in the stools in large numbers for up to six weeks after the start of the illness. At one time, poliomyelitis was by far the commonest cause of paralysis in young people and, for this reason, was known as 'infantile paralysis'.

Polio was also once a common cause of death, but the widespread use of oral vaccine has greatly reduced its incidence. Just as the dangerous viruses were once spread by direct faecal contamination of food by fingers, and by coughing, so the modified viruses in the oral vaccine are also spread. In this way, many more people acquire protection than those who have actually been given the oral vaccine.

Even in the unprotected, most cases of polio are mild, causing a brief, unidentified illness with HEADACHE, FEVER and sometimes VOMITING. But in some cases, this stage is followed by a more major illness, with severe headache, neck stiffness, high fever and progressive muscle weakness and paralysis. This reaches a maximum at the end of the first week of the severe symptoms and, thereafter, recovery is gradual.

Muscles which show no sign of movement by the end of a month are permanently paralyzed. If the upper part of the spinal cord or the brain stem are involved, death may occur from paralysis of respiration during the acute stage, unless some form of artificial respiration is used. The 'iron lung' was once the only way of saving the lives of those in this situation, but has now been replaced by better methods of maintaining the breathing.

Oral polio vaccine is completely successful in preventing such a catastrophe and should be given to everyone.

Port-wine stain

This blemish is an extensive, flat, reddish-purple birthmark (naevus) caused by a patch of widening of the smallest of the skin vessels, the capillaries. The medical term is a capillary haemangioma. The port-wine stain can often be treated by laser destruction of the dilated vessels or, if the skin is lax and the affected area not too extensive, by surgical removal. Sometimes a port-wine stain on the face or head is an outer sign of a more extensive and serious type of blood vessel tumour affecting the brain (the Sturge-Weber syndrome).

Powdery skin see CYSTIC FIBROSIS.

Precocious children see GIFTED CHILDREN.

Premature ageing see PROGERIA.

Prematurity

Several factors can cause, or are known to be associated with, prematurity in babies. These include:

- an unusually young mother – below 16 years of age
- a mother over 35
- too many pregnancies, too quickly
- maternal illness
- a previous premature birth
- cervical incompetence – cervix opens with abnormal ease
- excess of uterine fluid (polyhydramnios)
- premature rupture of the membranes
- maternal pre-eclampsia
- premature separation of the placenta
- maternal smoking
- excessive maternal alcohol intake
- maternal drug addiction
- maternal high blood pressure
- placental inadequacy
- twin or triple pregnancy
- abnormal attachment of the placenta
- infection in the uterus
- genetic defects

A premature baby is one born before 37 weeks of gestational life. Prematurity is not, however, primarily a matter of being born before the due date. Certainly, a baby born well before time will be premature, but it is essentially the baby's size that matters. Specialists are therefore inclined to define prematurity in terms of birth weight rather than in terms of the length of the pregnancy. Thus, a baby may be premature even if the pregnancy lasted for the full 40 weeks. Similarly, a baby born earlier than average may be of normal birth weight and development and would not be premature. A baby born at less than 37 weeks from the first day of the last menstrual period is called a 'preterm' baby. Unfortunately, about a third of preterm babies are also smaller than average for their gestational age.

Those whose birth weight is less than 2,500 g are usually referred to as 'low birthweight babies'. Those weighing less than 1,500 g are often called 'very low birthweight babies'. Babies born with a weight which is significantly low for the dates, are known as small-for-dates babies.

About 10 per cent of babies born are premature and about 1 per cent are born weighing less than 1,500 g. The average weight of a baby at birth is about 3.3 kg

(7 lb). There is, however, much natural variation and many babies are heavier than average because their mothers are heavy or diabetic.

Premature baby care units are nurseries staffed by medical and nursing personnel with special training and experience in the management of premature babies. Because of their ready tendency to hypothermia, premature babies are kept in temperature-controlled environments in incubators. These are designed to allow careful and continuous monitoring of all the important bodily functions.

The staff in premature baby care units are particularly careful about personal hygiene and wash their hands scrupulously before approaching their charges. Any member of staff who develops upper respiratory tract infections is automatically excluded from the unit. Masks are no longer considered essential, however.

Staff are also skilled in the feeding of premature infants and are very much aware of the dangerous tendency for such tiny babies to inhale liquid food. Many premature babies are fed exclusively by means of a fine, soft PVC tube that is passed through the nose and down into the stomach. Breast milk expressed from the mother's breasts may be used. Continuous feeding by this method may be used until the baby is mature enough to develop a suckling reflex. Vitamin supplements, folic acid and iron are usually given. Injections of vitamin K are given routinely to prevent a bleeding tendency.

Premature babies are more likely to have problems than full weight babies. In particular, they are apt to lose temperature very readily, are unusually prone to infection and have difficulty in swallowing and coughing. They are also especially prone to RESPIRATORY DISTRESS SYNDROME, RETROLENTAL FIBROPLASIA SUDDEN INFANT DEATH SYNDROME (cot death). See also BIRTHWEIGHT, IMMUNIZATION, IMMUNODEFICIENCY DISORDERS, INCUBATOR, NEONATOLOGIST.

Prickly heat

Repeated episodes of heavy sweating in conditions of high humidity and high temperature, as in the tropics, are liable to result in the itchy condition known popularly as 'prickly heat'. This condition, for which the medical term is miliaria rubra, is the result of sweat duct blockage. It may affect children in less extreme conditions, if they are unsuitably dressed. The blockage is thought to be due to excessive sogginess (over-hydration) of the skin. In the most severe forms, salt crystals may form in the sweat gland ducts, producing small blisters.

The condition features multiple small red bumps and a constant prickling or itching sensation from over-stimulation of the nerve endings. As acclimatization to the adverse conditions occurs, prickly heat usually resolves. Air conditioning, the choice of suitable clothing to encourage evaporation of sweat, and plenty of open-air swimming are all helpful.

Progeria

This is a very rare but extraordinary condition of accelerated ageing in which the usual processes of bodily decline and deterioration take place over the course of only a few years. Progeria occurs in two forms. In the Hutchinson-Gilford syndrome, the condition appears before the age of 4 and by 10 or 12 the affected child has all the physical characteristics of old age – lax, wrinkled skin, loss of hair, and all the other common degenerative changes, including widespread atherosclerosis. Death usually occurs about the age of 13, from coronary thrombosis or stroke.

Progeria occurring later, or Werner's syndrome, starts in late adolescence or early adult life and follows, over the course of about a decade, the same rapid progression to senility, with balding or greying hair, DEAFNESS, ARTHRITIS, CATARACT, loss of teeth, and ATHEROSCLEROSIS.

Little is known of the cause of progeria. Both the Hutchinson-Gilford syndrome and Werner's syndrome can be transmitted by recessive inheritance (see GENETICS – AN OUTLINE), but many occur as a fresh dominant mutation. Cultures of cells, such as the normally rapidly-reproducing skin fibroblasts, taken from children with progeria, undergo only a few cell divisions and then cease. Cell cultures from normal children produce 50 or more generations before reproduction stops.

Pseudohermaphroditism

In true HERMAPHRODITISM, which is excessively rare, the affected child has both male and female external genitalia, but in the somewhat commoner condition of pseudohermaphroditism, only those of one sex are present. There is, however, a congenital abnormality of the genitalia so that they resemble those of the opposite sex. Thus, a girl may appear to be a hermaphrodite because of an enlarged clitoris, which looks like a penis, and enlarged labia which resemble a scrotum. A boy with a very small penis and a divided scrotum, simulating labia majora, may also appear, wrongly, to be a hermaphrodite.

This condition is much commoner than true hermaphroditism. It is caused by excess male sex hormones in the female and deficiency of sex hormone in the male. These disorders are usually due to disease, but female virilization may occur from hormone therapy. Pseudohermaphroditism can usually be effectively treated.

Ptosis

The term 'ptosis' is an abbreviation for 'blepharoptosis' and means drooping of an upper eyelid. In children, ptosis is nearly always present at birth (congenital) and is due to a weakness of the thin, flat muscle that elevates the lid, as a result of a defect of the nerve that stimulates it. This is sometimes associated with a weakness of the muscle that turns the eye upwards – which is energized by the same nerve. The diagnosis of ptosis is obvious from the observation of the narrowing of the space between the edges of the upper and lower lids. When the child looks upwards, the upper lid on the affected side fails to rise as it should, and the child may corrugate the forehead in an attempt to raise the lid. The severity may vary greatly from cases to case – from a slight and barely discernible droop to total coverage of the front of the eye. The degree of droop

may also vary considerably in any one case.

Ptosis in childhood is not just a cosmetic problem: a lid that droops enough to cover more than half of the pupil of the eye is going to interfere seriously with the development of normal vision and, unless corrected urgently, is likely to lead to a lifelong defect of vision in the affected eye (see AMBLYOPIA). For this reason, ptosis should always be considered an urgent problem and an ophthalmologist (eye specialist) consulted. Surgical correction involves the shortening of the elevating muscle and is generally successful, unless the muscle is completely paralyzed. In that event, various lid sling procedures are possible so that the lid can be elevated by raising the eyebrows.

Puberty and adolescence

Puberty is the period of physical development during which certain physical changes occur in the body, leading to the child becoming sexually mature and capable of sexual activity and reproduction. Adolescence, on the other hand, is a social concept – the sometimes prolonged period of transition from childhood to adulthood. Puberty occurs during adolescence, but adolescence involves mental and

On average, at around the age of 10 in girls and 12 in boys, there is a striking growth spurt. The rate of growth increases to some 9 cm (3.5 in) per year in girls and over 10 cm (4 in) per year in boys. This prepubertal growth spurt affects different parts of the body at different times so that, for a while, the body may appear disproportioned. Growth acceleration affects first the feet, then the legs, followed by the trunk, and finally the face, especially the lower jaw. Because puberty occurs about two years later in boys than in girls, boys have a longer period of pre-adolescent growth spurt and tend to gain a significant advantage in height over girls.

emotional changes in addition to the those concerned with the reproductive function. Prior to puberty, children grow in body and mind but the changes that occur are only quantitative. At puberty, qualitative changes begin that fully differentiate relatively asexual girls and boys into women and men.

See introductory section (Teenage).

Punishment see MISBEHAVIOUR, SMACKING.

Puppy worm disease see TOXOCARIASIS.

Pyloric stenosis see CONGENITAL PYLORIC STENOSIS

Quinsy

This is an abscess between the capsule of the tonsil and the adjacent wall of the throat. Quinsy usually follows a severe attack of TONSILLITIS. The abscess is almost always on one side only, and the swelling appears above the tonsil, near the soft palate, so that the small floppy process of the soft palate (the uvula) is pushed across to the unaffected side. The throat is extremely painful and there is high fever, headache, and other signs of general upset. Speech is impaired and there is much salivation and dribbling. The neck lymph nodes are enlarged and tender.

ANTIBIOTICS, given at an early stage before the abscess has fully developed, may bring the infection under control, but once the quinsy is established they are of little value and surgical drainage is necessary. This is followed by rapid relief. When the condition has fully settled it is advisable to have the tonsils removed, to avoid recurrence.

Quintuplets

Quins are a group of five babies born in a single gestation. Prior to the introduction of 'fertility' drugs, to promote ovulation, triplets occurred once in 10,000 pregnancies and quadruplets once in 500,000. The incidence of quintuplets was too small to be assessed. Because the size of the baby is, in general, inversely proportional to the number in the gestation, the chances of survival drop sharply with increasing numbers. The survival of the Dionne quins, born in Canada in 1934, was a unique phenomenon, never before reported.

The Dionne quins arose from a single fertilized egg (ovum) which divided and separated three times, giving rise to six genetically identical individuals. The sixth fetus aborted spontaneously during the third month of the pregnancy. The five babies were, necessarily, all of the same sex and physical constitution, and this added greatly to their commercial value – a value successfully exploited for years.

Fertility drugs cause multiple pregnancies, not in this way, but by stimulating the ovaries to produce multiple ova, which may be fertilized separately. In this case, the siblings are genetically dissimilar. The risk of high multiple pregnancies is slight with the commonly used drug clomiphene, but is much greater when gonadotrophins are used to stimulate the ovaries. Quintuplet, sextuplet, septuplet and octuplet pregnancies are not uncommon when the latter drugs are used, but these fetuses are often too small at birth to survive. So far as *in vitro* fertilization is concerned, the Human Embryology Act (1990) imposes strict limitations on the number of embryos that can be implanted at one time.

R

Ramstedt's Operation see
CONGENITAL PYLORIC STENOSIS.

Rashes see CHICKENPOX,
CHILBLAINS, DERMATITIS,
GLANDULAR FEVER, HERPES
SIMPLEX, IMPETIGO, INSECT
BITES, LYME DISEASE, MEASLES,
MENINGITIS, NAPPY RASH,
RUBELLA, SCABIES, SCARLET
FEVER.

Reading difficulties see
DYSLEXIA, HYPERLEXIA.

Red birthmarks see STORKBITE.

Red blood cell fragility see
HEREDITARY SPHEROCYTOSIS.

Red eye

Surprisingly, when eyes look red, the redness is not in the eyeballs but in the thin,
transparent membrane which covers the
outside of the globe. This membrane is
called the conjunctiva and is normally
transparent, so that the white of the eye
shows through. But it contains a network of
tiny blood vessels which, in perfect health,
are too fine to be seen and it is when these
blood vessels enlarge, either temporarily or
permanently, that the conjunctiva becomes
red.

The conjunctiva is firmly attached to the
globe round the edge of the cornea and to
the insides of the eyelids, but elsewhere it
lies quite loosely on the eyeball so that the
eye is able to move freely. If you pull down
your lower lid, you will see that the conjunctiva forms a connection between the
globe of the eye and the lid. The same
thing happens at the upper lid, but here
the conjunctiva runs well back on the globe
before folding forwards to line the upper
lid. So the upper lid cul-de-sac is quite deep
and people sometimes 'lose' contact lenses
up there, but it is impossible for anything to
go right behind the globe.

Inflammation of the conjunctiva is called
conjunctivitis and this is one of the commonest known kinds of inflammation. The
conjunctiva is a very efficient, protective
seal between the deeper parts of the ocular
system and the outside world. But in ser-
ving this purpose it is exposed not only to
the great variety of germs that inhabit our
environment, but also to substances which
can cause allergy, irritating dusts, fluids
and aerosols, a variety of toxic or irritating
gases and a wide range of forms of radiation. Fortunately, the conjunctiva is capable
of repairing a good deal of the damage
done to it, but if the assault upon it goes
on too long, permanent changes – most
obviously shown as redness – can result.

Infective conjunctivitis is very common
in children. It is sometimes called 'pink eye'
and is usually nothing much to worry
about. It can be caused by any one of a
very wide range of germs which usually get
to the conjunctiva when children rub their
eyes with their fingers. Conjunctivitis starts
with a feeling of irritation in the eye, associated with redness, usually in one corner.
Often the lashes are gummed with dried
discharge and, especially on waking in the
morning, they may be so stuck together that
the lids can't be separated until the discharge is washed off. A small quantity of
pus may collect in the corner of the eye and
there may be small blobs of yellow mucus
in the tear film, especially down behind the
lower lid. Soon the whole of the conjunctiva
may be intensely inflamed and very red
and, if untreated, the condition may spread
to the other eye. Even if nothing is done,

most cases of simple conjunctivitis will clear up within a week or two, but recovery will be more rapid if ANTIBIOTIC eye drops or ointment are used as early as possible.

Note that, although mucus or other discharge may get on to the cornea and momentarily obscure vision, conjunctivitis itself never affects the vision. It is important for you to check that this is so with the child, by careful questioning. If the child with a red eye doesn't have clear vision when pus is removed by blinking or wiping with moist cotton wool, the matter is serious and specialist advice is needed. Similarly, although conjunctivitis may cause great discomfort, it never causes real pain in the eye. If an inflamed eye is painful – either a severe, dull ache or a sharp pain, as from a grain of sand pressing on the eye – the trouble is likely to be more serious than conjunctivitis and, again, the child needs the attention of a doctor.

Not all forms of conjunctivitis will clear up in a week or so. Some fairly common virus infections can produce severe redness with swelling of the conjunctiva, and even of the lids, which may persist for several weeks and cause the victim much concern. But, however severe or persistent, if the condition is one or other of the forms of conjunctivitis, it will eventually improve.

In babies, conjunctivitis may be associated with failure of the tear drainage duct to open up. In this case there will be overflow of tears and a tendency to pus and mucus production. A special case of infective conjunctivitis in newborn babies is infection caused by a disease such as gonorrhoea and acquired during birth from an infected mother. The gonorrhoea germ (*Gonococcus*) can cause havoc in the eye – even blindness, by perforation of the cornea – so it is important that any newborn baby with sticky or inflamed eyes should be urgently treated. The doctor will take a swab for identification of the organism and start effective antibiotic treatment at once.

Remember that any deterioration in vision, coming on rapidly in the presence of an inflamed eye, whether or not there is pain, is a matter of urgency and you should not delay in seeking advice. An eye specialist, by examining the child's eyes with a special instrument called a slit-lamp microscope, will have little difficulty in discovering what is wrong and he or she will at once arrange appropriate treatment. Your GP seldom has the necessary equipment to do this and if you make it plain that the child insists that vision has been affected, the doctor will appreciate the urgency and ensure that you are seen promptly by a specialist.

OTHER CAUSES OF RED EYE

Uveitis is an inflammation of the iris of the eye and of the focusing muscle that surrounds the root of the iris. Happily, it is rare in childhood except as a complication of juvenile rheumatoid ARTHRITIS (Still's disease). Uveitis causes redness of the eye, especially in the area around the edge of the cornea, a dull, aching pain, and blurring of vision. When an eye with uveitis is examined with a slit-lamp microscope, the fluid in the front chamber of the eye is slightly milky and clumps of cells have been deposited on the inside surface of the cornea. Often the inflamed iris will stick firmly to the front surface of the crystalline lens behind it and this can cause dangerous complications, by interfering with the drainage of fluid from the eye. The condition is treated by keeping the pupil widely dilated to avoid adhesions and by the use of steroid drops to control the inflammation.

Corneal ulceration usually causes fairly severe redness but there is also a powerful awareness of a foreign body sensation, so that the child is usually convinced that there is something in the eye. If the ulcer is near the centre of the cornea, vision will be severely affected and the situation is grave, but if the ulcer is near the margin, and can be healed before it spreads inward, all will be well.

An actual *corneal foreign body*, if very tiny, is unlikely to cause much redness, but a larger one, or one of an irritating nature will do so. Such a foreign body should, however, be easily seen, so the cause of the trouble will be obvious, and it can be removed.

Sub-conjunctival haemorrhage sometimes looks alarming but, in fact, of all the many causes of red eye, it is the least deserving of worry. As the name implies, sub-conjunctival haemorrhage is bleeding *under* the conjunctiva. The blood vessels of the conjunctiva are less well supported than other vessels of the same size elsewhere in the body. It is common for vessels of this size to bleed spontaneously, but when they do so in other parts of the body, we are quite unaware of what has happened, because they are concealed. When conjunctival vessels bleed, however, the released blood spreads out behind the transparent conjunctiva to give a very conspicuous redness, sometimes in a localized patch, but other times extensively. You can distinguish this from a conjunctivitis by looking closely at the affected area and observing that it is not caused by widened vessels but by a uniform patch of evenly distributed redness.

Sub-conjunctival haemorrhage, which is much commoner in adults than in children, is of no medical significance. Some people worry that it might indicate high blood pressure, or a disturbance of the blood or disease of the blood vessels. In 99 cases out of 100 it means nothing of the sort. Often it follows a sneeze or a bout of heavy coughing and occasionally it occurs while straining at some physical task. But in the majority of cases it happens for no obvious reason. Repeated haemorrhages from the same point in the conjunctiva may indicate a minor local abnormality or weakness in one of the conjunctival vessels – such as a small varicosity (local enlargement and swelling of the vessel with weakness of the wall) but this, too, is of no consequence and easily dealt with, if necessary.

The blood under the conjunctiva begins to be absorbed almost as soon as it has been released and, usually, the evidence of haemorrhage has disappeared within about 10 days. A very extensive haemorrhage may take longer to go away, but sooner or later, all of them will disappear, and you need give the matter no further thought.

Eye redness can also be caused by various forms of radiation, the most commonly encountered being the ultraviolet part of sunlight. This can be markedly damaging both to the skin and conjunctiva and can cause permanent changes in the tissues. In the case of the conjunctiva, these include chronic enlargement of the vessels and a thickening of the membrane, so that a fatty swelling bulges forward on either side of the cornea. The person concerned suffers a persistent irritative discomfort with a feeling as if there is 'sand in the eyes'. This takes many years to develop and so is not a problem likely to be encountered in children. But the point is that the damage starts in childhood and you should know about it.

Formerly, this was not considered to be a problem in temperate climates and it would still be an exaggeration to suggest that there is major danger from the ultraviolet component of sunlight in Britain. But there is clear evidence of a rise of conditions such as skin cancer, even in temperate areas, and this may possibly be related to damage to the ozone layer of the stratosphere. So unnecessary exposure to sunlight is not to be recommended, even in Britain. The eyes should be protected from unnecessary, prolonged exposure to the direct rays of the sun, especially in the middle of the day, when the ultraviolet radiation is most intense.

If you take your children skiing, be particularly careful. Snow reflects ultraviolet and the intensity is higher at higher altitudes. Snow blindness is a pure ultraviolet effect on the surfaces of the corneas. But much long-term damage can be done short of that. Suitable goggles should always be worn.

See also BLEPHARITIS.

Reflexes, primitive

Primitive reflexes are automatic movements made by newborn infants, in response to various stimuli applied to the body as a whole. These reflexes disappear during the first months of life, but provide useful guidance to the state of health of the developing nervous system.

They include:

- automatic closure of the hand around an object such as a finger (grasp reflex)
- sudden bending up of the legs and embracing movement of the arms in

response to a noise or to momentary lack of support to the head (Moro or startle reflex)
- the walking or stepping reflex, when the baby is held upright with its feet on the ground
- turning of the head and sucking actions when the cheek is stroked (rooting reflex)

The periods during which these responses are present are well known to paediatricians and the absence or undue prolongation of these primitive reflexes provides valuable clinical information about development. (See Child Development in introductory section)

Refractive errors

Children never complain of visual difficulty and vision must be properly tested if refractive errors are to be discovered. Defects in one eye only are especially difficult to detect because these are concealed from the child. It is, for instance, futile, during testing, to ask the child to use its hand to cover one eye at a time. When the good eye is 'covered' the child will instinctively, and unconsciously, peep through the fingers. Covering during testing must be done properly by an adult, using an opaque card, and the child's head must be held firmly to prevent turning that allows peeping. Children unable to read letters may be tested by the use of various kinds of cards. A common method involves the use of a card showing the letter E in various orientations and sizes. The child simply indicates which way the arms of the letter are pointing.

Children who fail an eyesight screening test should be seen by an ophthalmologist for a full ophthalmic examination and a formal refraction so that errors such as hyperopia, myopia, astigmatism and anisometropia (inequality in the optics of the two eyes) may be detected and glasses prescribed, if necessary. Many cases of one-sided visual defect are due to AMBLYOPIA. In a small minority of cases, visual defect is due to disease of the eyes or nervous system rather than to a refractive error.

MYOPIA

In myopia or short-sightedness, the focusing power of the eye is too strong so that the images of distant objects come to a focus in front of the retina. Rays from near objects, however, are diverging more when they enter the eye, and these focus further back, often on the retina. So a myopic child cannot see distant objects clearly, but sees near objects well. The condition is the result of a failure of the proper relationship between the curvature of the cornea, the length of the eye, and the power and position of the internal crystalline lens. To compensate for myopia, weakening (minus or concave) lenses are needed.

Myopia usually appears around puberty. It is rare for it to appear after body growth is complete. The earlier it starts, the higher the final degree is likely to be. Those whose myopia appears late in adolescence never develop high myopia. Because the condition is of dimensional origin, it is not surprising to find that it runs in families. Myopia is, in most cases, no more than a nuisance, calling for contact lenses or spectacles. But in the higher degrees there is a raised probability of eye trouble such as retinal detachment, retinal degeneration and bleeding (haemorrhages).

HYPERMETROPIA

In hypermetropia or long-sightedness, the corneal curve is too flat and/or the eye is too short. So parallel rays from a distant object have not converged enough by the time they hit the retina, and the image is blurred. In this case, however, use may be made of the power of accommodation to increase the convergence of the rays and allow distant objects to be clearly seen. Young people do this automatically, and without conscious effort, and are usually unaware that they are hypermetropic. Later in life, however, as the power of accommodation falls off, the hypermetropia becomes manifest and the vision is blurred both for near and distant objects.

In hypermetropia, the power of the cornea is inadequate so strengthening (convex or plus) lenses are needed in the glasses.

ASTIGMATISM

In astigmatism, the corneal curvature is not that of the surface of a sphere, but has a maximum curvature in one meridian (for example, that running from 12 o'clock to 6 o'clock) and a minimum curvature in the meridian at right angles (that from 3 o'clock to 9 o'clock). An astigmatic cornea thus has a range of focal lengths varying from a minimum, in the meridian of the steepest curve, to a maximum, in the meridian of the flattest. So if rays focused in one meridian produce a sharp image, those in the other will not. The effect is that the clarity of an object, as seen by an astigmatic eye, varies with its orientation. Horizontals may be clear while verticals are not, or *vice versa*. In many cases, the two principal meridia are not vertical and horizontal. They are always at right angles to each other, but may be set at any angle.

The degree of blurring of vision caused by astigmatism varies with the degree and type, but clarity can always be restored, either by suitable cylindrical spectacle lenses, set at the correct axis in the frames, or by contact lenses.

Refusal to defaecate see
CONSTIPATION.

Reimplantation, dental

This refers to the immediate replacement of a dislodged permanent tooth in its socket in the hope that it may be retained. No attempt should be made to reimplant primary teeth as this may damage the unerupted secondary tooth. The tooth must have a root to survive; a broken tooth cannot be reimplanted. The tooth should be thoroughly washed, and pushed back into the cavity, facing in the right direction, and held in place until a dentist can apply splinting. Success depends on various factors, but the sooner the tooth is replaced the better. Dental splinting, for several weeks, may be necessary. Parents squeamish about trying this should store the tooth in milk while the child is taken to a dentist.

Respiratory distress syndrome

This is a condition, affecting premature babies, of increased fluid in the lungs, so that the normal passage of oxygen into the blood is impeded and the lungs become stiffer. The fluid in the lungs comes from the blood and may clot, causing collapse of the air sacs and further reducing the passage of oxygen to the blood. Respiratory distress syndrome may occur in babies born before term whose lungs are immature and do not inflate fully after birth. This is the result of the deficiency of a substance known as a 'surfactant' which acts as a kind of detergent, or wetting agent, to lower the surface tension of the fluid in the lungs.

Reduced oxygen in the blood prompts faster breathing, but the increased stiffness of the lungs makes this much more difficult. The result is increasing distress. Fatigue of the breathing muscles leads to a worsening of the situation. Breathing becomes heavy and laboured. As the condition progresses, the skin becomes blue-tinged (CYANOSIS).

In the early stages, administration of oxygen by mask can raise the blood oxygen levels and his may be all that is required. If the condition worsens, a tube must be passed into the windpipe (trachea) and mechanical ventilation used to force oxygen into the lungs and inflate the air sacs, so that the volume of the lungs actually increases. The outcome depends on the severity of the condition and the effectiveness of treatment. It has recently been found that the outcome in babies treated with oxygen only can be substantially improved by giving them a single dose of surfactant extracted from minced pigs' lungs. The need for subsequent mechanical ventilation is greatly reduced in babies given surfactant.

In newborn babies, complications are common and respiratory distress syndrome still causes death in some premature babies.

Respiratory tract infections

Doctors refer to these so often that they call them 'URTIS' – upper respiratory tract infections. URTIs are usually caused by viruses and are seldom dangerous. They include common COLDS, TONSILLITIS, sore throat (pharyngitis), sinusitis, laryngitis and CROUP. They are all very common in children.

Most URTIs lead to nasal congestion and this causes distress, mouth breathing and, in babies, difficulty in both breast- and bottle-feeding. Nasal catarrh, with mucus accumulation, will cause similar problems. Cough, which is a constant feature of URTIs, should not automatically be treated, as the cough is part of the defensive mechanism of the respiratory system. But tiring and distressing coughing may helpfully be relieved in children over 1 year, who are not otherwise unwell, by a mild antihistamine and soothing (demulcent) mixture.

The widespread practice of treating URTIs with ANTIBIOTICS is generally deplored by experts justifiably alarmed that this will lead to a rapid increase in antibiotic resistance. On the other hand, streptococcal infections of the throat in children can lead to serious conditions such as RHEUMATIC FEVER and GLOMERULONEPHRITIS, and, in such cases, antibiotics are important.

Lower respiratory tract infections are, in general, more serious. They affect the breathing tubes (trachea and bronchi) and the lungs, and include acute bronchitis, acute bronchiolitis and various kinds of pneumonia.

Retinoblastoma

This is a tumour arising from the primitive cells which form the retina, some of which fail to develop normally and become malignant. It appears in the early years of life, usually before 3 years, affecting about one baby in 20,000, and often first shows itself as a visible whiteness in the pupil – the 'cat's eye' reflex. An eye affected in this way is usually blind and often develops a SQUINT. In about one-third of cases, both eyes contain the tumour.

Retinoblastoma may appear in more than one child in the same family and siblings should always be examined. It is a highly malignant tumour which can spread from the eye to the bony eye socket and along the optic nerve to the brain. It may also spread to remote parts of the body. Because of its high malignancy, early removal of the affected eye is often advised. If the tumour is present in both eyes, radiotherapy is usually applied to the less severely affected eye.

The possibility, however unlikely, of retinoblastoma makes it imperative that every baby with squint should be examined by an ophthalmologist.

Retrolental fibroplasia

This is a serious eye disorder that may affect premature babies who have been treated with high oxygen concentrations after birth. It appears within a few weeks of birth. When such babies are incubated or treated for RESPIRATORY DISTRESS SYNDROME, it is often necessary, as a life-saving measure, to provide them with oxygen at a concentration higher than atmospheric. The immature retinal tissues respond to this by closing off their blood vessels. When normal oxygen concentrations are resumed, these tissues now have an inadequate blood supply and bud out fronds of new vessels and strands of fibrous tissue. Fully mature tissues do not respond in this way to high oxygen concentrations.

The fibrous tissue may extend into the vitreous gel behind the lens, seriously interfering with vision and leading, later, to retinal detachment and other serious consequences. High myopia in one or both eyes is another common complication. Because of the range of complications, the condition is often called retinopathy of prematurity.

Recent advances in methods of directly monitoring oxygen levels in the blood of small babies have made it easier to maintain adequate oxygenation with a lowered risk of eye complications. Research, mainly done in Japan, has suggested that early freezing treatment can prevent retinal detachment in this condition.

Reye's syndrome

This is a rare disease of childhood in which swelling of the brain and severe liver inflammation (hepatitis) occur following infection with one of several viruses including CHICKENPOX, INFLUENZA, RUBELLA, HERPES SIMPLEX, and echovirus. Brain swelling causes uncontrollable vomiting, delirium, disorientation, fits, and rapid onset of stupor and coma. The liver disorder is also severe and there is reason to believe that the effect on the brain may be secondary to the liver damage.

Treatment is aimed at controlling brain swelling by steroids and drugs to withdraw fluid. Artificial ventilation may be needed. With increasing understanding of the condition and its management, the death rate from Reye's syndrome has dropped from about 50 per cent to about 10 per cent. Some children, unfortunately, suffer permanent brain damage.

Research has shown that Reye's syndrome is connected with aspirin-taking and the medical authorities in Britain and the United States initially advised that children suspected of having chickenpox or influenza should not be given aspirin. Some have gone further and have recommended that aspirin should *never* be given to children. The British pharmaceutical industry quickly accepted this advice, and paracetamol has replaced aspirin in paediatric painkillers. There is now an absolute veto on the use of aspirin in children suffering from fevers. Paracetamol has largely replaced aspirin as a painkiller in children.

Rhesus incompatibility

After the A, B, AB and O blood groups, the rhesus factor is the most important. The gene that makes a person rhesus positive is called D. This is present in 85 per cent of the population. Rhesus positive fathers may carry two D genes (homozygous) or only one (heterozygous) (See GENETICS – AN OUTLINE). All the offspring of homozygous fathers are rhesus positive. With a heterozygous father, each pregnancy will have a 50–50 chance of producing a rhesus positive baby.

When a rhesus positive father produces a rhesus positive baby in a rhesus negative mother, the baby's red blood cells will cause the mother to produce antibodies against them. The baby's red cells do not normally reach the mother's blood until labour so they are unlikely to cause serious harm in the first pregnancy. But in subsequent pregnancies, the levels of these antibodies in the mother's blood rise rapidly and soon reach a point at which they are able to destroy the red cells of the fetus.

In the most severe cases, the fetus dies in the womb, usually after the 28th week. If born alive, the child has deep JAUNDICE with an enlarged liver and spleen and bile-staining of the brain (KERNICTERUS). This can lead to paralysis, spasticity, LEARNING DIFFICULTY and defects of sight and hearing.

A badly affected baby can have an exchange transfusion, via the umbilical cord, as soon as it is born, or even while still in the womb. This corrects the anaemia and gets rid of the bilirubin. Exposure to intense blue light soon after birth assists in converting the bilirubin in the skin to a form which is harmless to the brain.

Rhesus negative women can be prevented from developing antibodies by being given an injection of anti-D gamma globulin within 60 hours of the birth of a rhesus positive baby. In order to protect future babies, this is done in all such cases. Gamma globulin is also given when there has been an abortion or if there is any other reason to believe that rhesus positive fetal blood may have gained access to the woman's circulation. The injection is also given if an amniocentesis shows blood-stained amniotic fluid.

Rheumatic fever

Happily, this distressing condition, which is usually related to poor living conditions, is now quite rare in Western societies. In spite of the name, rheumatic fever does not seriously affect the joints, and, although a passing ARTHRITIS does occur, this does not produce any permanent disability. Rheumatic fever is important because of the frequency with which it damages the heart; the commonest and most serious effect being scarring of the valves, with narrowing or leakage (incompetence). This may seriously interfere with the heart's action and severely affect health. Heart valve replacement may, eventually, be necessary. Medical students are traditionally told that rheumatic fever 'licks the joints, but bites the heart'.

The nervous system may also be involved, causing 'Saint Vitus' dance' (Sydenham's chorea) which features uncontrollable, jerky movements of the limbs and body and usually emotional upset. Rheumatic fever always follows a throat infection with a particular strain of *Streptococcus*. It can always be prevented by prompt treatment of the throat infection with ANTIBIOTICS. It seems that the antibodies produced by the immune system in response to the streptococci regard the joint linings and, particularly, the inner surface of the heart, as being so close to the streptococcal antigen that they should be attacked. This may be no more than an accident of similar chemical structure.

The early acute stage of rheumatic fever is treated with bed rest, aspirin, sodium salicylate and corticosteroids, after antibiotics have been used to destroy any streptococci present. Aspirin is, of course, not generally recommended for children under 12. But there is no absolute veto and as it is one of the most useful drugs in rheumatic fever and the latter is nearly always treated in hospital, its prohibition would be indefensible. Children who have had rheumatic fever should be protected from further damage by long-term preventive (prophylactic) penicillin, taken until they are about 20 years of age. Sydenham's chorea is helped by tranquillizer drugs and sedatives.

Rickets

This disorder, now very rare in the developed world, affects body calcium and phosphorus, mainly involves the bones, and is caused by vitamin D deficiency. This vitamin is necessary for the absorption of calcium from the intestine. Vitamin D is found in dairy products and fish oils. Vitamin precursors in the diet are also converted to vitamin D by the action of sunlight on the skin, and poorly nourished children, who for any reason are deprived of sunlight, are more likely to be affected.

Rickets involves diminished deposition of calcium in the bones and a consequent weakening and softening. The result may be:

- bowing of the legs
- pigeon breast deformity
- curvature of the spine
- increased tendency to bone softening and fracture

- squaring off and flattening of the skull
- delay in TEETHING
- softening of tooth enamel after eruption

Rickets is treated by adequate, but not excessive, doses of vitamin D and plenty of calcium-containing food, such as milk.

Ringworm

This is not a worm, but a fungus infection of the skin, properly called tinea. It is an infection of the skin by fungi, especially *Microsporum, Trichophyton* and *Epidermophyton* species, collectively known as dermatophytes. These fungi attack the dead outer layer of the skin, or the skin appendages – the hair and the nails – causing persistent and often progressively extending areas of scaling and inflammation.

The fungus starts as an enlarging reddish, slightly raised spot. Soon the skin first affected acquires resistance so the centre of the spot, heals, and returns to normal. The result is a gradually enlarging ring of fungus infection. This is how the condition acquired its popular name.

Tinea occurs most often in the moist areas of the body – the groins, armpits and feet, but can also affect the scalp and the nails. It is commoner in the tropics than in temperate climates. Antifungal treatment, either by ointments or tablets is effective, but may have to be continued for long periods.

Roseola infantum

This is a common but transient disorder of unknown cause, which affects toddlers. No virus has been isolated, but the disease has been transmitted by filtered blood. It is sometimes called 'sixth disease' (as it is an addition to the five common fevers of childhood). The condition features:

- high fever for three days
- sometimes a convulsion
- lymph node enlargement
- general upset

After two or three days, as the fever settles, a pink rash resembling that of RUBELLA appears. This is present only for a short time – often less than a day – and may easily be missed.

Roseola is almost always harmless and complete recovery is the rule.

Roundworms

These are common human intestinal parasites in underdeveloped countries. They are quite rare in Western societies. Even so, it is estimated that 98 per cent of the world's population either have a roundworm infestation or have had one at some time. As most have multiple worms, it follows that the roundworm population greatly exceeds the human population. The common roundworm has a lifespan of about a year and inhabits the small intestine. The females pass microscopic sized eggs in the faeces and, under suitable conditions, as in moist soil, these can survive for three years or more. Crops or hands are commonly contaminated by eggs and these are passed to other people. One unlikely-seeming vector is paper money; the fingers are commonly licked when money is being counted. Ingested eggs hatch in the small intestine, migrate to the lungs and return to the intestine by way of the air tubes and the gullet.

The commonest symptoms are abdominal discomfort and pain, NAUSEA, VOMITING, irritability, loss of appetite and disturbed sleep. These symptoms occur only if more than a few worms are present. In heavy infestations, of 500 to 1,500 worms, pneumonia or obstruction of the bowel may result.

Roundworms are easily got rid of by means of a drug such as piperazine.

Rubella (German measles)

This infectious disease is caused by a virus which infects the respiratory tract and spreads to local lymph nodes, especially those in the back of the neck. It causes a mild illness, swollen nodes and a scattered rash of slightly raised red patches. The disease is so mild that it often passes unnoticed. The natural infection produces lifelong immunity.

The importance of rubella is that, in pregnant women, viruses circulating in the blood can infect the fetus. Until this fact was known, rubella was a major cause of congenital heart disease and other malformations, blindness, DEAFNESS and LEARNING DIFFICULTY. The fetus is especially susceptible to the toxic effects of the virus during the first three months of pregnancy when the brain, the eyes, the ears and the heart are in early development.

Immunisation against rubella could eliminate this disease. All susceptible (seronegative) young girls and women of childbearing age should be vaccinated. But vaccination should never be done during pregnancy as the vaccine may affect the fetus. If there is a risk of pregnancy, effective contraception should be used for three months after vaccination.

S

Scabies

This is an infestation of the skin with the human scabies mite parasite *Sarcoptes scabiei*. The mite burrows in the skin, often on the hands or wrists, to lay eggs and feed on dead skin scales. Spread is by direct close contact and scabies, once acquired, usually spreads to other members of the family.

The infestation causes intense itching and constant scratching, with resultant damage to the skin and dispersion of the mite bodies. This promotes a severe local reaction (DERMATITIS). Treatment, with insecticide lotions, is highly effective, but all close contacts and all members of the family must be done at the same time.

Scalp blood clot in babies see
CEPHALHAEMATOMA.

Scalp swelling in babies see
CAPUT.

Scaly skin

Ichthyosis is a scaly, fish-like disorder of the skin, sometimes called 'fish skin disease'. *Ichthyos* is Greek for a 'fish'. The condition is usually genetically determined and present from birth. The skin is unable to form the normal waterproof horny outer layer, so that it cannot retain water and tends to dry out.

The treatment consists in soaking the skin, cleaning with aqueous cream or emulsifying ointment instead of soap, removing excessive scales by scrubbing or fine sandpapering, and the use of a protective and waterproof cream. Ichthyosis is always worse in cold weather when the low atmospheric humidity encourages water loss. Sufferers fare better in warm, moist climates. The condition often improves with age.

Scarlet fever

This is caused by a species of *streptococcus* that infects the throat and is passed on by coughs and sneezes or contaminated hands or food. Two to four days after contact there is fever. Sometimes the incubation period is increased to several days. There is tonsillitis, fever, abdominal pain and vomiting. The fever is at its peak on the second day and then falls to normal over the ensuing five days.

The tongue is at first coated white, then the coating peels off to leave a raw, 'strawberry' look. The rash quickly spreads all over the body. It consists of thousands of tiny scarlet spots which blanche briefly when pressed. The area round the child's mouth remains pale (circumoral pallor). After about a week the rash fades and the skin peels.

The complications of scarlet fever are usually more serious than the disease. They include middle ear infection (OTITIS MEDIA), sinusitis, mastoiditis, pneumonia, GLOMERULONEPHRITIS and RHEUMATIC FEVER. Fortunately, the *Streptococcus* is very sensitive to penicillin and this is usually given for 10 days to prevent complications.

Scissors gait see CEREBRAL PALSY.

Scoliosis see SPINAL PROBLEMS.

Seborrhoeic dermatitis

This minor skin problem affects very small babies. It appears as greasy, brownish scales, occurring in patches in more than one place – on the scalp and in areas of skin contact, such as in the groin, the armpits or behind the ears. The patches may also occur on the face and neck, and, unless severe, will usually respond to careful washing and drying in these areas. Soap and baby lotion may make the condition worse. Emulsifying ointment or olive oil can be used for cleaning.

Security object see introductory section (1 to 3 years).

Seizures or fits see EPILEPSY, CONVULSIONS.

Separation anxiety see introductory section (5 to 11 years).

Serious illness in childhood – how to recognize see introductory section (How to recognize serious illness)

Sex ambiguity see HERMAPHRODITISM, PSEUDOHERMAPHRODITISM.

Sexual abuse

Sexual abuse is likely to have a serious effect on development. As many as 100 children die every year in Britain from assault, and countless more lead lives of continual misery and fear. Sexual abuse is even commoner than other forms of assault. It is estimated that one girl in 10 and one boy in 15, under the age of 16, are sexually abused, usually by a father, stepfather or other resident of the house. Sexually abused children show precocious awareness of sexual matters and this may be evident in their language, play and drawings. They often show sudden changes in behaviour, such as loss of trust in parents, and they may openly talk about what has happened. Such allegations are usually true.

Sexually abused girls often sustain injuries to the genitalia; while the the anus can be damaged in either sex. They may have urinary tract infections or sexually transmitted diseases. The anal dilatation test – a tendency for the anus to open when the skin is gently pulled – is only one of many factors which doctors must consider in making up their minds in suspected cases. Sexual abuse is often followed by serious long term psychiatric effects and major difficulties in establishing proper sexual relationships and adjustments as an adult. Suicide is common many those who have been sexually abused.

Public awareness of child abuse has grown. Greater openness, school guidance, encouragement to report abuse, telephone helplines and counselling centres are all helping children have a better chance to defend themselves.

Short children

Body growth is influenced by many factors. Heredity is one of the most important. As a general rule, tall parents are more likely to have tall children. Certain genetic disorders, such as ACHONDROPLASIA, feature very short stature. Hormones, especially the growth hormone from the pituitary gland, can have a major effect. Deficiency of growth hormone in childhood causes DWARFISM and this can be treated by giving the hormone. Too much causes gigantism. Deficiency of thyroid hormones in childhood and sex hormones at puberty also leads to impaired growth.

The state of the early nutrition and of the general health are also important. Severe, long-term illnesses can limit growth as can the use of steroid drugs in childhood. General social and parental deprivation often leads to short stature.

Many parents of a short child simply live in hope that the child will outgrow its lack of stature and reach a normal height in adult life. To investigate this question, 453 children who were below the fifth centile (see PERCENTILE) at the age of 7 were followed up to the age of 23. None of these children had any disease or prolonged illness that would have accounted for their short stature. The results were interesting. In the case of the short girls, only 28.4 per cent of them became short women; and in the case of the short boys, only 31.6 per cent of them became short men. Having short parents did not seem significantly to increase the probability that children would be small as adults.

In boys, the fifth centile – a group near the bottom of the scale in height – was 111.9 cm (44 in) at age 7, and was 165.2 cm (65 in) at age 23. In girls it was 110.71 cm (43 in) at age 7 and 152.05 cm (60 in) at age 23.

The fact that a short child has two chances out of three of becoming an adult of more normal height may be relevant when considering whether or not growth hormone treatment is justified.

Short sight see REFRACTIVE ERRORS.

Shuddering attacks

Shuddering or shivering attacks in conditions of normal temperature can, rarely, occur in infants, and the tendency to such attacks may run in the family. They usually predict the benign condition of essential-familial tremor later in life. This form of shakiness is an unimportant, if occasionally embarrassing, condition which has a genetic basis and may produce an effect of nervousness. It does not progress to more serious disease and is usually temporarily relieved by alcohol. It may be suppressed by beta-blocking drugs such as propranolol.

Siamese twins

These are twins joined together at birth. The effect is extremely rare. Junction is usually along the trunk or between the two heads, at the front, back or sides. In some cases, organs are shared and this makes separation difficult or impossible. Sometimes, one twin is normal and the other is severely underdeveloped and relies on its sibling for nutrition. In such a case, it may be decided to remove the smaller twin in the interests of the other.

The name derives from the male twins Chang and Eng, born in Siam in 1811, and surviving until they were 63. Chang and Eng were joined face to face from breastbone to navel, but both married and each contrived to father several children.

Siamese twins are derived from a single fertilized egg and are monozygotic, identical twins with identical genes. In the normal case, at the time of the first division of the egg, the two resulting daughter cells either remain joined to produce one individual, or separate completely to produce two identical individuals, which then develop separately. In the case of Siamese twins, this separation is incomplete. The surprise is not that the phenomenon occurs, but that it should be so rare.

Sickle cell disease

Millions of Afro-Caribbean children carry one of the pair of genes for this condition and suffer little or no ill effects. In one in about 400, however, both genes are carried. This is called the homozygous state (see GENETICS – AN OUTLINE) and these children are at risk. Their red blood cells, which are abnormally shaped and fragile, may either clump together so that they block small arteries and veins, or may burst, causing severe ANAEMIA. These episodes are called sickle crises.

Small children with the disease fail to thrive and suffer JAUNDICE, anaemia and enlargement of the spleen. Later in childhood there may be:

- joint pain
- bone pain
- unusual tendency to infection, including pneumonia and meningitis
- septicaemia (blood poisoning)
- jaundice
- sickle crises

It is very important that the parents of these homozygous children should be aware of the fact that the children should wear an amulet and that they should be under the care of a hospital haematology department. All infants at risk should be screened at 4 to 8 weeks of age.

See also CHILDREN FROM OTHER COUNTRIES.

Sight problems see CONTACT LENSES, REFRACTIVE ERRORS, SPECTACLES, SQUINT.

Single parent families

High divorce rates and social acceptance of unmarried parenthood have led to an unprecedented rise in the numbers of one-parent families. Nearly 70 per cent of divorces involve children under 16. In the great majority of cases, the single parent is the mother, and the consequences are often serious hardship for both parent and child.

Parenthood makes enormous emotional demands, and these are normally limited or relieved by sharing. Partners, whether married or not, provide emotional support, advice, comfort, companionship, help in solving problems, and so on. None of this can be furnished by a young child or children, however loving. Single parents may have great difficulty in finding support of this kind and may try to rely on older children for it. Pubescent and adolescent children may thus have emotional demands made on them that they are not yet sufficiently mature to meet.

Parenthood also makes great physical demands. These are often quite enough to tire out a full-time, non-working mother. If there is no male partner to share them, and if the mother has to work to live, the purely physical stresses on a single mother may be overwhelming.

Single parents, especially if women, commonly also have to cope with serious economic difficulties. At best, ill-paid part-time work may be all that can be undertaken because of the necessity to look after young children. Shortage of money commonly precludes paying for carers. Only a small, albeit increasing, minority of single mothers are able to pursue a full-time career and to pay for nannies or others to take over from them many of the duties and responsibilities of parenthood. Even in these cases there may be serious conflicts between duty to the children and duty to the job. These conflicts are not, of course, limited to single parents but commonly arise whenever both parents pursue a professional career.

Single parenting may deprive male children of a male role model – something that many boys find essential. The result may be that, at least to some extent, role-modelling passes from the parents to some outside agency such as a teacher, an athletic coach, or even the leader of a street gang.

Parental exhaustion is very bad for the children and, if long-term, can interfere with development. This is because normal social and emotional development in the child can occur properly only is there is a full interplay and free responsiveness between parent and child. Parental exhaustion frustrates this, leads to irritability, frustration and anger and this may be vented on the children. These, in turn, withdraw emotionally from the parent. Night crying or SEPARATION ANXIETY may be consequences and these can be an added burden to an exhausted mother. Sadly, in some cases the final outcome is child abuse.

Single parents are sometimes people who, through inadequacy and other misfortune, have suffered great unhappiness and loneliness. Often they will cherish hopes that this unhappiness and sense of social failure may be relieved by parenthood. Regrettably, this is seldom the case, and these ambitions may lead such people even deeper into trouble.

This depressing account is no more than an attempt to face the facts of the matter and to highlight the special problems of single parents. Governments have not always been as sympathetic to the plight of single parents are they might have been and have been known to act on assumptions about single mothers that are not always justified. Few young people actively wish to be single parents; most of them are the victims of grave misfortune.

Sixth disease see ROSEOLA INFANTUM.

Skin blueness see CYANOSIS.

Skin circles see LYME DISEASE.

Skin cysts see DERMOID CYSTS.

Skin inflammation see DERMATITIS.

Skin mites see SCABIES.

Skin pallor

Skin colour depends on several factors including its thickness, the amount of pigment present in the form of cells containing the substance melanin, and, especially, the profusion and state of openness of the underlying small blood vessels. While it is true that extreme pallor may be caused by intense constriction of these blood vessels in the dangerous condition of surgical shock, this condition never occurs in otherwise healthy children, but only follows serious injury or grave illness. Similarly, ANAEMIA does not cause significant skin pallor unless it is severe enough to have other quite obvious effects.

The normal pinkness of the skin is simply a matter of how readily well-oxygenated blood in the small arteries can be seen through it. Sudden changes are common and these are due to sudden alterations in the degree to which the small blood vessels are open. A severe fright, for instance, may cause the face to become deathly pale simply because the blood vessels temporarily close down tightly under the influence of a sudden shot of adrenaline from the adrenal glands.

It follows from all this that skin pallor, by itself, has no medical significance. Much the same applies to 'dark rings under the eyes' which are due to the thinness of the skin of the lids and the profusion of the blood flow though the underlying veins. Contrary to the popular belief, this sign does not indicate any disorder whatsoever.

Skin problems see ACNE, ALLERGY, BIRTHMARKS, BOILS, BRUISING WITHOUT OBVIOUS CAUSE, CHILBLAINS, CAFÉ AU LAIT PATCHES, DERMATITIS, ECZEMA, IMPETIGO, INSECT BITES, JAUNDICE, LYME DISEASE, NAPPY RASH, RINGWORM, SCABIES, SCALY SKIN, STORKBITE, THRUSH, WARTS, PLANTAR WARTS.

Skull openings see FONTANELLE.

Sleeping problems

In certain aspects of their lives, children need regularity, rules and order. A recognized, relatively fixed bedtime is one of these. In families that are, for any reason, disorganized, this is likely to be impossible. Children also need rituals and one of these that makes for good sleeping habits is the ritual of bedtime washing, toothbrushing and story-telling before sleep. This pattern, once established, will set up a kind of conditioned reflex that greatly helps in promoting regular times for falling asleep. Unfortunately, in a badly organized family, in which children are allowed to stay up until they fall asleep in front of the TV, the children are likely to have sleep problems. So also is the child whose parents respond to resistance to going to bed by simply leaving the child alone. In this situation, regularity rules.

There are, however, many other reasons for sleep disturbances. A child with other behaviour disturbances is unlikely to fail to identify bedtime as an excellent opportunity to gain attention and cause parental anxiety. This is not primarily a sleep problem, as is apparent from the fact that such children, in their concern to maintain pressure on their parents, commonly fight strenuously to stay awake. When put to bed, such a child will usually cry. So long as there is no risk of danger to the child he or she should be left to cry. This can, at first, be relied on to last for about half an hour, but, as noisy night succeeds noisy night, the duration of the crying will lessen as the parents acquire hard-heartedness and confidence that no harm is being done. In many cases, the pattern is broken and the problem is solved within a week.

One of the most difficult situations to deal with is that of the child who goes off to sleep regularly at the proper time and with no fuss, only to wake in the middle of the night, full of beans and determined to play. In rare cases, the few hours of sleep such a child has had may well be his or her full physiological requirement, so that efforts to keep such a child in bed are fighting nature. Different children do require different amounts of sleep but very few will need as little as four or five hours. Many parents become anxious because they think a child who does not get a given amount of sleep, according to age, will suffer. There is no truth in this idea. Many lively and mentally active infants require less sleep than more placid children, and some of them actually need less sleep than their parents.

Most children showing the pattern of early waking simply require firm handling or, in extreme cases, behavioural training. If you are being driven to distraction, see your doctor and enquire about child guidance. Many parents of such children end up with the child sleeping alongside. Remember, however, that there are some physical factors that may keep the child awake. These include cough; the persistent itch of infantile ECZEMA; and the sore throat and tickle of upper respiratory tract infections. Babies should be checked for wet nappies.

Much sleep disturbance in children is due to NIGHT TERRORS. If this is happening frequently, you should consider what there is in the child's life that is promoting such intense and frightening dreams. It is easy for adults to fail to appreciate how terrifying some allegedly suitable television programmes can be for small children. It may also be necessary to investigate, either directly, or with professional help, irrational fears that the child may have. These can arise in the most seemingly innocent way – such as the observation of a dead bird or mouse. Fear of death is not unknown in young children.

About a quarter of all British children, of 1 to 2 years of age, regularly disturb their parents' sleep during the night. This usually starts at about the age of 9 months when the baby begins to realize that he or she is being left alone. A variety of approaches have been recommended – a clear indication, unfortunately, that none is completely satisfactory. They include:

- changing the domestic routine so as to reduce daytime naps
- sedatives for the child or the mother, or both
- leaving the child to cry
- attempts at behaviour modification

The latter involves methods such as rewarding the child for not disturbing the parent(s) or introducing a fixed bedtime ritual which conditions the child to stay quiet. Rituals are effective with children and should, preferably, involve both parents. They might include an agreement not to cry during the night. One important principle that should be constantly borne in mind is the ease with which conditioned reflex patterns of behaviour can be established. If an act on the part of the child, such

as crying, is routinely followed by a response from the parent, such as getting out of bed and picking up the child, it will not be long before the child will start crying for no other reason than to get the parent out of bed. The patterns may well be reinforced if the parent ignores the crying for a long time and then gives in to it. This is a no-win situation. After putting up with crying for a time, parents will often begin to be convinced that there is something genuinely wrong with the child. This induces anxiety, dispels sleep, and results in the inevitable response to the stimulus. In such cases, it may be best to respond on the child's first attempt rather than to potentiate the reflex by waiting a long time and then giving up and conforming.

Sedatives are widely used to quieten children who cry in the night but they work only while they are being given. They do not induce 'habits' of all-night sleep. They may be justified for short-term use when matters are reaching crisis proportions. The antihistamine drugs Vallergan (trimeprazine) or Phenergan (promethazine), or the hard-to-disguise, but highly effective chloral hydrate, are widely used to sedate children.

Smacking

This is a delicate subject in which discussion tends to be governed more by emotion than by reason and views are often extreme. There are those who hold that the current high levels of JUVENILE DELINQUENCY are due to the absence of parental discipline, and especially by the refusal to apply physical chastisement when it is badly needed. And there is probably as large a lobby who hold, with equal sincerity, that bad behaviour in the young is due to parental violence in the form of corporal punishment. Some authors insist that those who believe that smacking is justified in the interests of correcting behaviour, are guilty of child abuse. Abuse, they claim, is sanctioned and even approved in our society so long as it is described as childrearing.

These views are illogical and there is no reason to believe that either side of the argument is correct. Parental discipline is certainly important, but it is not a matter of physical violence. And just physical punishment of children in emotionally healthy family situations will not make children violent. Violent child abuse certainly can, and does, turn children into violent adults, but that is a different matter altogether. Moreover, normal parents do not develop a taste for child abuse by administering proper punishment to their children. Normal parents find it very distressing to have to inflict corporal punishment, however mild, on children, and hate doing so.

A High Court ruling in March 1994, held that it was lawful for a childminder to use corporal punishment on a child in her care so long as this was done with the consent of the parents. This ruling has caused anxiety in some people as it is thought that it may be seen by child abusers as justifying their actions.

Many parents, whose affection for their children cannot be questioned, and who could never, under any circumstances be described as child abusers, will, on occasion and after painful consideration, smack their children. These parents hold that there are occasions on which smacking, formally applied as an unequivocal punishment for seriously unacceptable behaviour, is not only allowable but, in the long-term interests of the child, desirable. It goes without saying that punishment of this kind is very seldom applied and that its application is a major event, justified only by such activities as habitual lying, stealing money or destroying property. It also goes without saying that the child must be in no doubt as to the reason for the punishment and that the nature of the smacking should be such as never to cause any physical harm to the child.

A widely held, and sensible, view is that in a loving context, in which the child never doubts the parent's affection and permanent support, corporal punishment can be, and commonly is, perceived by the child as a clear sign that he or she has committed a grave offence. This offence is seen to be something the punishing parent takes very seriously and is deeply concerned about. The child will also perceive that the inflicting of the punishment is distressing to the parent. This perception can be extraordinarily influential on a child and it will fortify the child's awareness of the gravity of the crime of which he or she has been guilty.

Most children are happiest with clear rules and with no doubt as to the limits allowed. When this is the case, transgression of the limits is seen by them to be an event justifying punishment. If the relationship with the parent is a healthy one, the child will not resent punishment.

Following the High Court ruling of 1994, a panel of over 150 doctors was asked to respond to questions on the matter. On the question whether the ruling was correct, 71 per cent voted YES, 23 per cent voted NO and 6 per cent could not make up their minds. On the question whether premeditated smacking as a regular form of discipline was more acceptable than a last resort smack when the parent had lost his or her temper, 46 per cent voted YES, 44 per cent voted NO and 11 per cent were undecided. And on the question whether the court ruling would endanger the welfare of some children by increasing the risk of abuse, 67 per cent voted NO, 20 per cent YES and 14 per cent didn't know.

Although the questions posed and answered in the box do not directly address the issue of whether or not smacking should be illegal, it is fairly clear from the doctors' answers that a considerable majority of them would reject this proposition.

See also MISBEHAVIOUR, CHILDREN AND VIOLENCE.

Small head see MICROCEPHALY.

Smoking

Smoking is the 'chief, single, avoidable cause of death in our society and the most important public health issue of our time' (US Surgeon General). Regrettably, smoking is still highly prevalent among children Almost 30 per cent of boys and girls in the age range 11 to 15 years, smoke regularly.

Consistently, more girls than boys smoke. The 1994 Office of Population Census and Surveys check of children's smoking confirmed that the percentage of British boys and girls aged 11 to 15 who were smoking regularly in 1994, was the highest ever recorded. Many younger children also smoke regularly or occasionally. Of those who start smoking when they are 11 to 12, about two-thirds continue to smoke and are regular smokers four years later.

There can be very few young people unaware, at least in a general way, that cigarette smoking is dangerous and damaging. What is it that makes so many of them act so gravely against their own interests? Peer pressure is an important factor and a force very difficult for young people to resist. Two-thirds of teenage smokers report that they were induced to take their first cigarette by friends. Many of them require little or no pressure to conform. Handing out cigarettes is, to many, an important social act that promotes solidarity with a group. Many perceive smoking as a norm within a group; others smoke as an act of rebellion.

Another important factor is cigarette advertising. This specifically targets young people. Now that so many of their customers in the Western world have been killed off, the cigarette manufacturers are concentrating on the young of the Third World. One major cigarette manufacturer sold 499 billion cigarettes world wide during the first nine months of 1995 and is enjoying rising sales in countries such as China, Brazil, Sri Lanca and Indonesia. Over this period, their profits were £1.2 billion – 34 per cent higher than in the same period the year before. This company is now extending its cigarette activities to new markets in Russia, Ukraine, Uzbekistan and Cambodia. The World Health Organization has noted that although cigarette consumption has dropped 10 per cent since 1970 in developed countries, it has risen by 67 per cent over the same period in Third World countries.

Cigarette manufacturers insist that, to quote one of their spokespersons: 'The notion that we play any role in increasing tobacco usage is fanciful'. But it seems, on the face of it, improbable that the industry would spend £100 million a year on promotional activities if it did not expect to increase usage. Assuming that the current rate of cigarette consumption continues, some 10 million people will die from tobacco-related diseases in 30 years' time. The amount of ill-health caused by them is incalculable.

Young people continue to smoke because it is always easy to find reasons or excuses for continuing to do what one wants to do. This is called rationalization and it is a common element in human psychology. Rationalizations about smoking adopted by young people include that:

- it is a form of addiction that can't be broken
- the doctors don't really know what they are talking about
- the evidence about smoking and health is purely statistical
- grandfather smoked all his life, and lived to be 95, hale and hearty. What I do is nothing to do with other people
- it's my life

and so on.

Rationalizations have nothing to do with logic, although they often possess a kind of pseudo-logic. For many children, the social factors in smoking seem far more important than the, to them, largely theoretical dangers to health. Because these dangers are not immediately apparent, they are easily brushed aside. And once a new smoker has come to enjoy the little personal treat that a cigarette allows, the impulse to repeat the act of self-gratification becomes hard to resist.

Smoking is a mild form of drug addiction. In children and young people who have not had time to establish a prolonged habit, 'withdrawal symptoms' usually last just a week or two. Cutting down, as a means of gradually giving up, is a waste of time. Some people claim to have been helped by substitutes, such as dummy cigarettes, nicotine chewing gum and patches, and so on. It is doubtful, however, how much value these are in the long-term. Most of these will not be suitable for children and adolescents.

In 1994, the British government spent about £10 million in attempts to prevent smoking. The receipts from tax on tobacco sales in the same period were, however, about £8,643 million. Over £100 million of this was from the illegal sale of cigarettes to children under 16.

See also PASSIVE SMOKING.

Solid food see introductory section (Baby Care).

Solvent abuse

This is the term given to deliberate inhalation of the vapour from various solvents for the narcotic effect. Substances used include:

- any solvent-based commercial adhesive
- volatile cleaning fluids
- lighter fuel
- petrol
- paint-thinner solvents
- marking ink
- anti-freeze
- nail-varnish remover
- butane gas
- toluene

Usually, a small quantity of the solvent is poured into a polythene bag which is held tightly against the nose and mouth.

The effects of 'glue sniffing'

These are generally intoxicant, with loss of full awareness of the surroundings, loss of coordination and muscle control and, sometimes, hallucinations. Unconsciousness may occur and death may result from asphyxiation, inhalation of vomit, or accident. Many cases of brain, liver and kidney damage have occurred, especially in children who have become addicted.

The practice is often performed in groups and many youngsters take to it as a result of peer pressure. For many, however, glue sniffing episodes are merely experimental and are not repeated. Children must, however, be made to understand that this is a lethal activity that kills many young people each year.

Sparkly loss of vision see HEADACHE.

Spastic paralysis see CEREBRAL PALSY.

Spectacles

Many children hate wearing glasses and it is common for behavioural problems to arise when parents, on the advice of opticians, insist that they do. Reasonable parents dislike any form of imposition without reasonable explanation, but often feel hopelessly uninformed on this matter. They are also concerned that damage to their children's vision may result if glasses are not worn.

After the age of about 8 years, glasses are needed only by those who cannot see clearly without them. However poor the vision, no harm is done to the eyes if glasses are not worn or if the prescription is incorrect. The worst that can happen is a feeling of discomfort, strain or dissatisfaction and, in cases of myopia, severe hypermetropia and severe astigmatism, difficulty in seeing the blackboard clearly at school and the resulting educational disadvantage (see REFRACTIVE ERRORS).

During the period from birth to 8, however, glasses may be critically important, not primarily for purposes of seeing clearly, but to allow the full visual function to develop normally. The full link-up between the eye and the brain is not present at birth and is not complete until about the age of 8, and this link-up will not occur unless young children form sharp images on their retinas. This is why glasses may be important in childhood for the long-term quality of vision. Any focusing errors, or differences in focus between the two eyes, present in young children, may result in the failure of full neurological link-up with the brain and the production of a form of defective vision known as AMBLYOPIA.

Ophthalmologists and skilled opticians can determine the refraction in a small child, without any more cooperation than that the eyes are kept open. In cases of extreme difficulty, it may be justified to give a child a general anaesthetic, but this is rarely necessary. Children accommodate so strongly that it is often necessary to use drops which temporarily paralyse the accommodation before doing the test. This will always be done in children found to have squints. Atropine is generally used, other drugs seldom being strong enough to prevent this powerful focusing.

Speech problems

These may result from DEAFNESS, emotional upset, developmental delay, lack of stimulation or from psychological or physical difficulty in articulating speech. Articulation problems may be due to CEREBRAL PALSY or to abnormalities of the mouth, such as CLEFT PALATE or poor alignment of the teeth.

STUTTERING usually starts in childhood, almost always before the age of 8 and persists in about 1 per cent of the adult population. Temporary stuttering is common in children of 2 to 4 years. About half those whose stutter continues after the age of 5 will have a permanent stammer. Stuttering is commonest in males, twins, and left-handed people. The cause is disputed, but it is generally believed to be a psychological problem and it can usually be improved or cured by speech therapy.

Speech difficulties must be assessed by comparison with the average child, but it must be emphasized that the range of normality at any age is wide. By the age of 6 to 10 months most babies can coo and babble. Babbling peaks at about 1 year and is then gradually replaced by meaningful words. The average toddler of 18 months has a vocabulary of between 20 and 50 words, depending largely on how well the child is encouraged, at this stage, to talk by hearing normal speech from parents and other children rather than baby noises.

Up to about 18 months, infants understand many more words than they can speak – often well over 100 words. But around the end of the second year there is usually a sudden considerable increase in the power of expression. Vocabulary and the ability to form sentences increase rapidly. If the child clearly falls well behind these, rather arbitrary, standards, help is probably needed.

The treatment of speech problems depends on the cause. When possible, deafness must be corrected at the earliest opportunity. Hearing aids may be needed. Cleft palate should be repaired as soon as the child is mature enough. STUTTERING usually disappears without treatment but severe cases may require speech therapy. Children with developmental speech problems can also often be helped by speech therapy.

Spider-like fingers

Doctors call this arachnodactyly and it is the most obvious feature of a rare, autosomal dominant, inherited condition called MARFAN'S SYNDROME.

Spina bifida

This is a developmental defect in which the rear part of one or more of the bones of the spine (vertebrae) remain incomplete. As a result, the spinal cord, which runs down through a series of holes in the vertebrae, is relatively unprotected in the affected area. In the 1970s, the incidence of spina bifida was about 1.5 per 1,000 births in southern England and about 4 per 1,000 in South Wales and Ireland. By 1991 it had fallen sharply to 0.15 per 1000. The reason for this is partly the discovery that the condition can be prevented by taking supplementary folic acid before conception and during the first 12 weeks of pregnancy. Women with a previously affected baby should take 5 mg a day; others should take 0.4 mg daily. Unfortunately, many women who would benefit do not take this vitamin, which is recommended by the Department of Health.

There are three degrees of severity and seriousness. In spina bifida occulta, the condition is hidden and unsuspected and usually discoverable only on X-ray. In the next more serious group, the coverings of the cord (the meninges) pass back through the opening to form a cyst-like swelling (a meningocoele). In the worst case, the spinal cord itself is exposed. This is called a myelocoele and there is usually paralysis of the legs and loss of sensation. There is often an associated HYDROCEPHALUS and subsequent brain damage.

Spina bifida, especially if severe, is easily diagnosed before birth, by amniocentesis, alpha-fetoprotein estimation and ultrasound examination. In severe cases, detected early in pregnancy, the option to terminate the pregnancy may be considered. Surgery to correct the defect may be performed soon after birth.

Spinal problems

Postural curvature is the commonest problem. Backward curvature in the back region is called KYPHOSIS and a sideways 'S' curvature is called scoliosis. These are usually the result of poor habits of standing and can often be checked if children are constantly encouraged to 'walk tall'. Scoliosis can be due to a congenital abnormality of the spinal bones (vertebrae), but this is a rare cause. It is also a feature of various neurological problems or MUSCULAR DYSTROPHY. Treatment may involve the use of a plastic or plaster jacket. Sometimes surgery is needed.

Bone disease, such as tuberculosis, is now uncommon but can cause severe spinal deformity by collapse of one or more vertebrae. Wry neck (see TORTICOLLIS) can cause severe distortion of the upper part of the spine. SPINA BIFIDA is most important for its effects on the nerves within the spine. Spondylolisthesis is a slipping of one vertebra on another, usually in the lowest part. This can cause severe lower back pain. 'Slipped disc' is rare in children but can occur.

Spinal twisting see KYPHOSIS.

Squint

Only one eye is aligned on the object of interest in the condition of strabismus. If the other eye is directed too far inward, the condition is called convergent squint, and if too far outward, divergent squint. Occasionally, one eye will be directed upward or downward, relative to the fixing eye. This is called vertical squint.

Squint may be present at birth (see below) but most commonly starts in early childhood. This usually occurs because the brain mechanisms that allow fusion of the images from the two eyes into one (binocular vision) have not yet developed fully at a time when new stress factors begin to operate. The most important of these is hypermetropia, a focusing error in which the relaxed lens system of the eye is not strong enough to bring the image to a focus on the retina (see REFRACTIVE ERRORS). Hypermetropia forces the child to exert strong accommodation to see clearly and the result is a convergent squint. The strong accommodation actually prompts the brain to turn the eyes in. But the child is trying to look at an object further away, so one eye remains straight while the other turns in.

Such a squint causes double vision and, to overcome this, the brain immediately rejects the signals from the deviating eye. From that moment on, visual development stops in the squinting eye, and the result, unless effective treatment is given, is a severe and permanent defect of vision in that eye, known as AMBLYOPIA. By the age of 7 or 8 years the whole system has firmed up and nothing can be done to correct amblyopia after this age. The earlier amblyopia is treated, the easier it is to correct.

The treatment involves stopping the child from making this excessive accommodative effort by prescribing a full spectacle correction for the hypermetropia. This is one of the cases in which SPECTACLES are sight-saving. After glasses have been prescribed, management will usually be undertaken by an orthoptist (see ORTHOPTICS). The 'lazy' (amblyopic) eye has to be forced to make a seeing effort. This is done by covering up the good eye (patching or occlusion) for varying periods, until vision is restored to its former level in the squinting eye. At this stage, the squint will often alternate from one eye to the other. This is an encouraging sign and a muscle balancing operation at this stage will often complete the cure. But glasses must still be worn at least until the neurological control system is fully mature and stable.

Babies do not acquire coordinated control over their eye movements until about three months or so after birth. During the first three months there may be occasional crossing of the eyes but the eyes will often be straight. By six months the eyes should be able, at all times, to align accurately on the object of interest. From birth, eye movements, although not necessarily coordinated, should be unrestricted. A persistently fixed inturning of one or both eyes is abnormal and should be reported at once. Similarly, inability to turn either eye outwards beyond the straight ahead position, is abnormal and requires professional attention. This inability may be concealed by the child turning his or her head, but if the head is secured and the attention directed to an interesting object, the failure of out-turning of the eyes may be demonstrated.

Stammering see STUTTERING.

Sticky eye

This is a popular term for infective conjunctivitis with pus formation. See RED EYE.

Stiff neck see NECK RIGIDITY.

Steroids in childhood

Steroids are powerful drugs and, given by mouth or injection in large doses, are often life-saving in critical conditions. Doctors will never hesitate to use steroids if a child's life or future health are at risk, and steroids are an appropriate form of treatment.

It is when steroids are used for less serious conditions that contention arises. Large doses of steroids can:

- cause children to stop growing
- cause premature hairiness and acne
- interfere with the immune system so that severe infections may occur
- interfere with the body's healing processes
- precipitate diabetes

- cause loss of bone protein and calcium (osteoporosis)
- dangerously reduce the body's normal safety response to severe injury or surgery

The latter effect may persist for as long as two years after stopping the drug. Children on large doses of steroids must carry a steroid card giving details.

None of these effects is caused by steroids used by inhalation for ASTHMA.

Stings, bee

Bee venom contains highly irritating protein substances. These cause a local area of blanching surrounded by a red swelling. The black sting may be seen in the centre of the swelling and, to avoid possible injection of further venom, this should be removed by a careful scraping action rather than by pulling. Use a credit card or a blunt knife. Eyebrow tweezers are liable to ensure that the full dose of venom is acquired by the child. Antihistamine or cortisone skin cream, or even an ice cube, will reduce pain.

Over 100 simultaneous stings would be needed to provide a potentially lethal dose, but it should be remembered that people who have been stung before may have become hypersensitive. In such cases, a single sting may provoke a serious, even fatal, reaction. This is called anaphylactic shock. Fortunately, it is rare in children. Also dangerous are stings on the inside of the throat. These may occur from bees floating on the surface of drinks. Stings in this area are liable to cause such severe swelling of the tissues around the vocal cords that the breathing is cut off. If this happens, life can be saved only by cutting into the windpipe (trachea) centrally, just above the notch of the breast bone. This procedure is called TRACHEOSTOMY.

It is for consideration whether older children and adolescents known to have suffered an anaphylactic reaction should be provided with a sealed syringe of adrenaline for emergency use. If you are worried, discuss this with your doctor.

Stool-holding see CONSTIPATION.

Storkbite

One in three newborn babies have small pinkish-red skin blemishes around the eyes and at the nape of the neck. These are called 'storkbites' or salmon patches, and those on the face nearly always disappear in the first year of life. They are actually benign tumours of tiny blood vessels (haemangiomas) and are entirely harmless. Salmon patches on the neck may, however, persist.

Strabismus see SQUINT.

Strawberry tongue see SCARLET FEVER.

Strep throat see STREPTOCOCCAL INFECTIONS.

Streptococcal infections

These are infections caused by bacteria of the genus *Streptococcus*. These are common bacteria causing disease in children and are responsible for TONSILLITIS, pharyngitis, SCARLET FEVER, IMPETIGO, erysipelas, endocarditis and urinary tract infections. In addition to causing infections, streptococci can give rise, by an immunological process, to the more serious conditions of RHEUMATIC FEVER and GLOMERULONEPHRITIS.

Stuffy nose see NASAL CONGESTION.

Stunted growth see GROWTH DISORDERS.

Stuttering

A condition, common in childhood, that features intermittent inability to produce smooth and normal speech. Stuttering almost always starts before the age of 8 and tends to be worse in conditions of stress, or when the affected child is in a conspicuous situation. It does not occur during singing and is usually absent when the child speaks to an animal.

> ### Principal features of stuttering
> - uncontrollable blocking of speech with long pauses
> - repetition of the first letter of words
> - difficulty with certain consonants, especially 'b' and 'p'
> - increased severity with stress, excitement or embarrassment
> - grimacing or tic-like movements of the head, neck and limbs
> - reduced severity on relaxation
> - severity greater when using the telephone, sometimes less
> - freedom from stuttering in relaxed company
> - stuttering is absent while singing lyrics

Stuttering is not caused by any organic disorder and appears to be the result of habits acquired during early speech learning. The great majority of stutterers achieve normal speech by the end of adolescence, but a small percentage remain severely affected and this can be very disabling. Mild stuttering in a child need cause no great concern. It is common and will pass. Severe stuttering is a major social disadvantage for a child and attempts should be made to deal with it. In such a case you should consult your doctor. Try to analyze the circumstances that bring on the stuttering and, if possible, avoid them. Remember that a stuttering child has a low threshold of emotional tension.

Speech therapy is highly effective in treating stuttering and should be started as soon as the condition is established, no matter how young the child.

Styes

Styes and BOILS are essentially the same – infections in the root of a hair with development of a small abscess. In the case of styes, the infection is around the root of an eyelash. Like other hair follicles, eyelash follicles contain one or more tiny sebaceous glands, which produce an oily lubricating substance called sebum. Infection of the sebaceous glands, usually with the bacteria called staphylococci, is the cause of styes.

Bacteria reach the follicles from the outside and when they multiply they produce powerful poisons – toxins – which inflame and damage local tissue, causing redness, swelling and pain. Millions of defensive white cells are attracted to the site from the blood and most of these are killed while attacking the bacteria. The accumulated bodies of these cells are called pus and this forms as a 'yellow head' around the base of the eyelash.

Once a stye has formed there is really nothing to be done but to wait for it to settle down – which it will do in a week or so. In many cases, if your child will allow it, you can hasten recovery by taking hold of the lash at the point of the yellow head with eyebrow tweezers, and pulling it out. This will discharge the pus and reduce the pain. But it calls for resolution in both parent and child and should not be tried unless there is a very obvious yellow head through which the lash passes.

Styes tend to recur because the number of bacteria on the skin of the lids makes spread of infection to adjacent lash follicles likely. You can prevent this by applying an antibiotic eye ointment to the lid margins two or three times a day for two or three weeks.

Sudden infant death syndrome (SIDS or 'cot death')

This is the name given to the sudden unexplained death of an apparently well baby. The child, not more than a few months old, is found dead in the cot and no apparent cause can be found, even by a detailed postmortem examination. The sudden infant death syndrome is now the third most common mode of death for infants between 1 month and 1 year of age, after major congenital abnormalities and severe prematurity. Each year, about 1,500 babies die in Britain in this way and the distress to parents and relatives is incalculable.

In spite of agonized public concern and intensive study, the causes remain unknown. From ancient times, cot deaths have been attributed to suffocation from 'overlying' by the mother, and countless women have been unjustly accused of causing the deaths of their infants in this way,

either accidentally or intentionally. But in more recent years it has become apparent that sudden death commonly occurs in a baby sleeping alone.

The unexpected death of a baby affects boys more often than girls and is commoner in winter than in summer. Premature babies are at greater risk. Maternal smoking during pregnancy and narcotic addiction or alcoholism are associated with a higher incidence. Breast-fed babies are less often affected than bottle-fed babies.

Many theories have been put forward to account for the deaths of these babies. These include:

- over-soft bedding, in which the baby's face becomes buried
- high environmental temperatures causing heat stroke
- the fear paralysis reflex, brought on by separation from the mother, especially in the dark
- sensitivity to cow's milk
- botulinum poisoning
- unnoticed chest or bowel infection

None of these has been accepted as a major cause, although all have been implicated in some cases. It is now universally accepted that a major causal factor in cot death is the former common practice of wrapping babies up tightly *and laying them to sleep face down*. The abandonment of this practice has led to a marked reduction in the tragedy. This is not, of course, the sole factor. Some experts believe that some cot deaths result from a transient disorder of the nerve control of breathing and heart beat.

In most cases of sudden infant death syndrome, death occurs during sleep and without any suffering on the part of the child. But the effect on the family is devastating and close support is needed. Inevitably, the sense of loss is compounded by feelings of guilt and remorse for real or imagined failure to anticipate danger. This is seldom justified. Counselling and supportive visits from others who have suffered the same kind of bereavement are helpful in making the necessary adjustment to the prospect of having further children. Such help is available from local health authorities and from Cruse-Bereavement Care.

Sugar in urine see DIABETES.

Suicide of a young person

Suicide by children is, fortunately, rare, but the figures for suicide in young people – teenagers, especially – have increased steadily over the past 30 years or so. In the USA, suicide is now the third commonest cause of death in young men in their late teens and early twenties. This suggests that strong social factors are operating on these young people – factors unlikely to be directly the responsibility of parents. In at least half the cases of adolescent suicide, there is clear evidence of psychiatric illness.

Bereavement following suicide is probably worse than any other. On top of all the usual factors the bereaved person almost always suffers a terrible sense of guilt and, in many cases, has to live with the spoken, implied or imagined criticism of others. When there is a suicide, most people feel that someone has to be at fault, and society will usually attribute blame to the person closest to the deceased. The result is much worse than just the absence of sympathy – it may be frank accusation. The reaction to this is, understandably, severe, and whether the accusation is accepted or, as is more usual, denied, there is likely to be a serious interference with mourning.

The sense of guilt may be terrible to bear. Suicide, by a loved dependent, seems to imply rejection of parental love, or suggests that love was not recognized. It suggests that all the previous efforts of the parents, now rendered futile, were considered of no value by the young person. And it blasts all the hopes for the future which had been invested in the child. So there is, inevitably, a dreadful sense that there was no real understanding between the parent and the one who has died, and, with it, the agonizing questions about how this could have come about. Naturally, the older person feels that he or she should have seen some indications of what was happening, and should have been able to do something to prevent it.

If you are the parent of a child who has committed suicide, you will, time and time again, have asked yourself the apparently unanswerable question: why? There is little consolation for such a tragedy, but it may help if you can understand how this tragedy may have happened.

Many suicides are not intended to succeed and do so accidentally. Sometimes, after a few sleeping tablets have been taken, there is a stage of disorientation in which the person concerned can go on taking more in an automatic fashion. Deaths by falling, even if staged as suicide attempts, may still be accidental. 'Suicide gestures' by hanging are very dangerous and many of these end in disaster.

Suicide gestures are usually intended to draw the attention of parents or others to the plight of the young person, but tragically, communication between such young people and their parents is often so poor that this is the only way some of them have to express their distress at their sense of their own unimportance. And, tragically, too, parents often have so little insight into the minds of their children that they have no idea of what is going on. If you feel that this kind of situation was behind the suicide, and wonder whether you are to blame, remember that the causes of failure of communication between the generations are much too complex to be attributed to any one person.

Communication failure is related, among other things, to differing attitudes and values. People can only react according to their own values and opinions, and young people can hardly be expected to share those of a different generation. Young people, today, are the products of very different influences from those of older generations. These include a vast input of information from television and popular magazines, and much of this influence may be in conflict with the formed values of older people. So, to the age-old classic failure of communication between the generations, has been added a new factor, and of this you are, to some extent, the victim.

Sunburn

Sunburn is the damaging or destructive effect of solar ultraviolet light on the skin. Sunburn is more likely to occur in children unaccustomed to exposure to bright sunlight and in those with minimal skin pigmentation. Carefully graduated exposure, for periods starting with no longer than 15 minutes a day and increasing progressively as the skin pigmentation builds up, can prevent sunburn.

It should be remembered, however, that even if sunburning does not occur, all intense sunlight is damaging to the skin and may have permanent undesirable effects. The elastic collagen of the skin is changed, causing permanent loss of elasticity and wrinkling. The DNA of deep epidermal cells may be altered so that tumours such as rodent ulcers (basal cell carcinomas), squamous carcinomas and malignant melanomas become more likely to occur later in life. See MELANOMAS.

Sunscreens and protective clothing can effectively minimize skin damage, but people in tropical and sub-tropical areas are well aware of the advantages of remaining indoors.

Sunken eyes see DEHYDRATION.

Swallowing and breathing problems see TRACHEO-OESOPHAGEAL FISTULA.

Swollen glands

This is the popular term for enlargement of the many lymph nodes that are concentrated in the groins and armpits, at the sides and back of the neck, and at the elbows and behind the knees. These are not glands, but are units in the immune system that help to limit the spread of infection. Lymph node enlargement occurs with any infection in the area drained by the local lymph vessels. Generalized enlargement is a feature of many conditions including:

- GLANDULAR FEVER
- other virus infections
- tuberculosis
- brucellosis
- TOXOPLASMOSIS
- LEUKAEMIA
- lymphomas
- KAWASAKI DISEASE

You should never delay in reporting any suggestion of a general enlargement of lymph nodes.

T

Taking blood in children

Blood tests, of which there are many, are so important that it is often necessary to take samples of blood. Children are no exception to this and parents are often alarmed at the prospect. The first thing to be said is that the concern about this is nearly all imaginary. Adults who have experienced blood sampling by an expert will vouch that the experience is almost entirely painless. It is, however, important that the person who takes the blood is, in fact, experienced. Those most skilled in the procedure are the nurses and technicians in haematology departments who have done it many thousands of times and who know all the tricks.

Sometimes only a drop of blood is needed. In babies, this is usually obtained by a quick stab to the side of the heel with a special sterile lancet. In older children, the stab is usually made in the thumb. If a larger quantity of blood is needed, a fine, very sharp needle must be inserted into a vein. This is done after the veins have been caused to swell by temporary compression of the limb above the site of puncture. The child is held in the parent's arms and the head turned away. A nurse will usually hold the arm or leg. The child is likely to be told that he or she is to have a 'little scratch' and will then get a 'big bandage'. In babies, it is sometimes necessary to pass a fine needle into a vein on the scalp.

Talipes see CLUB FOOT.

Tantrum see introductory section (1 to 3 years).

Tapeworms

Infestation with these worms is rare in Britain. Tapeworms are ribbon-like populations of joined flatworms, which grow from a small common head equipped with hooks or suckers which it uses to attach itself to the lining of the bowel. The body of the worm is composed of segments of increasing size, each of which is a separate individual containing both male and female reproductive organs. Tapeworms extend to about 4 metres in length and have 800 to 1,000 segments. The younger, smaller segments release sperm which fertilize the eggs contained in the older segments.

Segments with developing embryos break off and are passed in the faeces. If these are eaten by an animal (the intermediate host), the larvae develop, travel to the animal's muscles and form cysts. Pork meat containing tapeworm cysts is called 'measly pork' and if this is eaten, undercooked, the worm is released in the intestine, attaches itself, and the life cycle is continued.

Tapeworms can be eliminated fairly easily with suitable drugs.

Tay-Sachs disease

This recessive genetic disorder (see GENETICS – AN OUTLINE), is very rare in the general population but occurs more frequently amongst Ashkenazi Jews. It appears in the early months of life and leads to blindness, deafness, progressive dementia, seizures, paralysis and death, usually before the age of 3 years. The condition is due to the absence of an essential enzyme which breaks down a substance called ganglioside, present mainly in the nervous system. It is the accumulation of this material that is so damaging.

Unfortunately, there is no treatment for Tay-Sachs disease so it is very important for carriers or possible carriers to have GENETIC COUNSELLING. Antenatal diagnosis by chorionic villus sampling can be done and, if the diagnosis is confirmed, termination of pregnancy can be offered.

Tearing see WATERING EYE.

Teeth care

Tooth decay (dental caries) is one of the commonest minor problems of childhood. Although it is preventable, well over 90 per cent of British children develop it before the age of 15. Some parents think that caries of the primary teeth doesn't matter because the teeth are to be replaced. The fact is, however, that children who suffer decay of the primary teeth are much more liable than average to have caries of the permanent teeth. This is because there is no reason why the factors that caused primary tooth caries should not persist. It is true that caries occurs more readily in the primary than in the secondary teeth.

The avoidance of caries requires knowledge and determination. The facts are quite straightforward (see TOOTH DECAY) but the inculcation of proper habits of teeth care in children may be less easy. Unfortunately, children are really not much concerned with what happens to them later in life. Warnings about requiring dentures may, however, justify your insistence that children do their brushing and flossing regularly and properly.

Disclosing agents used once or twice can be effective in demonstrating to children the acidic plaque deposits that are eating away at the enamel of their teeth. Toothpaste should be fluorinated, especially in areas where the water has a low fluoride content.

Toothbrushes should always have multi-tufted synthetic (nylon) filaments. These retain their flexibility and elasticity and do not absorb water. They are cleaner than other forms of brush bristle. Avoid 'hard' brushes which can quickly lead to serious tooth abrasion. Select 'medium' or 'soft' texture brushes, but ensure that the bristles are springy. Brushes should be renewed regularly, well before they begin to show signs of tiring. Teeth should not be brushed in a side-to-side manner as this is inclined to abrade the necks. Working up-and-down, from gum to free edge and back again, is better, but probably best of all is a small, circular scrubbing action, with the emphasis on the areas, front and back, where the teeth meet the gums. The grinding and biting surfaces of teeth should also receive attention. It is of no consequence how the teeth are brushed, however, if the method fails to remove plaque. The use of a disclosing agent *after* brushing can be revealing in mores senses than one. Techniques may have to be amended to achieve good plaque removal.

Electric toothbrushes are probably the most effective way of cleaning teeth. They have a reciprocating, oscillating action that allows good access to the spaces between the teeth and provide a method of cleaning that is almost impossible to reproduce manually. Children can reasonably be expected to do a proper job of cleaning using these devices; this is not always so with cheaper methods. It is still necessary, however, to ensure, by using a disclosing agent, that plaque is being properly removed.

The only way plaque can be removed from the areas between the teeth is by the use of dental floss. In very young children, however, flossing can be distressing and can damage the gums. It is therefore reasonable to defer the regular use of floss until some gum recession has occurred and there is a visible space between the necks of the teeth.

Children should be taught what sugar does to teeth and should be brought up to recognize that residual sugar on the teeth, from any source (including non-sweet carbohydrates) should be an indication for tooth cleaning. The secret is to establish in the child a feeling of discomfort after eating until the teeth have been cleaned. Once this habit (see HABIT FORMATION) is fully formed, the problem has been cracked.

See also TOOTH ABSCESS, TOOTHACHE.

Teeth grinding

Habitual, rhythmic grinding or clenching of the teeth is called bruxism. This is common in children and usually occurs during sleep. Bruxism while awake generally implies some emotional problem. The contraction of the muscles that clench the jaw can be observed in front of the ear. Sometimes bruxism is performed unconsciously. It may also result from an unsatisfactory alignment of the upper and lower teeth MALOCCLUSION.

In most cases bruxism does little harm, but in severe cases it can lead to wearing away or loosening of the teeth, and pain and stiffness in the jaw joint. Occasionally it is necessary to protect the teeth during sleep with a dental bite plate.

Teething

The time of appearance of the milk (primary) teeth is very variable. Some babies are actually born with one or more teeth, much to the alarm of the breast-feeding mother. Others still have no teeth by 1 year. Both extremes are normal and need cause no concern. In most cases, the first teeth – the central incisors (biting teeth) – appear around 6 to 9 months, followed, in a month or two, by the other incisors. Around 10 to 16 months, the first molars (grinding teeth) appear and at 16 to 20 months, the canine (tearing teeth) appear. The second molars usually erupt sometime between the second and third years of life.

Teething causes gum tenderness, some pain, and dribbling and the baby will spend much time investigating his or her mouth. Teething can certainly lead to fractiousness and crying, but this is seldom a serious problem. Other conditions may cause these symptoms which may be wrongly attributed to teething. Evidence of undue distress should lead to investigation. There is, however, no truth in the general belief that teething causes a range of disorders such as infection, fever, rashes, diarrhoea or convulsions. If a child becomes unwell during teething, it is essential not to dismiss the problem as 'just teething'. Full medical investigation is mandatory.

Teething powders and chewing rings should be avoided. Aspirin is now out because of REYE'S SYNDROME, but a suitable dose of a paracetamol preparation can be a great comfort to all concerned. A mild local anaesthetic preparation, with an astringent to reduce salivation, may be helpful.

Teeth overlap see
MALOCCLUSION.

Television and violence see
CHILDREN AND VIOLENCE

Temper tantrums see
introductory section (1 to 3 years).

Testicle, disorders of

The testicles develop in the abdomen and descend into the scrotum soon before birth. It is not uncommon for one, sometimes both, to fail to descend. Testicles remaining in the abdomen become sterile and should be brought down surgically during infancy. Sometimes the testicle has partly descended, but remains in the (inguinal) canal in the groin through which it normally descends. Again, correction is necessary if fertility is to develop. An undescended testicle is more liable to develop cancer later.

Inflammation of the testicle (orchitis) is fairly common as a complication of MUMPS. Torsion of the testis is the acutely painful condition in which the spermatic cord becomes twisted within, or just above, the scrotum. The veins in the spermatic cord are soon occluded and the return of blood obstructed. There is great swelling, tenderness and bruising. Early surgical correction is necessary if fertility, in the affected testicle, is to be preserved. The other testicle may be secured, as a precaution.

Testicle surgery see
ORCHIDOPEXY.

Tests of fetal health

A number of tests and examinations can be performed during pregnancy to ensure that all is well with the growing fetus. A short account of the most important of these follows:

Alphafetoprotein is a protein synthesised in the fetal liver and intestine and present in fetal blood. Small quantities are passed into the womb fluid (amniotic fluid) and are subsequently swallowed by the fetus. Some gets into the mother's blood, by way of the placenta. The levels of alphafetoprotein rise as the pregnancy advances, and can be measured from the third month onward. If the levels are greatly raised this may indicate that the fetus has SPINA BIFIDA or absence of the brain (anencephaly), and further investigation becomes urgent. Ultrasound scanning and amniocentesis (see below) should be done. Levels may also be raised in certain fetal kidney and bowel abnormalities, in multiple pregnancy, and in threatened or actual abortion. Confusion sometimes occurs and the levels may seem abnormally raised if there has been a mistake in the pregnancy dates.

AMNIOCENTESIS

Amniocentesis is an important method of obtaining information about a fetus and about the probability of the future development of genetic disorder. It is usually done between the 16th and 20th weeks of pregnancy. Routine amniocentesis is usually recommended for women over 35, because at that age the risk of the procedure causing miscarriage (see below) is about the same as the risk of the fetus having DOWN'S SYNDROME. In other cases, amniocentesis is done if there is any special reason to suspect trouble.

An area of the abdominal wall is anaesthetized with an injection of local anaesthetic. Ultrasound scanning is then used to ensure that a needle can be passed safely through the wall of the abdomen and straight through the wall of the womb into the amniotic fluid in which the fetus is floating. A sample of fluid is then sucked out with a syringe. Because this fluid contains cells shed from the skin of the fetus and various substances secreted by the fetus, samples obtained can be of the greatest importance for diagnosis. Every fetal cell contains a complete set of the DNA of the fetus.

Amniocentesis provides information directly about the likelihood of a number of conditions, such as rhesus factor disease, congenital absence of the brain (anencephaly) and RESPIRATORY DISTRESS SYNDROME. Alphafetoprotein levels in the amniotic fluid can give reliable information on the likelihood of congenital defects in the spinal cord and column (spina bifida). Levels in the mother's serum are also measured routinely. Cells from the amniotic fluid are grown in tissue culture so that chromosomal analysis can be done after three or four weeks. In this way, Down's syndrome, and a great range of other genetic diseases, can be diagnosed before birth. It is possible to detect CYSTIC FIBROSIS, factor VIII and factor IX types of HAEMOPHILIA, Duchenne MUSCULAR DYSTROPHY, THALASSAEMIA, SICKLE CELL DISEASE, antitrypsin deficiency and PHENYLKETONURIA.

Amniocentesis is not entirely without risk and should not be done without good reason. It may cause abortion if done early. It may damage the afterbirth (placenta) or the fetus, and may cause bleeding into the amniotic fluid. The risk of fetal death from amniocentesis is as high as 1 per cent. Sexing of the future child is certainly not a justification for the procedure, and the practice of amniocentesis followed by abortion of a fetus of the unwanted sex, is considered reprehensible by the medical profession. The Indian government made this illegal in August 1994.

Such early methods of detection of serious or potentially serious major disorders give parents the option of an early termination of the pregnancy. They also sometimes provide the opportunity for early treatment of the disorder while the fetus remains in the womb.

CHORIONIC VILLUS SAMPLING

An alternative to amniocentesis is chorionic villus sampling. This has the advantage that it can be done earlier – some eight to 10 weeks after fertilization. There are, however, risks (see below). The principle is simple.

At an early stage the embryo differentiates into two parts, one becoming the future individual and the other developing into the placenta ('afterbirth'). The part that forms the placenta starts out as finger-like processes called chorionic villi which burrow into the wall of the womb to come into close association with the mother's blood vessels. These villi are formed by division of the original fertilized ovum and thus have exactly the same chromosomes, including any possible genetic abnormality, as the embryo. Any defect in one will be present in the other.

A small sample of chorionic villi can be obtained in one of two ways. It can be sucked out with a syringe through a fine, flexible tube passed through the vagina and the neck of the womb (cervix), and guided to the site of the placenta under ultrasound scanning control. Or it can be obtained by passing a needle through the abdominal wall. Cells obtained in this way can be cultured and chromosome analysis done. Should abnormalities be found, many mothers find it easier to accept termination at this early stage.

Chorionic villus sampling is not entirely without risk. In about one case in 500 there is serious infection, and the rate of miscarriage (spontaneous abortion) is raised by the procedure. If performed through the cervix, the rate of fetal loss may be as high as 10 per cent. Done through the abdominal wall, fetal loss is about 6 per cent. But that may be a small price to pay for the opportunity to detect conditions like DOWN'S SYNDROME, CYSTIC FIBROSIS, THALASSAEMIA and many other conditions caused by chromosomal abnormalities in patients in high risk groups.

ENDOSCOPY

Endoscopy is the direct visual examination of any part of the interior of the body by means of an optical viewing and illuminating instrument. In this context, the instrument is introduced through a small surgical incision made for the purpose in the wall of the mother's abdomen. The endoscope then passes through the wall of the womb and into the womb fluid. The fetus can then be inspected directly and abnormalities noted.

Much use is made of endoscopes by obstetricians for examining the fetus in the womb. This is called fetoscopy. In addition to examining and photographing the floating fetus, the doctor can take samples of fluid for alphafetoprotein and other estimations and can also take blood samples and biopsies. Fetoscopy allows direct confirmation of suspected physical fetal abnormalities. It carries a slight risk of causing abortion, but in cases in which there is a high probability of inherited disease or gross physical abnormality, this risk is usually considered worth taking.

ULTRASOUND

Ultrasound scanning, unlike X-rays and CT scans, does not involve any potentially dangerous radiation. In ultrasound scanning, a beam of 'sound' – of a frequency of about three to 10 *million* cycles per second – is projected into the body. Whenever it meets a surface between tissues of different density, echoes are created and these return to the source. The time taken to do so depends on the distance. The ultrasound waves are produced by feeding short pulses of alternating current, at the frequency desired, to a piezoelectric crystal in the scanner head. The electrical variations cause the crystal to vibrate at the same frequency. Piezoelectric materials have the property of working in both directions: they change shape when electricity is applied to them, but they also generate electricity if their shape is distorted. So the returning echoes cause the crystal to act as a microphone and this, in turn, generates a tiny electric current. The length of time between the emitted pulse and the returning echo is a measure of the distance to the interface. Any device which converts one mode of energy into another is called a *transducer* and this is the term used for the scanner head.

The returning echoes are correlated, in a computer, with the corresponding angle of the beam, and this enables a two-dimensional picture to be built up. The quality of resolution is much less good than CT scans or MRI (magnetic resonance imaging) but, so far as is known, ultrasound, of the intensity and frequency used in scanning, is completely harmless. There are no recorded instances of any damage being caused and millions of pregnant women, and their fetuses, have had scans with no apparent indications of harm. A report in the *Lancet* in October 1993, however, suggested that women who had repeated examinations of a type known as continuous-wave Doppler flow studies, might produce babies which, on average, were slightly smaller than those of women who had not had repeated ultrasound examinations. The authors did not suggest that this method of examination, which provides valuable information on the flow of blood in the placenta, should not be used. They advised, however, that repeated examinations of this type should be limited to women in whom the information obtained was likely to be of clinical benefit.

Routine ultrasound screening significantly reduces birth mortality, mainly through the early detection of fetal abnormalities. Ultrasound can detect twins, can confirm that the fetus is of a size appropriate to the stage of pregnancy, can detect major fetal abnormalities, such as absence of the brain (anencephaly) and spina bifida. It can even measure the rates of blood flow through the heart valves and the large arteries of the fetus and can sometimes detect certain forms of congenital heart disease. The position of the afterbirth (placenta) can be determined and trouble from malposition, such as placenta praevia, anticipated. Ultrasound is also used to facilitate amniocentesis, fetal blood sampling, chorionic villus sampling and fetoscopy (see above).

Under ultrasound control, fetal blood samples can be obtained through a fine tube, and analyzed to detect coagulation disorders, infections, haemoglobin abnormalities and immunodeficiency disorders. Antibody levels in the blood can provide indications of infections such as RUBELLA and TOXOPLASMOSIS. Biopsy specimens can be taken for pathological examination. Exchange blood transfusion in rhesus disease can be done in the uterus, drug treatment given, and even certain forms of surgery performed – all under ultrasound visualization.

Tetanus

This is a serious infection of the nervous system. The organism which causes it is found in cultivated soil and manure and gains access to the body by way of penetrating wounds, which may be small and seemingly trivial. Tetanus is now rare in Britain, but is very common in babies in some of the less well developed countries, often as a result of infection of the umbilical cord.

The tetanus organism produces a powerful toxin which triggers off violent spasms in muscles. The chief early sign is a spasm of the chewing muscles, causing great difficulty in opening the mouth – hence the name of 'lockjaw'. This spasm spreads to the muscles of the face and neck producing a snarling, mirthless smile. The back muscles then become rigid and, in severe cases, the back becomes strongly arched backwards. Spasms of contraction occur every few minutes and increase in severity over the course of a week. There is also fever, difficulty in swallowing, severe stiffness of the limbs, sore throat and headache. Death from exhaustion or from asphyxia in the course of convulsions, is common.

Tetanus is treated with tetanus antitoxin and large doses of antibiotics. Spasms are controlled by Valium (diazepam), given into a vein. It may be necessary to maintain the patient under general anaesthesia for several days. Tetanus is a terrifying ordeal and much reassurance is necessary. It is easily prevented by safe immunization with tetanus toxoid. All children should have this protection as a matter of routine.

Thalassaemia

This heading covers a range of conditions featuring genetically-induced abnormal haemoglobin in the red blood cells. They mainly affect people of Mediterranean and South-East Asian origin. Haemoglobin is the pigment in red blood cells which transports oxygen. The thalassaemias lead to unduly rapid breakdown of the cells and severe ANAEMIA. The haemoglobin abnormality can take various forms, but all are due to the inheritance of a abnormal gene or an abnormal gene pair (see GENETICS – AN OUTLINE). One gene causes a minor disturbance, but inheritance of both genes causes a much more serious type. Thalassaemia major features:

- very severe anaemia
- breathlessness
- easy tiredness
- JAUNDICE
- enlargement of the spleen

These symptoms are caused by the anaemia and the reduced oxygen-carrying capacity of the blood. The body responds by attempting to produce more red cells in the bone marrow and this may cause characteristic enlargement of bones, such as 'bossing' of the skull in children. Thalassaemia major may require transfusion of normal blood cells so as to allow normal development. Accumulation of iron in the body, from red cell breakdown, must also be treated, or this will cause complications, including cirrhosis of the liver.

Thalassaemia minor is much less serious and usually causes little or no trouble. It may, however, lead to a mild anaemia. Its importance is that it is the heterozygous form of the recessive disease and people who carry the gene should certainly be aware of it, especially if contemplating becoming parents.

Thalidomide effect

The drug Distaval – the trade name for thalidomide – was widely advertised as the safest sedative yet produced, and was prescribed to millions, including many women in early pregnancy. In 1961, it was found to be linked with a syndrome of severe congenital malformation featuring especially gross stunting of the limbs, which were often replaced by short flippers (PHOCOMELIA). Research then showed that the drug was interfering with the normal development of the fetus early in pregnancy. About 10,000 babies with such deformities were born, half of them in Germany, where the drug was most widely used, and these unfortunate people are now coping as well as they can with severe disabilities.

This tragedy prompted much stricter governmental control on the testing and safety of new drugs, all of which are now checked for any tendency to interfere with fetal development, as well as for other hazards.

Threadworms

These are the commonest worm parasite of children in temperate areas. At least 20 per cent of all children are affected at any one time. The mature female worm is about 1 cm long, white, and with a blunt head and a fine, hair-like, pointed tail. The male is shorter and is rarely seen, as he remains in the intestine.

The pregnant female worms, moving on the skin around the anus to deposit their eggs, cause a strong tickling sensation. The child scratches and the eggs adhere to the fingers and nails. These are then transferred, either directly to the mouth to cause re-infestation, or, by way of toys, blankets, etc., to other children. The eggs can survive for three weeks. Diagnosis is easy, as the worms are readily seen and may appear on the faeces. In cases of doubt, Sellotape can be applied to the skin around the anus to pick up eggs, which can then be identified microscopically.

It is unlikely that threadworms ever do any real harm except to disturb the sleep of children and the sensibilities of fastidious parents. If reinfestation is avoided, the problem will disappear within a month. Ointments may be used to allay the anal itching and there are various effective de-worming drugs, such as mebendazole, piperazine or pyrantel. The usual remedy in children over 5 is a sachet of piperazine stirred into a drink. Younger children get half this dose. Treatment of all the members of the family is necessary.

Throat abscess see QUINSY.

Thrush

Persistent rashes in the nappy area encourage secondary infection with thrush. *Candida* infection (candidiasis) is common in babies and the fungus may be present in the bowel. Rashes lasting for over two weeks in spite of apparently satisfactory management, should arouse the suspicion of thrush and you should seek medical advice.

Candida thrives best in darkness when the temperatures are right and especially when there is a good supply of carbohydrate for its nutrition. So thrush of the female vulva is particularly common if there is diabetes, in which there is sugar in the urine. A urine test is essential in all such cases. Thrush is easily recognized. There is persistent itching or soreness and sometimes a burning pain on contact between urine and affected areas. Inspection shows characteristic white patches, rather like soft cheese, with raw-looking inflamed areas in between.

Thrush is treated with azole preparations such as clotrimazole (Canesten) or miconazole (Daktarin). The oral preparation fluconazole (Diflucan) is not recommended for children.

Thumbsucking

This is a fairly harmless habit, common and normal in young children, which may safely be ignored unless persisted in after the age of 6 or 7 years, when it may lead to some forward displacement of the central teeth (incisors). In this case, the child may require orthodontic treatment and possibly the use of a dental appliance at night.

Tics

These are repetitive, twitching movements occurring at irregular intervals and always at the same site. Simple tics occur in about a quarter of all children and usually disappear within a year. They are three times as common in boys as in girls and are absent during sleep and when the child is deeply absorbed. Like STAMMERING, they are made worse by stress and by observation. A small proportion persist into adult life and most of these are minor. Some, however, become so severe and widespread as to call for medical assistance. Such major tics occasionally affect the diaphragm, causing a grunting sound.

Tics do not indicate any organic disorder, but reflect a psychological disturbance. They can be controlled by an effort of will, but as they appear to release emotional tension, such control is unpleasant. See also GILLES DE LA TOURETTE SYNDROME.

Tight foreskin see
CIRCUMCISION.

Tongue-tie

Tongue-tie is a rare defect in which the soft partition under the tongue (the frenulum) extends too far forward and is too tight, thereby limiting tongue movement. This may affect speech, but is easily corrected simply by snipping the frenulum.

Tonsillectomy

This is the surgical operation for the removal of the tonsils. The tonsils serve a useful purpose in defending a common portal of entry to the body against infection. In so doing, they become inflamed and enlarged, but this is not now considered justification for removing them unless the attacks are frequent and severe or prolonged, or are causing complications such as obstruction to breathing or swallowing. The condition of QUINSY is also a reason for removing the tonsils.

Tonsillectomy is done under general anaesthesia. The mouth is held open by a ratchet 'gag' and each tonsil is grasped, in turn, by forceps and separated from its bed by blunt dissection and minimal cutting. Bleeding from the raw areas left is sometimes a problem, and it is occasionally necessary to tie off a small bleeding artery. Rarely, severe bleeding occurs some hours after the operation. Tonsillectomy is followed by a period of severe discomfort, especially on swallowing, but this settles in two or three weeks.

Tonsillitis (inflammation of the tonsils)

Acute tonsillitis is often caused by a (species of *Streptococcus*, but may be caused by many other germs. The tonsils become swollen and red and the surfaces may show spots of pus. The lymph nodes in the neck, just behind or under the angle of the jaw, are swollen and tender to the touch. There is sore throat, pain on swallowing, headache, fever, which may be very high in young children, and a feeling of unwellness. Constipation and earache are common. The tongue is often furred and the breath unpleasant. There may be slight difficulty in opening the mouth and thickened speech.

Complications of tonsillitis are uncommon, but may include abscess behind the tonsil (QUINSY), abscess in the back of the throat, middle ear infection (OTITIS MEDIA) and blood poisoning (septicaemia). Streptococcal tonsillitis may be complicated by RHEUMATIC FEVER and the kidney disorder GLOMERULONEPHRITIS.

Tonsillitis responds well to ANTIBIOTICS and these should always be given if the infection is suspected of being streptococcal. Recurrent, severe or complicated tonsillitis may justify TONSILLECTOMY.

Tonsil surgery see
TONSILLECTOMY.

Tooth abscess

This is a late complication of neglected TOOTH DECAY (dental caries). Infection, which has gained access to the root canal of the tooth, causes an inflammation in the tissues surrounding the tip of the root, leading to local tissue destruction and a collection of pus. The abscess may involve the bone of the socket. There is pain, especially on biting and chewing, and the surrounding gum is usually inflamed, tender and swollen. There may be swelling of the face and fever.

Often a tooth abscess will spread sideways under the gum to cause a 'gumboil' and if this opens and discharges into the mouth, the pain will be relieved. Sometimes treatment of the abscess requires removal of the tooth so that the abscess can drain, but it is often possible to save a tooth by drilling down through it into the abscess to release the pus and then to treat with ANTIBIOTICS and root filling. Antibiotics alone are of no value in the treatment of established abscesses.

Toothache

Pain in a tooth is usually from TOOTH DECAY (dental caries) in which the hard enamel or the underlying dentine has been breached so that infecting organisms have reached the central pulp and caused inflammation. The pulp contains sensory nerves and it is the stimulation of these that causes the pain. Toothache is very common in children.

Caries reduces the thickness of the hard material between the exterior and the tooth nerve and leads to undue sensitivity to cold, heat, acid materials or even to sweet substances. In the presence of caries, all of these can cause toothache. Toothache can also be caused by a broken tooth or by inflammation of the supporting tissue around a tooth

(periodontitis). The roots of the upper teeth project into the sinuses (maxillary antra) in the cheeks and inflammation in these sinuses can cause toothache.

Toothache is a symptom indicating that something is wrong, probably with one or more teeth. Neglect will usually lead to a worsening of the situation and possibly to the loss of an otherwise reclaimable tooth. Toothache is an indication for an immediate visit to a dentist.

Tooth decay (dental caries)

This is damage to the enamel and underlying dentine of teeth so that cavities form. If neglected, these will allow infection to reach the pulp of the teeth and destroy the internal blood vessels and nerves on which the survival of the teeth depend.

A small proportion of people who do not regularly brush their teeth appear, nevertheless, to be immune to dental caries. But the majority who, by neglecting brushing and flossing, allow plaque to develop, will eventually lose all or most of their teeth. Plaque contains bacteria which act on sugary (carbohydrate) food residues to produce acid, and it is this which causes the caries, by eating into enamel and dentine. Proper brushing after meals and the use of dental floss, will prevent the accumulation of plaque and the further stage of calculus formation. Regular dental inspection will ensure that plaque is revealed, calculus removed by scaling and early cavities cleaned and filled. Fluoride is protective.

Dental caries is always avoidable. See also TEETH CARE.

Toothpaste

Toothpaste contains a fine abrasive powder, such as chalk and a little soap or detergent. Together, these assist in the removal of plaque. It also contains some flavouring, often peppermint, and some sweetening agent and, ideally, a fluoride salt. Many dentifrices also contain a chemical to coagulate protein in the tooth tubules and desensitize them to acids and temperature changes.

Tooth replacement see
REIMPLANTATION, DENTAL.

Tooth straightening see BRACE,
DENTAL; ORTHODONTICS.

Torticollis

Commonly known as 'wry neck', this condition features persistent or permanent twisting of the neck and an abnormal head position. Common causes of torticollis include:

- damage at birth to one of the main longitudinal muscles of the neck so that it is shortened and the head tilted to one side
- whiplash injury to the neck with painful muscle spasm
- lack of balance in the eye muscles so that a tilt is needed to avoid double vision
- severe scarring and shortening of the skin of the neck

The treatment of torticollis depends on the cause. Congenital muscle shortening from injury should be corrected by early stretching and perhaps operation, otherwise permanent lack of symmetry of the skull and face may result. Skin contractures call for plastic surgery procedures and eye balance problems for squint surgery. Muscle spasm from injury will usually settle with rest and time.

Tourette's syndrome see GILLES
DE LA TOURETTE SYNDROME.

Toxocariasis

Infestation with the juvenile forms of the common puppy worm *Toxocara canis*. The condition is largely confined to children who come into contact with puppy fur and contaminated soil. London parkland has been shown to be extensively and uniformly contaminated with *Toxocara* worm eggs deposited by dogs.

When the eggs are swallowed they hatch in the intestine and the juveniles penetrate the wall of the bowel to gain access to the bloodstream. They are carried to every part of the body and can remain alive in the tissues for many weeks where their movement produces tracks of haemorrhage, inflammation and dead cells. Eventually they die, and at the sites of death, small abscesses and collections of fibrous tissue and new blood vessels (granulomas) occur. In some cases, live juveniles may remain walled up for years only to resume their migration at a later date.

The migration of the juvenile worms causes a transient illness known as visceral larva migrans. There is fever, pallor, lassitude, loss of appetite and weight, and often cough and wheezing. Rarely, epileptic seizures – usually of the petit mal type (see ABSENCE ATTACKS) – may occur. POLIOMYELITIS and heart muscle inflammation (myocarditis) have been described.

Human infestation is commoner than has been supposed, for many cases are free of symptoms. Surveys have shown that in some groups of children (black youngsters in the southern states of the USA), up to 25 per cent have antibodies to *Toxocara*. White children in the same areas show a prevalence of about 5 per cent. Whether or not symptoms occur is determined by the number of live eggs swallowed and by the resistance of the child.

The chief interest has been in those comparatively few cases in which the eye has been involved. If a juvenile worm happens to lodge in the layer of blood vessels behind the retina, and dies, the result is a tumour-like mass at the back of the eye which may cause great damage to vision. In addition, the mass may be mistaken for the highly malignant RETINOBLASTOMA. In the past, many children's eyes were removed because toxocariasis was not recognized for what it was and the clinical appearances could not be distinguished from this form of cancer. This tragedy is now rare, as toxocariasis is now well understood and tests, such as the ELISA test, can point to the correct diagnosis. Taken in combination with other clinical and laboratory findings, this test now enables doctors to make the diagnosis with considerably more confidence.

Treatment of eye involvement is a difficult problem, and if severe damage has been done to the eye at the time of diagnosis, little of benefit can be done. Steroids may be used to try to minimize the inflammatory damage. Laser or photocoagulation has been used to kill the juvenile worm and to prevent its migration to the more important central area of the retina.

Prevention is, of course, better than cure. Many puppies are infested *in utero* and require de-worming, with the anti-worm (anthelmintic) drug piperazine adipate, at two, three, four and eight weeks after birth, and then twice more between three and six months. Thereafter, one further dose is desirable. Pregnant bitches should also be repeatedly treated with the same drug. As the eggs can survive for years in soil, all dog faeces should be collected and destroyed. It has been proposed that special dog exercise areas should be set aside in parks, from which children would be excluded, and both parents and children should be aware of the dangers associated with puppies. Eating earth (PICA) should be discouraged.

Toxoplasmosis

This is an infection with the microscopic organism *Toxoplasma gondii*, often acquired before birth, but sometimes passed on by domestic cats or acquired by eating undercooked meat from infected animals. The organism infects all known mammals and most of us have antibodies to it. Although the infection is common, it is comparatively rare for the disease to manifest itself. Toxoplasmosis can, however, affect the nervous system, especially the eye, and is a cause of permanent damage to the retina, causing a blind spot of variable size, which may enlarge at intervals throughout life. The condition should not be confused with TOXOCARIASIS, which is a worm infestation, also capable of affecting the eye.

In most cases, the infection causes no symptoms or observable effects, as the immune system is capable of controlling it and preventing significant damage. Antibodies, however, operate less efficiently in the internal tissues of the eye than elsewhere, and damage to the retina and the underlying layer (the choroid) is fairly common. Recurrences, each of which tends to cause further permanent damage to the retina, are a feature of the condition. But it is only when the central (macular) part of the retina is involved that loss of vision is apparent.

Apart from eye damage, toxoplasmic infection sometimes causes widespread lymph node enlargement in people with apparently normal immunity. The node enlargement may be accompanied by fever, headache, malaise, muscle and joint aches, and liver enlargement. When heavy infection occurs before birth, the fetus, which has little immunological protection, often suffers extensive damage to the nervous system and elsewhere, and miscarriage or stillbirth is common. For the same reasons, toxoplasmosis in people with immune deficiency, either from AIDS or other cause, may be a severe disorder, with tissue destruction in the brain, lungs and heart caused by the rapidly spreading organisms. About 10 per cent of patients with AIDS suffer a severe encephalitis (brain inflammation) from toxoplasmosis.

Ocular toxoplasmosis is treated with pyrimethamine, an antimalarial drug, used in conjunction with sulphadiazine or another similar sulpha drug.

Tracheitis

This is inflammation of the lining of the windpipe (trachea), usually as an extension of an infection of the throat or voice box (larynx). It is also commonly associated with bronchitis. Tracheitis is usually caused by a virus infection but some cases are due to organisms susceptible to ANTIBIOTICS. It causes CROUP in young children.

Tracheitis causes pain in the upper part of the chest, hoarseness, sometimes wheezing, and a painful dry cough. In very small children there may be some risk of asphyxia. This was a common cause of death when tracheitis was caused by DIPHTHERIA. Treatment involves antibiotics, if appropriate, the use of soothing inhalations and sometimes drugs to control ineffective coughing. Most cases settle without treatment.

Tracheo-oesophageal fistula

This fortunately rare condition is an abnormal connection between the windpipe (trachea) and the gullet (oesophagus), occurring as a birth defect due to an abnormality of development. Swallowing is impeded and food may enter the trachea so that the baby is at risk from choking, asphyxia, pneumonia and collapse of the lungs.

The condition is often associated with other congenital defects and, unless of a very mild degree, calls for early surgical correction.

Tracheostomy

This is a life-saving operation in which an artificial opening is made in the windpipe (trachea) and a tube inserted, through which breathing may continue until the normal airway can be restored. It is often carried out as an emergency when life is threatened by obstruction to the airway. Tracheostomy is also commonly performed on children unable to breathe spontaneously, so that the respiration can be maintained artificially by an air pump.

The operation is preferably performed in theatre under general anaesthesia and with the usual full aseptic routine. Respiration and inhalation anaesthesia are maintained through a cuffed tracheal tube until the trachea is opened. A short transverse incision is made in the lower part of the neck between the notch at the top of the breastbone and the prominence of the Adam's apple. This is carefully deepened until the narrow central part of the thyroid gland is reached. This may be cut through or pulled out of the way to reveal the cartilage rings of the trachea. A cut is made in the second or third ring, or a small flap is cut and folded downwards. The curved tracheostomy tube is now inserted and oxygen can be given through it. Because it readily becomes blocked with dried secretions, the tracheostomy tube is double-lined. The inner lining may be removed regularly for cleaning and then replaced. The outer part has flanges by which the tube can be secured in place with tapes tied round the neck.

There is an alternative to tracheostomy that is often used in an emergency. This is called cricothyrotomy and it enables a child with a totally blocked airway to be kept alive for up to half an hour while preparations for a formal tracheostomy are arranged. The equipment for this is simple and it is available in every Accident and Emergency department and in most medical facilities. It consists of a narrow, flexible 12 or 14 gauge tube, called an over-the-needle cannula, that is fitted snugly over a sharp needle. The child is usually unconscious so it is easy to feel for the membrane on the front of the neck immediately below the thyroid cartilage and above the narrower cricoid cartilage. The needle is attached to a syringe and is simply pushed through this membrane exactly in the midline. As this is being done, the syringe plunger is pulled back. As soon as the tip enters the windpipe it becomes possible to draw air into the syringe and the needle is pushed no further. The needle is then slowly pulled out as the cannula is advanced into the trachea. A Y-shaped connector is now attached to the cannula and one end of this is connected by tubing to an oxygen supply. The other end is covered for inspiration and uncovered for expiration.

Travel sickness see MOTION SICKNESS.

Trisomy

The chromosomes occur in 23 matched and identifiable pairs. Trisomy is the condition in which there are three, instead of two, of a particular chromosome. This is always serious and has effects varying from death of the fetus in the womb (uterus) to a range of structural abnormalities affecting parts such as the heart, the face, the skeleton or the brain.

The commonest form of trisomy is trisomy of chromosome number 21. This causes DOWN'S SYNDROME. Trisomy can be detected by chromosome analysis.

Trisomy 21 syndrome see DOWN'S SYNDROME.

Turner's syndrome

This is an uncommon genetic disorder affecting females and caused by a sex chromosome abnormality. The normal female has two X (sex) chromosomes; in most females with Turner's syndrome one of the X chromosomes is missing. Sometimes both X chromosomes are present, one being normal and the other defective. Turner's syndrome may also result from an abnormal distribution of sex chromosomes occurring in normal females at the time of one of the early cell divisions. In this case, some cells have the normal number and some not. This is called MOSAICISM. Unlike Down's syndrome, Turner's syndrome is not affected by maternal age.

Girls with Turner's syndrome feature:

- shortness of stature
- webbed neck skin
- misshapen ears
- increased outward angulation at the elbows
- underdevelopment of the uterus, vagina, and breasts
- lack of pubic and axillary hair
- absence of the menstrual periods
- Localized narrowing of the largest artery in the body (COARCTATION OF THE AORTA)
- abnormalities of the eyes and of the bones
- usually some degree of LEARNING DIFFICULTY

Attempts have been made to increase growth with anabolic steroids or growth hormone, but these are liable to cause the growing bone ends to fuse prematurely and so ensure DWARFISM. Coarctation of the aorta can, and should, be treated by early surgery.

Twins

Twins are two offspring from a single pregnancy. The incidence is about one in 90 pregnancies. Twins may be identical, if they both arise from one fertilized egg (ovum), or non-identical, if two separate eggs are separately fertilized by separate sperm.

Twins developing from a single egg are called monozygotic or monovular twins and have identical genetic material. They occur if the fertilized egg separates completely, at an early stage of development, into two embryos, each of which then proceeds to develop normally. Very rarely, this division occurs too late so that separation is incomplete, resulting in SIAMESE TWINS. Monozygotic twins are both nourished by the same single placenta. They may differ in size at birth, but are always of the same sex and appearance.

Dizygotic or binovular twins imply the release of more than one egg from one or both ovaries. Each egg is fertilized by a different sperm. Apart from age, they have no more in common than any pair of siblings and may be of the same or of different sexes. Each dizygotic twin has its own placenta. Some families have a history of dizygotic twins.

Twitching and grimacing see TICS.

Umbilical cord

This is the life-line that connects the fetus to the placenta. It contains two arteries and one vein. The fetal heart pumps blood along the arteries to the placenta to pick up oxygen and nutrients, and this blood returns to the fetus by way of the vein. After birth the cord is tied and cut. The stump usually falls off by the 10th day leaving a clean yellow scar that becomes the navel. Watch out for reddening around the scar as this suggests infection. This should be reported at once. ANTIBIOTICS may be needed.

Umbilical hernia

This is common in Afro-Caribbean babies, who may have a protrusion at the navel resembling a small elephant's trunk. The cause is a weakness in the abdominal wall, at the navel, caused by a slight separation of the two central longitudinal muscles, allowing a knuckle of small intestine to protrude under the skin and push it forward. The conventional treatment is to push the hernia back and keep it in with a coin wrapped in a cloth. This is likely to push the muscles further apart, and should not be done. Fortunately, most umbilical hernia correct themselves without treatment. In rare cases a surgical repair may be necessary.

Undescended testicle see
CRYPTORCHIDISM.

Unequal limb growth see
DYSCHONDROPLASIA.

Upper respiratory tract infection (URTI)

This group includes any infection of the nose, throat, sinuses and larynx. RESPIRATORY TRACT INFECTIONS are amongst the commonest of all illnesses, especially in young children, the most familiar being the common COLD, sore throat (pharyngitis), TONSILLITIS, sinusitis, laryngitis and CROUP.

Urinary disorders

The commonest urinary infection is cystitis. This is more prevalent in females than in males because of readier access of germs by way of the much shorter urine tube (urethra). About 1 per cent of newborn babies develop a urinary infection. Urinary infection in babies and young children should arouse the suspicion of congenital abnormalities of the urinary tract.

Cystitis causes frequency of urination and urgency and a burning pain on passing urine. There may be fever and general upset, especially if the infection spreads up to the kidneys. 'Reflux' of infected urine back up the ureters to the kidneys is abnormal and suggests a congenital defect. Unexplained fever in children may be caused by urinary infection and the urine should always be checked.

Urgency or frequency does not necessarily imply infection. It is more often caused local by irritation from shampoos, bubble baths, biological washing powder residues on underclothes, fabric softeners, tight garments, emotional stress and THREADWORMS.

Obstruction to urinary outflow can occur in small boys with very tight foreskins. CIRCUMCISION may be necessary.

Other urinary tract disorders include GLOMERULONEPHRITIS and Wilms' tumour. See KIDNEY DISORDERS IN CHILDREN.

Uveitis see RED EYE.

V

Vaginal discharge

A thick, white vaginal discharge is often seen in newborn babies for the first 14 days or so. Sometimes this is tinged with blood. This is a normal effect and is due to the loss of the mother's oestrogen hormones which passed to the fetus via the placenta during the pregnancy. Once these have gone, the vagina becomes normally colonized by organisms.

In older little girls, inflammation of the vagina (vaginitis) is common and causes discharge and itching. Most cases are caused by infection, especially with the *Candida albicans* fungus which cause THRUSH. Gonorrhoea may affect little girls who are especially susceptible because of the thinness of the vaginal lining. The usual source of infection in infantile gonococcal vaginitis is the mother, and infection may be acquired during birth. *Trichomonas vaginalis* infection is uncommon in children but may affect adolescents, especially the sexually active.

Vaginal discharge is also sometimes caused by a foreign body which has been pushed into the vagina and retained.

Vernix

Properly called vernix caseosa, this is the layer of greasy material, fine hairs and skin scales with which fetuses and newborn babies are covered. Vernix is easily washed off after birth and does not recur.

Verruca (Wart)

It is widely believed that verrucas occur only on the soles of the feet (see PLANTAR WART). These are, however, only one of the several varieties of verruca (wart) affecting any part of the skin.

Vision – defective from birth

CATARACT present at birth (congenital cataract) – is often caused by maternal German measles (rubella) early in pregnancy, or less often, to the effects of drugs taken by the mother during the early weeks when the eyes of the fetus were developing. DOWN'S SYNDROME is commonly associated with cataract as are various rare hereditary conditions. GALACTOSAEMIA is a condition in which the infant is unable to break down galactose into simpler sugars so that it accumulates in the body. Unless a galactose-free diet is given, cataract is inevitable.

Vision problems see CATARACT, REFRACTIVE ERRORS, SPECTACLES, VISION – DEFECTIVE FROM BIRTH.

Vitamin K controversy

Babies deficient in vitamin K – which is necessary for normal blood clotting – have a small risk of brain damage or even death from the bleeding disorder known as haemorrhagic disease of the newborn. At the same time, vitamin K, given by intramuscular injection, is said, on generally accepted statistical evidence, to be associated with a doubling of the risk of the development of various cancers later in childhood.

Haemorrhagic disease may occur as late as the sixth week of life and in half of these late cases bleeding occurs into the brain. The discovery of the relatively frequent occurrence of late haemorrhagic disease of the newborn in the 1980s led to increased use of vitamin K and this was most commonly given by intramuscular injection so as to ensure full protection. The vitamin can be given by mouth but the effect is less certain and the levels of the vitamin in the blood do not remain at the same high level provided by the injection. It is thought that the injected vitamin forms a depot in the muscle from which it is gradually released.

When the reports of the association between the injections and the increased risk of cancer were published, there was a major shift towards giving the vitamin by mouth. This has caused problems because three doses have to be given at intervals. In the case of exclusively breast-fed babies, the third and last dose must be given at the four to six week check. Studies have shown that more than 60 per cent of babies in one London unit did not get the third dose.

The controversy has been heightened by the view that vitamin K is inherently unlikely to be the cause of the increased risk of cancer; some other substance, such as phenol, present in the injection, would be a more probable cause. Some doubt has also been cast on the validity of the original research that showed the connection. Other epidemiological studies have not confirmed the association.

Vomiting

Vomiting is a sign of some particular disorder. There is always a cause and this should, if possible, be found and removed. It is usually preceded by severe nausea, sweating, excessive salivation, pallor and slowing of the heart rate.

Vomiting may result from allergic sensitivity to various foods, undue distention of the stomach from overeating, severe indigestion, APPENDICITIS, or peritonitis. Infection of the intestine, as in FOOD POISONING, or heavy ROUNDWORM infestation, commonly causes vomiting. Bowel obstruction, from causes such as CONGENITAL PYLORIC STENOSIS or telescoping of the bowel (INTUSSUSCEPTION) will, unless relieved, inevitably lead to vomiting.

Vomiting is also an important sign of a rise in the pressure within the skull from any cause such as brain tumour, ENCEPHALITIS, or HYDROCEPHALUS. These may cause unexpected, forcible, 'projectile' vomiting, often without nausea. Cyclical vomiting is a condition, tending to run in families, which causes recurrent attacks of vomiting and headache. It often starts in childhood and is associated with migraine.

W

Waddling gait see HIP, CONGENITAL DISLOCATION OF.

Walking problems

Nine out of 10 children are walking by 15 months. Infants still making no attempt to walk by this age may possibly be suffering from developmental delay and should be seen by a doctor.

Abnormal walking may be due to CERE-BRAL PALSY, CONGENITAL DISLOCATION OF THE HIP, or other hip disorders such as Perthes' disease, MUSCULAR DYSTROPHY, severe spinal problems, or foot deformities, such as CLUB FOOT.

Warts

Warts are very interesting to children, annoying to parents, and badly understood. They occur when a small patch of cells at the base of the outer layer of the skin is forced to overgrow by the presence of a virus, called a papillomavirus. They can occur anywhere on the skin. The medical term for a wart is 'verruca', wherever it may occur. They are uncommon in babies but very common in older children.

Warts are harmless and only matter because of their appearance. They are commonest on the hands and often last for years. Half of all new warts go away in a month or two without treatment. If they persist, wait until the child is old enough to put up with the treatment without too much distress. The exception is a wart on the sole of the foot (PLANTAR WART). These get pressed in by the weight of the body and are particularly troublesome.

Warts are removed by freezing with liquid nitrogen, burning with an electric cautery under anaesthesia, or by the use of salicylic acid or other lotions. One should always consider whether treatment is justified.

Watering eye

Because the tube that carries surplus tears down from the eye into the nose often remains obstructed at birth, it is common for babies to have a persistently watering eye. And because bacteria are not carried away with the tears, infection of the upper part of the tear duct (the lacrimal sac) is also common. This may cause a swelling below the inner corner of the eye and an accumulation of pus between the lids. Pressure with the finger-tip on the skin just inwards of, and below, the inner corner of the eye may overcome the blockage, and this should be done repeatedly. If the problem persists for more than about three months, you should consult your doctor. In some cases it is necessary to pass a fine metal probe down the tear duct to clear the obstruction. This must be done under anesthesia.

Water on the brain see HYDROCEPHALUS.

Weaning see introductory section (birth to 1 year).

Weight problems

Patterns in eating may be established early in life and fat mothers probably unconsciously encourage habits of excessive intake in their children. This is more plausible than the suggestion that obesity – which is an acquired feature – is hereditary. It has also been suggested that infant obesity, from excessive intake, leads to the production of an increased number of fat cells in the body, and that the number of fat cells remains constant after childhood. If this is true, the obese have more cells to fill than the non-obese and are faced with an almost insuperable problem in keeping thin. The idea has been disputed by some experts.

Fat mothers usually have fat babies and these tend to turn into fat adults. Although body weight varies with height and with skeletal shape and bulk, the largest variation in body weight in Western societies is the amount of fat storage. Excess fat storage is dangerous, but the effects are seldom seen in childhood. Parents should, however, be aware of these as defective eating and EXERCISE habits are laid down in infancy and childhood. Obese adults suffer from:

- high blood pressure
- diabetes of the 'maturity-onset' variety
- increased incidence of cancers of the breast, womb, ovaries and gall-bladder in women
- increased incidence of cancer of the colon, rectum and prostate gland in men
- orthopaedic problems, such as osteoarthritis and foot trouble
- depression
- a sense of social disadvantage and unattractiveness
- reduced life expecting

Efforts should therefore be made, at all costs, to avoid obesity, and the time to start is in infancy. Mothers should never inflict their own eating habits on children and should never use food for any purpose other than nutrition. Children should be allowed to eat only at meal times.

Whipworm infestation

Infestation with *Trichuris trichiura*, an intestinal parasitic worm, universally found in underdeveloped areas. The adult worms are 2.5 to 5 cm long and have a whip-like appearance, the 'tail' being the head. In the male worm, the 'handle' of the whip is also spiralled. Each pregnant female lays about 2,000 eggs a day and these survive in moist soil contaminated with faeces. In conditions of poor hygiene and sanitation, the eggs readily find their way into the mouths of children and others.

Whipworms inhabit the lower bowel and usually cause no trouble, but in very large infestations with hundreds of worms, there may be a wasting diarrhoea which, in children suffering from MALNUTRITION, may be serious. The characteristic barrel-shaped eggs are easily identified in the stools, by microscopy, and treatment with mebendazole (Vermox) will drive out the worms. The real solution, of course, is to improve, if possible, the social conditions.

White hair in childhood see
ALBINISM.

White cat's eye pupil see
RETINOBLASTOMA.

White pupil see CATARACT.

Whooping cough

This is an acute, highly infectious, disease occurring almost exclusively in children under 5 years of age and spread by droplet infection. It is also known as pertussis. The early, infectious stage cannot be distinguished from a cold, so epidemics commonly occur in susceptible children.

The disease, which can be very distressing, lasts for about six weeks. After the first week of two of cold symptoms, the characteristic cough begins and the number of paroxysms of coughing varies from two or three to as many as 50. These bouts are commoner at night. The child is seized by an uncontrollable succession of short, sharp coughs, so insistent and rapid in sequence that there is no time to draw breath between them. The lungs thus become almost emptied of air and the cough sequence is followed by a long, deep inspiration which often features a whooping sound. The child may turn blue from CYANOSIS. The final paroxysm in a series is often followed by VOMITING. The process is exhausting to child and parent alike. Children who become blue should be treated in hospital.

Whooping cough may lead to pneumonia, collapse of part of a lung, epileptic seizures from lack of oxygen in the brain, ulceration of the central membrane under the tongue and pushing out (prolapse) of the rectum. The ANTIBIOTIC erythromycin, given early, shortens the course of the illness, but antibiotics are of little value once the coughing stage has been reached, unless secondary infection occurs. Effective cough suppressants are available. Vomiting may interfere with nutrition, but food is usually retained if given immediately after vomiting.

In very rare cases, whooping cough vaccine is believed to have caused brain damage, but there is no doubt that, on a statistical basis, whooping cough is much more dangerous than vaccination against the disease. Brain damage can result from whooping cough. Most doctors advise that this disease should be prevented by active IMMUNIZATION of all infants, from 3 months of age unless the child is suffering from any other acute illness or shows an adverse reaction to the first injection of the vaccine. Decisions may be difficult in the case of children with a history of brain damage or seizures or a family history of EPILEPSY. In these, the risk of vaccination may be higher, but so may be the risks of whooping cough. Babies under 3 months should be protected, as far as is possible, from contact with children who may be infected with whooping cough.

Wind

Greedy or hungry babies often succeed in swallowing air along with their feeds and this air becomes compressed by the normal bowel action (peristalsis) and may cause colic, pain and much crying. It often leads to regurgitation of food, much to the annoyance of the parent who has to clean up, and may also feel obliged to replace losses. Traditional burping methods help, but many parents will ask for something more reliable.

Dill water, a gentle carminative, may be useful, as may dimethicone which is a silicone polymer oil, useful as a skin barrier cream or ointment base, but used here to reduce surface tension and allow froth to coalesce, so that it may more easily be expelled from either end.

Witches' milk

Surprisingly, the breasts of newborn babies sometimes produce milk. The reason is interesting. Throughout the pregnancy, the output of the milk-promoting hormone, prolactin, by the mother's pituitary gland has been rising steadily. At the time of birth, peak concentrations of this hormone are circulating freely in the mother's blood. Some of this hormone enters the baby's blood through the placenta and acts on the baby's breasts in exactly the same way as it acts on the mother's. The baby, however, produces no prolactin of its own and the effect soon wears off.

Wry neck see TORTICOLLIS.

Yellow skin see JAUNDICE.

GLOSSARY

The terms in this short medical dictionary have been selected for their relevance to children and to supplement the information in the main body of the encyclopedia.

abdomen, acute any serious internal intestinal problem.

abrasion, dental wearing away of the teeth. This may result from over-enthusiastic scrubbing with hard toothbrushes or from tooth-grinding (bruxism).

abscess a localised collection of pus following an infection.

abscess, dental a collection of pus at the root of a tooth.

accident-prone more than normally liable to accidental injury. Many active children are accident-prone from heedlessness or from lack of awareness of danger.

accommodation the act of focusing the eyes.

achalasia a swallowing disorder from spasm of the gullet.

Achilles tendon the prominent tendon above the heel.

achondroplasia a genetically-caused form of dwarfism.

acne a skin disorder involving the oil-producing glands. Most cases occur in adolescents, but infantile acne is not uncommon.

acrocyanosis blueness of the hands and feet from poor circulation.

actinic pertaining to sunlight. Actinic skin damage and actinic-induced skin cancers are on the increase.

acuity, visual clarity of seeing.

acute of sudden onset, severe, and of short duration. Compare 'chronic' which means persistent or long-lasting.

Adam's apple the bump on the front of the neck caused by the voice box (larynx).

adenitis inflammation of glands or lymph nodes.

adenoidectomy removal of the adenoids.

adenoids masses of lymph tissue at the back of the nose.

adhesion a sticking, or healing, together.

adipose tissue fat.

adrenal glands the glands, on top of each kidney, which produce steroid hormones and adrenaline.

adrenal hyperplasia, congenital enlargement and overactivity of the adrenal glands, present at birth.

adrenaline an adrenal hormone which helps the body to cope with highly stressful emergency situations.

adrenogenital syndrome premature sexual development and male changes in girls.

aetiology cause.

aggression a tendency to attack or assault, physically or in words.

airway the vital route of air from the atmosphere to the lungs.

airway obstruction any partial or total blockage of the airway.

albinism a genetically caused lack of body colour.

albumin an important blood protein.

albuminuria albumin in the urine suggesting kidney disease.

alignment, dental the proper relationship of the teeth to each other.

allergy an abnormal sensitivity to any substance, contact with which causes various symptoms.

allopathy orthodox medicine.

alopecia baldness, patchy or total.

amaurotic familial idiocy a serious genetic disorder causing blindness and learning difficulty.

ambidexterity able to use either hand with equal facility.

amblyopia loss of clear vision due to disuse rather than organic disease.

amelogenesis imperfecta a hereditary tooth defect causing brown mottling.

ametropia a defect of eye focusing – long sight, short sight or astigmatism.

amphetamine a powerful stimulant of the nervous system.

ampicillin a widely used antibiotic drug. Also called Penbritin.

amputation, congenital born with a limb, or part of a limb, missing.

anaemia less than normal oxygen-carrying haemoglobin in the blood.

anaemia, aplastic anaemia due to failure of blood production in the bone marrow.

anaemia, iron-deficiency anaemia due to insufficient iron in the diet, or to excess blood loss.

anal dilatation an unreliable test for child sexual abuse.

anal stenosis abnormal narrowing of the anus. Sometimes called anal stricture.

angioedema local allergic swellings of the skin. Also called urticaria or hives.

anisometropia a difference of focus in the two eyes.

anthelmintic drugs drugs used to get rid of worms.

antibiotic drugs drugs used to combat infection with bacteria.

anticonvulsant drugs drugs used to prevent or control epileptic fits.

antidiarrhoeal drugs drugs used to treat diarrhoea.

antihistamine drugs drugs used in allergic conditions or as sedatives.

antipyretic drugs drugs to control fever.

antitussive cough prevention or checking.

antiviral drugs drugs used to combat virus infections.

anuria absence of urine from cessation of production.

anus the outlet canal for faeces.

anus, imperforate closure over of the anus, present at birth.

aorta the main artery of the body.

aortic incompetence failure of the main outlet valve of the heart.

aortic stenosis narrowing of the main outlet valve of the heart.

aperient a gentle laxative.

Apgar score a system of assessment of the condition of a newborn baby, done in the first five minutes of life.

appendicectomy removal of the appendix.

appendicitis inflammation of the appendix.

appendix the short, worm-like tube connected to the start of the large intestine.

arachnodactyly spider-like fingers. A feature of Marfan's syndrome.

ascariasis roundworm infestation.

ascorbic acid vitamin C.

asphyxia suffocation.

aspiration sucking out fluid or accidentally breathing in fluid or solid matter.

asthma a disease affecting the ability to breathe easily.

astigmatism a focusing error caused by lack of even curvature of the cornea (the outer lens of the eye).

asymptomatic free of symptoms.

atopy a tendency to allergies such as asthma, eczema and hay fever.

atrium one of the upper chambers of the heart.

atrophy shrinkage or wasting of an organ or a bodily tissue.

audiogram a graph of the hearing sensitivity.

audiometry the method of testing hearing.

aura a strange feeling which warns that an epileptic or migraine attack is coming.

auriscope an instrument for examining the inside of the ear.

auscultation listening to the chest, or other part, with a stethoscope.

autism a condition in which a child is unable to form normal relationships with others.

autoimmune disorders diseases caused by an attack, by the body's immune system, on parts of its own body.

axilla the armpit.

bacillary dysentery an acute infection of the bowel, featuring diarrhoea, colicky abdominal pain, fever, blood and pus in the stools, and dehydration.

bacteria germs. Single-celled, microscopic, living organisms occurring in countless numbers almost everywhere. Bacteria produce powerful poisons that damage cells and cause disease.

bacterial encephalitis inflammation of the brain caused by bacteria.

bacterial meningitis see MENINGITIS.

bacterium the singular of BACTERIA.

bacteriuria bacteria in the urine. The presence of 100,000 or more disease-producing bacteria per millilitre of urine indicates a urinary tract infection.

bad trip a popular expression for a highly unpleasant reaction to a hallucinogenic drug. Such reactions may recur months later without further exposure to the drug.

balanitis inflammation of the bulb (GLANS) of the penis.

balanoposthitis inflammation of the glans of the penis and of the foreskin (prepuce).

bandage a binder. A strip of woven cotton, wool, plastic, rubber or other material wrapped firmly round any part of the body for a variety of reasons. Bandages may be non-stretch or elastic, conforming or otherwise, adhesive or plain.

barium meal an X-ray examination enhanced by the use of the insoluble barium sulphate, usually in the form of a liquid suspension.

barotrauma injury resulting from changes in atmospheric (barometric) pressure as in aircraft flight. Barotrauma mostly affects the ear-drums when there is obstruction to the eustachian tubes.

bar reader a device used in orthoptics consisting of a narrow, opaque strip fixed between the child's eyes and the printed page, so that different parts of the page are occluded from each eye. The method is used to promote binocular vision.

barrier creams creams used to protect the skin against environmental hazards such as dirty nappies or ammoniacal urine.

barrier nursing local isolation of a patient with an infectious disease so as to avoid spread.

basal meningitis meningitis affecting primarily the membranes covering the base of the brain.

bat ear a minor disfigurement of childhood in which the ears are larger and more protruding than usual.

battered-baby syndrome the clinical condition of a baby or young child who has been assaulted.

B cells one of the two main classes of lymphocytes – white cells found in the blood, lymph nodes and tissue – which, with other cells, form the immune system of the body.

BCG bacille Calmette-Guérin, a modified form of the tubercle bacillus, used to stimulate a protective immunological response from the body.

belly button a slang term for the navel (umbilicus).

benign opposite of malignant. Mild, not usually tending to cause death.

biceps muscle the prominent and powerful muscle on the front of the upper arm which bends the elbow and rotates the forearm outwards.

bilateral involving or affecting both sides. In the case of paired organs, bilateral means affecting both of them.

bile the dark greenish-brown fluid secreted by the liver, stored and concentrated in the gall bladder, and ejected into the duodenum to assist in the absorption of fats.

biliary atresia a congenital disorder in which the larger branches of the bile ducts are so narrowed that the bile cannot escape and the baby becomes severely jaundiced with enlargement of the liver.

biliousness an inaccurate term for the feeling of nausea and flatulence associated with minor dyspepsia or any other mild stomach upset.

bilirubin the coloured substance in bile derived from the breakdown of haemoglobin in effete red blood cells at the end of their 120-day life.

binocular vision simultaneous perception with both eyes.

binovular of twins, derived from two separate eggs and thus non-identical.

biopsy a small sample of tissue, taken for microscopic examination, so that the nature of a disease process can be determined.

birth injury an injury sustained during birth.

birthmarks benign tumours of skin blood vessels, including the temporary strawberry marks, port-wine stains (capillary haemangiomas) and the conspicuous cavernous haemangiomas.

Bitot's spots foamy white patches in the conjunctiva at the corners of the eyes, strongly suggestive of vitamin A deficiency.

blackhead an accumulation of fatty sebaceous material in a sebaceous gland or hair follicle, with oxidation of the outer layer, causing a colour change.

blackout a common term for any temporary loss of vision or consciousness.

Blalock's operation a palliative operation performed for the relief of Fallot's tetralogy in very young babies.

blepharitis inflammation of the eyelids.

blepharoptosis a drooping eyelid. Usually called 'ptosis'.

blepharospasm uncontrollable winking or sustained tight closure of the eyes.

blood count determination of the number of red and white blood cells per millilitre of blood.

blood culture incubation of a sample of blood in a suitable culture medium to grow bacteria for purposes of identification.

blood vessel any artery, arteriole, capillary, venule or vein.

blue baby a baby with an inadequate amount of oxygen in the blood, resulting in cyanosis.

boil an infection of a hair follicle which has progressed to abscess formation.

bonding the formation of a strong relationship, particularly that between a mother and her newborn child.

bone marrow the substance contained within bone cavities. The marrow cells form all the cells of the blood, both red and white.

bone marrow biopsy a sample of marrow usually taken from the crest of the pelvis.

bone marrow transplant a means of providing a recipient with a new set of blood-forming cells from which a continuing supply of healthy new red and white blood cells can be derived.

booster a dose of a vaccine, given at an interval after the primary vaccination, to increase the effect.

borborygmi bowel noises.

bottle-feeding the alternative to breast-feeding for babies. Formula milk contains none of the valuable antibodies present in the mother's milk.

bowel the intestine.

bow legs bandy legs or genu varum.

brace an orthodontic appliance used to correct malposition of the teeth by exerting pressure in the desired direction, or an externally worn leg support.

brain fever a common term for encephalitis.

breast-feeding the normal, and best, method of providing baby nutrition.

breast pump a device used to relieve engorged and painful breasts of excess milk, or to remove milk for use later.

breath-holding attacks a form of infantile blackmail imposed on indulgent parents by determined and manipulative young children.

bronchial pertaining to any part of the branching system of breathing tubes (the bronchial tree).

bronchitis acute or chronic inflammation of the lining of a bronchus.

bronchoconstriction contraction of the circular muscles in the walls of the bronchi, so narrowing the bore of the tubes and restricting air entry.

bronchodilatation widening of the bore of a bronchus by relaxation of the circular muscles in its wall.

bronchus a breathing tube. A branch of the windpipe (trachea) or of another bronchus.

bruise the appearance caused by blood released into or under the skin.

bruxism habitual grinding or clenching of the teeth, often to the point of wearing away the enamel and eroding the crowns.

buccal relating to the cheek.

buck teeth undue protrusion of the central upper teeth. This can readily be put right by orthodontic treatment.

buphthalmos enlargement of the corneas resulting from abnormally raised pressure within the eyes at birth (congenital glaucoma).

———

cachexia a state of severe muscle wasting and weakness occurring in the late stages of serious illness.

caesarian section an operation to deliver a baby through an incision in the abdomen, performed when natural delivery is impracticable or dangerous, or urgency is necessary.

calcium a mineral present in large quantity in the body, mainly in the form of calcium phosphate in the bones and the teeth, but not in the nails.

cancrum oris a disease affecting grossly malnourished and neglected children in which infection, ulceration and progressive tissue destruction occur around the mouth until large areas of both cheeks and nose are eaten away.

Candida albicans the common thrush fungus.

candidiasis thrush. Also known as candidosis.

canthus the corner the eye where the upper and lower eyelids meet. In epicanthus, the upper lid margin curves over to conceal the canthus.

caput succedaneum a boggy (oedematous) swelling of a baby's scalp seen for a period after birth and caused by sustained scalp pressure against the edges of the widened (dilated) cervix. The caput disappears within hours or days.

cardiopathy any heart disorder or disease.

cardiovascular relating to the heart and its connected, closed circulatory system of blood vessels.

carminative having the power to relax muscle rings (sphincters) so as to release gas and relieve flatulence. A drug having this property.

cartilage gristle. A dense form of connective tissue performing various functions in the body, such as providing a supportive tissue in which bone may be formed during growth.

casein a protein derived from milk.

cataract opacification of the internal focusing lens of the eye. This may be congenital.

caul a persistent amnion membrane covering the baby's head at birth.

cavus a foot deformity in which the longitudinal arch is greatly exaggerated.

cephalhaematoma a collection of blood between a baby's skull and the overlying membrane, usually resulting from unavoidable injury sustained in the course of a difficult forceps delivery.

cerebellum the smaller sub-brain lying below and behind the cerebrum. The cerebellum is concerned with the coordination of information concerned with posture, balance and fine voluntary movement.

cerebral palsy spastic paralysis.

cerebrum the larger, and most highly developed, part of the brain. It contains the neural structures for memory and personality, cerebration, volition, speech, vision, hearing, voluntary movement, all bodily sensation, smell, taste and other functions.

cervical pertaining to a neck. This may be the neck of the body or the neck of an organ such as the womb.

cervical incompetence the inability of the inner opening of the neck of the womb to remain properly closed. This is a cause of repeated, painless, spontaneous abortions around the fourth or fifth month of pregnancy.

chemosis collection of fluid under the conjunctiva covering the white of the eye so that it balloons forward.

child abuse active assault or physical or emotional neglect of a child.

child guidance the skilled management of problems such as solitariness, anxiety, phobias, serious learning difficulties, persistent bedwetting, sleep disturbances or persistently aggressive behaviour.

cholesteatoma a tumour-like mass of cells, shed by the outer layer of an infected eardrum, which relentlessly invades the middle ear through a perforation in the drum, to cause serious internal damage.

chorea an involuntary, purposeless jerky movement, repeatedly affecting especially the face, shoulders and hips. Popularly called St Vitus' dance.

choreiform resembling chorea.

chorionic villi the finger-like projections from the chorion into the wall of the womb at the site at which the placenta is developing.

chorionic villus sampling removal, by way of a fine tube or needle, of a small part of the tissue in process of forming the placenta. This has the same DNA as the embryo, so allows gene analysis and may give very early warning of inherited disease.

chromosome analysis examination of stained chromosomes in a stage at which they are widely separated and easily visualized.

chromosomes the coiled DNA structures, present in all body cells, which carry the genetic code for the construction of the body.

chronic lasting for a long time.

circumcision surgical removal of the male foreskin (prepuce) or of parts of the female external genitalia.

clavicle the collar bone.

cleft lip and palate a developmental defect caused by the failure of full fusion together of the processes which grow out from the front end of the primitive tube-like structure of the body to form the face.

cleidocranial dysostosis a congenital disorder featuring defective bone formation in the collar bones (clavicles) and the skull.

coarctation of the aorta a congenital narrowing of a short section of the main artery of the body, the aorta.

codliver oil an extract of the liver of the codfish, rich in vitamins A and D.

coeliac disease an intestinal disorder caused by intolerance to the protein gluten in wheat and rye.

colon the large intestine.

colostrum the yellowish, protein-rich, milk-like fluid secreted by the breasts for the first two or three days after the birth of a baby. Colostrum contains large fat globules and a high content of antibodies.

coma a state of deep unconsciousness from which the affected person cannot be aroused even by strong stimulation.

combined immune deficiency disease a condition in which both main classes of immune system cells, the T cells and the B cells, are absent. The effect is a severe, and usually fatal, inability to resist infection.

complementary feeding bottle-feeding of a baby primarily nourished from the breast.

complication an additional disorder, or new feature, arising in the course of, or as a result of, a disease, injury or abnormality.

compound fracture a bone break with perforation of the skin.

concussion a 'shaking-up' of the brain, from violent acceleration or deceleration of the head, causing unconsciousness lasting for seconds to hours.

congenital present at birth. A congenital disorder need not be hereditary, although many are.

congestion an abnormal collection of fluid, often blood, in an organ or part. Congestion is the result of some other disease process, such as infection or heart failure, and will usually settle when the cause is removed.

conjunctiva the transparent membrane attached around the cornea, covering the white of the eye and curving back over the inner surfaces of the eyelids.

conjunctivitis inflammation of the conjunctiva.

conservative treatment treatment that avoids extreme or radical measures but which aims to maintain or improve the state of the patient.

constipation unduly infrequent and difficult evacuation of the bowels.

consultant highly qualified and selected specialist doctor who practises without supervision.

contraindication anything which makes a proposed or possible form of medical treatment undesirable or dangerous.

convalescence the period of recovery following an illness, injury or surgical operation. The process of such recovery.

convulsion a fit or seizure.

cornea the outer, and principal, lens of the eye through which the coloured iris with its central hole (the pupil) can be seen.

cover test a test for squint (strabismus).

cradle cap a type of seborrhoeic dermatitis occurring in infants and consisting of thick, yellow, greasy, crusted scales on the scalp. It is easily treated.

cretinism a condition caused by thyroid underaction from severe iodine deficiency early in life.

cross-eye the popular term for strabismus or squint.

croup inflammation and swelling of the main air tubes to the lungs (laryngotracheobronchitis) affecting young children and causing difficult, harsh, noisy and painful breathing and a typical 'barking' cough.

cryptorchidism undescended testicle.

cyanosis blueness of the skin from insufficient oxygen in the blood.

cyclical vomiting periodic attacks of vomiting in children with no discernible cause.

cystitis inflammation of the urinary bladder caused by infection.

---

dacryocystitis inflammation of the tear sac (lacrimal sac) which lies in the eye socket (orbit), between the inner corner of the eye and the nose.

dandruff a popular term for pityriasis capitis, a condition featuring scaliness of the scalp from flakes of dead skin.

debility lack of strength due to loss of muscle bulk and reduction in the efficiency of the heart and respiratory system from disease or disuse.

defaecation voluntary or involuntary emptying of the rectum so as to relieve oneself of accumulated faeces.

deficiency diseases the large range of conditions resulting from the lack of any of the essential nutritional elements, such as protein, vitamins or minerals, or from the body's inability to digest, absorb or utilize these.

dehydration a reduction in the normal water content of the body.

delayed speech failure of development of speech by the end of the second year of life.

delirium a mental disturbance from disorder of brain function caused by high fever, head injury, drug intoxication, drug overdosage or drug withdrawal.

deltoid muscle the large, triangular 'shoulder-pad' muscle which raises the arm sideways.

deltoid ligament the strong triangular ligament, on the inner side of the ankle, which helps to bind the foot to the leg.

Denis Browne splints splints used to correct club foot (talipes equinovarus) in infants.

dental caries tooth decay.

dental floss strong, often waxed, thread used to remove plaque from around the necks of the teeth and discourage dental caries.

deoxyribonucleic acid DNA.

dermatitis inflammation of the skin from any cause.

diagnosis the art and science of identifying the disease causing a particular set of clinical signs and symptoms.

diarrhoea the result of unduly rapid transit of the bowel contents so that there is insufficient time for reabsorption of water to firm up the faeces.

Dick test a test of susceptibility to scarlet fever.

diplopia double vision.

disclosing agents stains that reveal plaque on the teeth to encourage regular toothbrushing and flossing.

disease any abnormal condition of the body or part of it, arising from any cause. A specific disorder that features a recognizable complex of physical signs, symptoms and effects.

drug abuse the use of any drug, for recreational or pleasure purposes, which is currently disapproved of by the majority of the members of a society.

ductus arteriosus a short shunting artery lying, during fetal life, between the main artery to the lungs (pulmonary artery) and the main artery to the body (aorta).

dwarfism abnormal shortness of stature.

---

earache pain arising from the external ear passage, the ear-drum, the space between the drum and the inner ear (the middle ear) or, rarely, the inner ear.

ear-drum the freely mobile membrane that separates the inner end of the external auditory canal (the meatus) from the middle ear.

ecstasy a popular name for the drug 3,4-methylenedioxymetamphetamine (MDMA), a hallucinogenic amphetamine with effects that are a combination of those of LSD and amphetamine.

eczema a skin disorder featuring itching, scaly red patches and small fluid-filled blisters which burst, releasing serum, so that the skin becomes moist, 'weeping' and crusty.

egg the ovum or female reproductive cell (gamete).

Ehlers-Danlos syndrome a genetic disorder in which the skin is abnormally elastic so that it may be greatly stretched.

embryo an organism in its earliest stages of development, especially before it has reached a stage at which it can be distinguished from other species.

emergency any sudden crisis, calling for urgent intervention to avoid a serious outcome.

encopresis faecal incontinence or soiling not due to organic disease or involuntary loss of control, but resulting from deliberate intent.

endemic occurring continuously in a particular population.

endocrine system the group of hormone-producing glands.

enema the introduction of various fluids, solutions or suspensions into the rectum to treat constipation, to assist in X-ray or endoscopic examination, or to administer drugs or nutrients.

entropion inward curling of the margin of an eyelids so that the lashes tend to rub against the eye.

enuresis bedwetting. The involuntary passage of urine, especially during sleep.

enzyme a biochemical catalyst that enormously accelerates a chemical reaction.

epidemic the occurrence of a large number of cases of a particular disease in a given population, within a period of a few weeks.

epiphora running over of tears as a result of failure of the normal tear drainage into the nose.

epiphysis the growing sector at the end of a long bone.

epistaxis nose bleed.

erythroblastosis fetalis the type of severe anaemia with jaundice caused in babies by rhesus factor incompatibility.

eustachian tube a short passage leading backwards from the back of the nose, just above the soft palate, on either side, to the cavity of the middle ear.

Ewing's tumour a very malignant bone cancer affecting children up to the age of about 15.

exchange transfusion the treatment given urgently to all babies with severe haemolytic disease of the newborn (erythroblastosis fetalis) from rhesus incompatibility with the mother.

exophthalmos protrusion of an eyeball.

exotropia divergence of the lines of vision of the two eyes. Divergent squint.

expressing milk removal of excess milk from tight and uncomfortable breasts by simulating with the fingers the action of the baby's gums.

---

facial pertaining to the face.

faecalith fecal matter that has become so hard as to resemble a stone.

faeces the natural effluent from the intestinal tract.

fainting temporary loss of consciousness due to brain deprivation of an adequate supply of blood and thus oxygen and glucose.

familial occurring in some families but not in others, as a result of genetic transmission.

family therapy the treatment of behavioural and emotional problems in an individual by involvement of the whole family in the treatment process.

fascia tendon-like connective tissue arranged in sheets or layers under the skin, between the muscles and around the organs, the blood vessel and the nerves.

fatigue physical or mental tiredness.

febrile pertaining to, or featuring, a fever.

febrile convulsion a seizure or fit caused by a sudden rise in temperature.

femoral pertaining to the thigh or the thigh bone (femur).

fertilization the union of the spermatozoon with the egg (ovum) so that the full complement of chromosomes is made up and the process of cell division, to form a new individual, is started.

fetal alcohol syndrome the group of damaging effects caused to the growing fetus by sustained high levels of alcohol in the mother's blood during pregnancy.

fetal asphyxia the serious condition of deprivation of oxygen to the fetus from interference with its blood supply.

fetal distress observable changes in the fetus during pregnancy or, more often, labour, caused mainly by an insufficient oxygen supply via the placenta.

fetus the developing individual from about the eighth or tenth week of life in the womb until the time of birth.

fever elevation of body temperature above about 37°C, taken in the mouth.

fibrous tissue a simple, strong structural or repair tissue consisting of twisted stands of collagen and laid down by cells known as fibroblasts.

first degree burn a mild, fully recoverable degree of burning causing only redness of the skin.

fistula an abnormal communication between any part of the interior of the body and the surface of the skin, or between two internal organs.

flat foot the condition in which the normal longitudinal arch of the foot has collapsed.

fontanelles the gaps between the bones of the vault of the growing skull of the baby and young infant that can be felt, as soft depressions on the top of the head, by gentle pressure with the fingers.

food additives substances, numbered in thousands, added to food for purposes of preservation, appearance, flavour, texture or nutritional value.

food allergy sensitivity to one or more of the components of normal diets.

foramen a natural hole in a bone for the passage of a nerve, artery or a vein or other anatomical structure.

forceps delivery delivery of a baby assisted by traction on the head with obstetrical forceps after the neck of the womb (cervix) is fully widened (dilated).

foreskin the prepuce or hood of thin skin that covers the bulb (glans) of the penis.

fragile X syndrome a major genetic disorder caused by a constriction near the end of the long arm of an X chromosome.

frequency an informal term referring to the condition in which urine is passed more often than normal (frequency of urination).

frontal pertaining to the forehead or to the frontal bone.

frontal sinus one of a pair of mucous membrane-lined air spaces of variable size lying behind and above the level of the eyebrows.

funnel chest a condition in which the breastbone is hollowed backwards, especially at its lower end.

———

gag a device used by dental and other surgeons to keep the mouth wide open and permit oral treatment.

gait the particular way in which a person walks.

galactosaemia a genetic disorder due to the absence of an enzyme necessary for the breakdown of milk sugar (galactose) to glucose.

gallows traction a method of treating fractures of the thigh bone (femur) in young children. Skin traction is applied to both legs and the child is suspended from a beam so that the buttocks are just clear of the bed.

gamete a cell such as a sperm or ovum.

gametogenesis the production of gametes.

gamma globulin a protein, one of the five classes of immunoglobulins (antibodies). Gamma globulin, or immunoglobulin G (IgG), is the most prevalent and provides the body's main antibody defence against infection.

gangrene death of tissue, usually as a result of loss of an adequate blood supply.

gargoylism the effect of one of a number of X-linked or autosomal recessive disorders of metabolism that cause coarsening of the features, excessive hairiness and often learning difficulty.

gastric pertaining to the stomach.

gastroenteritis inflammation of the lining of the stomach and the small intestine from infection with germs.

gene the physical unit of heredity, represented as a continuous sequence of bases, arranged in a code, in groups of three, along the length of a DNA molecule (nucleic acid).

general practitioner a doctor who does not specialize in any particular branch of medicine but who treats a wide variety of relatively minor medical conditions and is able to discern those conditions requiring specialist attention.

generic drug a drug sold under the official medical name of the basic active substance.

genetics the branch of biology concerned with the structure, location, abnormalities and effects of the genes.

genome the complete set of chromosomes, together with the mitochondrial DNA, containing the entire genetic material of the cell.

genu valgum knock-knee.

genu varum bow or bandy legs.

germ a popular term for any organism capable of causing disease.

German measles rubella.

gigantism excessive body growth. This is usually the result of an abnormal production of growth hormone by the pituitary gland in childhood.

gingivitis inflammation of the gums.

glans the acorn-shaped bulb at the end of the penis or the small piece of erectile tissue at the tip of the clitoris.

glaucoma a rise in the pressure in the fluids within the eye of sufficient degree to cause internal damage and affect vision.

glomerulonephritis inflammation of the kidneys.

glossitis inflammation of the tongue.

glue ear secretory otitis media.

glue sniffing solvent abuse.

goitre enlargement of the thyroid gland from any cause.

gonads the sex glands. The ovaries in the female and the testicles in the male.

greenstick fracture a type of long bone break common in children, in which the fracture is incomplete, the bone being bent on one side and splintered on the other.

grey baby syndrome a dangerous condition of acute failure of the blood circulation caused by the antibiotic chloramphenicol.

grommet a short tube used to secure and maintain drainage of the middle ear, through the ear-drum, in cases of 'glue ear'.

growing pains a popular medical fiction. Growth is never painful.

growth hormone the hormone, somatotrophin, produced by the pituitary gland, that controls protein synthesis and hence the process of growth.

gullet the common term for the oesophagus.

gumboil an abscess in the gum and the outer bone covering (periosteum) arising from a spread of infection from a decayed tooth.

Guthrie test a sensitive test for phenylketonuria that can be done on the newborn baby.

gynaecomastia the occurrence in the male of breasts resembling those of the sexually mature female.

———

haematemesis vomiting blood.

haematoma an accumulation of free blood anywhere in the body, that has partially clotted to form a semi-solid mass.

haematuria blood in the urine.

haemoglobin the iron-containing protein that fills red blood cells and links readily to oxygen.

haemoglobinopathies a group of inherited diseases in which there are specific abnormalities in the haemoglobin molecule. The group includes sickle cell disease and the thalassaemias.

haemolysis destruction of red blood cells by rupture of the cell envelope and release of the contained haemoglobin.

haemolytic pertaining to haemolysis.

haemolytic anaemia a form of anaemia arising from haemoglobin loss as a result of increased fragility of red blood cells.

haemoptysis coughing up blood.

haemorrhage bleeding.

handicap any physical, mental or emotional disability that limits full, normal life activity.

hare lip a lay term for the appearance caused by a badly repaired cleft lip.

heart failure the condition in which the heart is no longer capable of pumping a sufficient volume of blood to meet the body's needs for oxygen and nutrition.

heart rate the number of contractions of the pumping chambers of the heart per minute.

Henoch-Schönlein purpura a bleeding disorder, mainly affecting children and caused by an allergic (anaphylactoid) reaction.

heredity the transmission from parent to child of any of the characteristics coded for in the chemical sequences on DNA known as the genes.

hermaphroditism the rare bodily condition in which both male and female reproductive organs are present, often in an ambiguous form.

hernia abnormal protrusion of an organ or tissue through a natural or abnormal opening.

heroin babies babies who have received a regular morphine dosage via the placenta before birth and who show withdrawal signs after birth.

histology the study of the microscopic structure of the body.

humerus the long upper arm bone.

hydrocephalus 'water on the brain' – an abnormal accumulation of cerebrospinal fluid within, and around, the brain.

hygiene the study of the promotion of health.

hyperextension 'over-straightening' of a joint beyond its normal limits.

hyperflexion bending beyond the normal limits.

hyperpyrexia body temperature above 41.1°C (106°F).

hypervitaminosis one of a number of disorders that can result from excessive intake of certain vitamins, especially vitamins A and D.

hypospadias a congenital abnormality of the penis in which the urine tube (urethra) opens on the underside of the organ, either at the neck of the bulb (glans) or further back.

———

iatrogenic pertaining to disease or disorder caused by doctors.

icterus an alternative term for JAUNDICE.

identical twins twins derived from the same egg (ovum) which, after the first division, has separated into two individuals. Identical twins thus have the same genetics.

ileum the third part of the small intestine lying between the jejunum and the start of the large intestine, the caecum.

immunization the process of conferring a degree of protection or immunity against infection or the effects of infection.

immunodeficiency disorders any one of a number of congenital or acquired conditions in which the body's immunological system of defence against infection, foreign material and some forms of cancer, is defective.

immunoglobulins antibodies.

immunosuppressant drugs drugs which act on any part of the immune system of the body, so as to interfere with the normal reactions to the presence of any antigen.

imperforate having no opening. Used of a structure normally having an opening, as of an imperforate hymen or anus.

incidence the number of new cases of an event, such as a disease, occurring in a particular population during a given period. Incidence is usually expressed as so many cases per 1000, or per 100,000, per year.

incision a surgical cut made to achieve access or to allow discharge of unwanted material such as pus.

incisor one of the four central teeth of each jaw, with cutting edges for biting pieces off food.

incontinence loss of voluntary control of one or both of the excretory functions.

incubation period the interval between the time of infection and the first appearance of symptoms of the resulting disease.

incubator a piece of equipment providing a closed, controllable environment in which optimal conditions may be established for the nutrition, growth and preservation of premature babies.

infant mortality the number of infants per thousand live births who die before reaching the age of 1 year.

infectious mononucleosis glandular fever.

inferior situated below.

inflammation the response of living tissue to injury, featuring widening of blood vessels, with redness, heat, swelling and pain. Inflammation also involves loss of function and is the commonest of all the disease processes. It is expressed by the ending '-itis'.

informed consent the formal agreement to a surgical or medical procedure by a patient or parent who has been adequately briefed on what is proposed and who is fully aware of all reasonably possible side-effects or complications.

inguinal pertaining to the groin.

inhalers devices for delivering medication in aerosol, vapour or powder form to the bronchial tubes and lungs, especially for the treatment of asthma.

inoculation immunization or vaccination.

intensive care the application of close and continuous monitoring of the condition of patients in a critical or unstable condition who are liable to die suddenly unless certain danger signs are detected early and appropriate action taken.

interventricular septal defect an abnormal congenital opening in the wall (septum) between the two lower chambers (ventricles) of the heart. One of the 'hole in the heart' disorders.

intraocular pressure the hydrostatic pressure within the otherwise collapsible eyeball necessary to maintain its shape and permit normal optical functioning.

intravenous within a vein or into a vein. Intravenous injection of a drug achieves rapid action.

intussusception the movement of a length of bowel into an adjacent segment, in the manner of a telescope.

in vitro occurring in the laboratory rather than in the body. Literally, 'in glass'.

in vivo occurring naturally within the body.

ischaemia inadequate flow of blood to any part of the body.

---

jaw winking an inherited condition, also known as the Marcus Gunn syndrome, in which there is a drooping eyelid (ptosis) that retracts suddenly and momentarily when the mouth is opened wide or the jaw is moved firmly to one side.

Jehovah's Witnesses a widespread religious group who interpret certain passages in the bible, which they take as a literal record of God's word, as a prohibition of blood transfusion. Many have died after refusing critically needed medical treatment. Most doctors respect this view except when it is applied to young children.

jejunum the length of small intestine lying between the duodenum and the ileum and occupying the central part of the abdomen.

jugular pertaining to the throat or neck.

jugular veins the six main veins that run down the front and side of the neck, carrying blood back to the heart from the head.

junk food a popular term for highly refined and processed, readily assimilable and palatable food with a low level of roughage. Junk food has a high calorific value but is often low in vitamins and minerals.

juvenile delinquency criminal behaviour by a young person.

---

karyotype the individual chromosomal complement of a person or species, or the chromosomes of an individual set out in a standard pattern.

keloid an abnormal healing response causing scars that are markedly overgrown, thickened and disfiguring. Keloids are commoner in black people than in white.

keratin a hard protein (scleroprotein) of cylindrical, helical molecular form, occurring in horny tissue such as hair and nails and in the outer layers of the skin.

keratoconus a growth disorder (dystrophy) of the cornea causing central peaking or conicity and affecting vision.

kerion a localized boggy swelling on the scalp with oozing of pus and serum from the hair follicles. Kerion is a reaction to fungus infection of the scalp (tinea capitis) and is self-curing.

kernicterus jaundice of the brain resulting from rhesus factor disease in babies.

kidneys paired, reddish brown, bean-shaped structures lying in pads of fat on the inside of the back wall of the abdomen on either side of the spine, just above the waist. The kidneys filter the blood, remove waste material and adjust the levels of essential chemical substances to keep them within necessary limits. In so doing, they produce a sterile solution called urine.

kidney failure the stage in kidney disease in which neither organ is capable of excreting body waste products fast enough to prevent their accumulation in the blood.

kidney transplant the insertion of a donated kidney into the body and connection of its blood vessels to the host vessels and its ureter to the host bladder.

kilocalorie the amount of heat needed to raise the temperature of a kilogram of water by 1°C. This has been the standard nutritional unit of energy for years, but is now being replaced by the kilojoule. 1 kcal = 4.2 KJ.

kiss of life mouth-to-mouth or mouth-to-nose artificial respiration.

Klinefelter's syndrome a male bodily disorder caused by one or more additional X (sex) chromosomes. This has a feminizing effect.

Koplik's spots tiny white spots, surrounded by a red base, occurring on the inside of the cheeks and the inner surface of the lower lip during the incubation period of measles.

kwashiorkor a serious nutritional deficiency disease of young children resulting from gross dietary protein deficiency with a high intake of carbohydrate of low nutritional value.

kyphoscoliosis an abnormal degree of backward curvature of the dorsal spine (kyphosis) combined with curvature to one side (scoliosis).

kyphosis an abnormal degree of backward curvature of the part of the spine between the neck and the lumbar regions.

---

labyrinth the cavities of the internal ear, comprising the vestibule, semicircular canals and the cochlea.

labyrinthitis inflammation, usually as a result of an influenza or mumps virus infection, of the part of the inner ear responsible for balance.

lacrimal pertaining to the tears, to their production and to their disposal.

lacrimal canaliculus one of four tiny tubes that carry tears from the inner corners of the four eyelids to the lacrimal sac.

lacrimal gland the tear-secreting gland lying in the upper and outer corner of the bony eye socket (orbit), and opening by many small ducts into the upper cul-de-sac of the conjunctiva behind the upper lid.

lactation the secretion and production of milk in the breasts after childbirth.

lanugo the short, downy, colourless hair that covers the fetus from about the fourth month to shortly before the time of birth. Similar hair sometimes grows on girls with anorexia nervosa.

laparoscopy direct visual examination of the interior of the abdomen, through a narrow optical device (endoscope), passed through a natural orifice or a small incision in the abdominal wall.

laparotomy an exploratory operation performed for purposes of diagnosis.

larynx the 'Adam's apple' or voice box.

latent present but not manifest. Not yet having an effect.

lateral of, at or towards the side of the body.

laughing gas a popular term for the anaesthetic drug nitrous oxide.

Laurence-Moon-Barogt-Biedl syndrome a rare genetic disorder featuring learning difficulty, extra toes or fingers, and a retinal degeneration – retinitis pigmentosa – that may progress to blindness.

Lesch-Nyhan syndrome a rare X-linked recessive disease of boys in which a severe over-production of uric acid causes gout, cerebral palsy, learning difficulty, chorea and compulsive self-mutilating biting.

lesion a useful and widely used medical term denoting any injury, wound, infection, or any structural or other form of abnormality anywhere in the body.

leucocyte any kind of white blood cell.

leucocytosis an increased concentration of white cells (leucocytes) in the blood other than one caused by one of the leukaemias.

lice small, wingless, insect parasites of humans.

ligaments bundles of a tough, fibrous, elastic protein called collagen that act as binding and supporting materials in the body, especially in and around joints of all kinds.

ligature any thread-like surgical material tied tightly round any structure.

listeriosis an infection with the organism, *Listeria monocytogenes*, which is found in most meats, poultry, fish, crustaceans and in soft cheeses and various pre-cooked foods.

liver the largest organ of the abdomen occupying the upper right corner and across the midline to the left side. The liver receives chemical substances in the blood, especially in the nutrient-rich blood from the intestines, and processes these according to the needs of the body. It takes up the products of old red blood cells and converts these into bile. It breaks down toxic substances into safer forms including urea, which is excreted in the urine.

liver failure the end stage of severe liver disease in which liver function is so impaired that it cannot meet the metabolic needs of the body.

liver transplant the introduction of a donated liver or liver segment into the body of a person suffering from liver failure.

livid black or bluish-black discolouration from accumulation of free blood in the tissues.

lobe a well-defined sub-division of an organ.

loins the soft tissue of the back, on either side of the spine, between the lowest ribs and the pelvis.

lordosis an abnormal degree of forward curvature of the lower part of the spine.

lumbar relating to the loins and lower back.

lumbar puncture passage of a needle between two vertebrae of the spine, from behind, into the fluid-filled space lying below the termination of the spinal cord.

lungs the paired, air-filled, elastic, spongy organs occupying each side of the chest. The function of the lungs is continuously to replenish the oxygen content of the blood and to afford an exit path from the blood for carbon dioxide and other unwanted gases.

lymph tissue fluids drained by the lymph vessels and returned to the large veins.

lymph gland the incorrect term for a lymph node. These are not glands, although commonly so described, even by doctors.

lymph nodes small oval or bean-shaped bodies, up to 2 cm in length, situated in groups along the course of the lymph drainage vessels.

lymphocytes specialized white cells. Part of the body's immune system.

———

macula lutea the yellow spot in the centre of the retina on which the image of the point of greatest visual interest falls when something is observed.

magnetic resonance imaging (MRI) an important method of body scanning offering a degree of resolution of detail unequalled by any other method.

malaise a vague general term for feeling unwell.

malignant a term usually applied to cancerous tumours, but also used to qualify unusually serious forms of various diseases tending to cause death unless effectively treated.

malingering pretending to suffer from a disease, or the simulation of signs of disease, so as to gain some supposed advantage.

malnutrition any disorder resulting from an inadequate diet or from failure to absorb or assimilate dietary elements.

mammary gland the breast.

mandible the lower jaw bone.

Marfan's syndrome a rare autosomal dominant genetic disorder involving weakness of structural collagen protein.

marijuana the dried leaves, flowers or stems of various species of the hemp grass *Cannabis*, especially *Cannabis sativa, Cannabis indica* and *Cannabis americana*.

mastoid bone a prominent bony process which can be felt behind the lower part of the ear.

mastoiditis inflammation of the mastoid air cells from infection usually spread from an otitis media.

meatus any passage or opening in the body.

meconium the thick, greenish-black, sticky stools passed by a baby during the first day or two of life.

medial situated toward the midline of the body.

mediastinum the central compartment of the chest.

medicated of soaps, shampoos, lotions, confections, etc., containing a drug or other medication.

melaena blackening of the stools by altered blood that has been released into the bowel from bleeding.

melanin the body's natural colouring (pigment) found in the skin, hair, eyes, inner ears and other parts.

menarche the onset of menstruation. Compare menopause.

meninges the three layers of membrane that surround the brain and the spinal cord.

meningioma a tumour of the cells of the meninges.

meningism a collection of signs and symptoms, such as headache, stiff neck and fever, suggestive of meningitis, but occurring in the absence of a positive diagnosis of the condition.

mesenteric adenitis inflammation, probably from virus infection, of the lymph nodes in the mesentery. The condition is common in children and can be very difficult to distinguish from appendicitis.

metacarpal one of the five long bones situated in the palmar part of the hand.

metatarsal one of the five long bones of the foot lying beyond the tarsal bones and articulating with the bones of the toes.

micturating cystogram an X-ray taken while the subject is actually urinating.

middle ear the narrow cleft within the temporal bone lying between the inside of the ear-drum and the outer wall of the inner ear.

minerals chemical elements required in the diet, usually in small amounts, to maintain health.

mitosis the division of a cell nucleus to produce two daughter cells having identical genetic composition to the parent cell.

moon-faced pertaining to the full-cheeked, hamster-like appearance caused by excessive doses of corticosteroid drugs or by excessive production of the natural adrenal cortical hormone in Cushing's syndrome.

morbilli measles.

mortality rate the ratio of the total number of deaths from one or any cause, in a year, to the number of people in the population.

mucous membrane the lining of most of the body cavities and hollow internal organs such as the mouth, the nose, the eyelids, the intestine and the vagina.

mucus a slimy, jelly-like material, chemically known as a mucopolysaccharide or glycoprotein, produced by the goblet cells of mucous membranes.

murmur a purring or rumbling sound of variable pitch heard through a stethoscope, especially over the heart or over a narrowed or compressed artery.

muscle a tissue consisting of large numbers of parallel elongated cells with the power of shortening and thickening so as to approximate their ends and effect movement.

mutation any persisting change in the genetic material (DNA) of a cell.

mutism inability or refusal to speak.

myopia short-sightedness.

———

NAD nothing abnormal detected.

narcotic a drug which, in appropriate dosage, produces sleep and relieves pain.

nasal pertaining to the nose.

natal pertaining to birth or to the buttocks.

navel the depressed scar in the centre of the abdomen left when the umbilical cord drops off and the opening into the abdomen heals.

neonatal pertaining to a newborn baby.

neonate a newborn baby.

neoplasia the process of tumour formation.

neoplasm a collection of cells, derived from a common origin, often a single cell, that is increasing in number and expanding or spreading, either locally or to remote sites. A tumour.

nephrectomy surgical removal of a kidney.

nerve a pinkish-white, cord-like structure consisting of bundles of long fibres (axons) of nerve cells and fine blood vessels held together by a connective tissue sheath.

nervous breakdown a popular and imprecise term used to describe any emotional, neurotic or psychotic disturbance ranging from a brief episode of hysterical behaviour to a major psychotic illness such as schizophrenia.

nervous system the controlling, integrating, recording and effecting structure of the body.

neuralgia pain experienced in an area supplied by a sensory nerve as a result of nerve disorder, that results in the production of pain impulses in the nerve.

neuritis inflammation of a nerve.

neurofibromatosis a genetic disease of dominant inheritance or caused by new mutations, featuring multiple soft tumours of the fibrous sheaths of nerves in the skin and elsewhere.

nit a louse egg.

nocturnal emission spontaneous ejaculation, with orgasm, occurring during sleep, often at the climax of an erotic dream.

nocturnal enuresis involuntary urination during night-time sleep. Bedwetting.

notifiable disease any disease, especially a communicable condition, required by law to be reported to a central medical authority by the doctor who diagnoses it.

nutrient anything that nourishes. Any physiologically valuable ingredient in food.

nutrition the process by which substances external to the body are assimilated and restructured to form part of the body or are consumed as a source or energy. Also, the study of the dietary requirements of the body.

———

obesity excessive energy storage in the form of fat.

oedema excessive accumulation of fluid, mainly water, in the tissue spaces of the body.

oesophagus the gullet.

olfactory pertaining to the sense of smell.

oncology the study of the causes, features and treatment of cancer. An oncologist is a cancer specialist.

ophthalmia neonatorum eye inflammation occurring in the newborn baby as a result of infection acquired during birth.

ophthalmologist a doctor who specializes in the eye and its disorders.

oral pertaining to the mouth.

orchitis inflammation of the testicle.

orthodontics the dental specialty concerned with the correction of irregularities of tooth placement and in the relationship of the upper teeth to the lower (occlusion).

orthopaedics the branch of surgery concerned with correction of deformity and restoration of function following injury or disease of the skeletal system and its associated ligaments, muscles and tendons.

orthoptics a discipline, ancillary to ophthalmology, concerned mainly with the management of squint (strabismus) in childhood and the avoidance of amblyopia.

orthoptist a person trained in the diagnosis of inapparent squint, in the measurement of the angle of squint, in assessing the visual acuity in young children and in the ability to determine the degree to which the child is able to perceive simultaneously with the two eyes (binocular vision).

Osteogenesis imperfecta (fragilitas ossium) a congenital brittle bone disease associated with blueness of the whites of the eyes due to unusual thinning of the sclera.

OTC over-the-counter. This refers to drugs or other remedies that may be purchased from a pharmacist without a doctor's prescription.

oxycephaly a skull abnormality causing the head to assume a conical or peaked appearance.

oxygen a colourless, odourless gas, essential for life.

---

paediatrics the medical specialty concerned with all aspects of childhood diseases and disorders, and with the health and development of the child in the context of the family and the environment.

paedophilia recurrent sexual urges towards a prepubertal child by a person over the age of 16 and at least five years older than the child.

paramedic any health care worker other than a doctor, nurse, or dentist.

paraphilia any deviation from what is currently deemed to be normal sexual behaviour or preference.

parenteral nutrition intravenous feeding.

parotid glands the largest of the three pairs of salivary glands.

passive smoking inhaling cigarette smoke exhaled by others.

patella the knee cap.

pathogenic able to cause disease.

penis the male organ of copulation containing the urethra through which urine and seminal fluid pass.

perinatal pertaining to the period immediately before and after birth.

perineum that part of the floor of the pelvis that lies between the tops of the thighs.

peritoneum the double-layered, serum-secreting membrane that lines the inner wall of the abdomen and covers, and to some extent supports, the abdominal organs.

peritonitis inflammation of the peritoneum.

persistent foramen ovale failure of the hole in the wall between the two upper chambers of the heart to close fully at birth.

petechiae tiny, flat red or purple spots in the skin or mucous membranes caused by bleeding from small blood vessels.

pH an expression, widely used in medicine, of the acidity or alkalinity of a solution.

phagocyte an amoeboid cell of the immune system that responds to contact with a foreign object, such as a bacterium, by surrounding, engulfing and digesting it.

phalanges the small bones of the fingers and toes. Fingers have three phalanges; the thumbs and big toes have two.

pharynx the common passage to the gullet and the windpipe from the back of the mouth and the back of the nose.

phimosis tightness of the foreskin (prepuce) of such degree as to prevent retraction.

phlebitis inflammation of a vein.

phocomelia a major, congenital limb defect featuring absence of all long bones, so that the hands or feet are attached directly to the trunk and resemble flippers. Spontaneous cases of phocomelia are rare but the condition occurred in many children whose mothers were given thalidomide early in their pregnancy.

physiology the study of the functioning of living organisms, especially the human organism.

pigeon chest a deformity in which the chest is peaked forward, seen in people who have suffered from severe asthma from infancy.

pigeon toes a mainly cosmetic defect in which the leg or foot is rotated inwards.

pigmentation colouration of any part of the body, especially the skin.

pituitary gland the central controlling gland in the endocrine system.

placebo effect the temporary alteration in a patient's condition, following treatment, which is due exclusively to expectation rather than to the treatment.

plantar wart an ordinary wart (verruca) occurring on the sole of the foot and forced into the skin by pressure from the weight of the body.

plastic surgery any surgical procedure designed to repair or reconstruct injured, diseased or malformed tissue so as to restore normal appearance and function.

pneumonia inflammation of the lower air passages (bronchioles) and air sacs (alveoli) of the lungs.

prognosis an informed medical guess as to the probable course and outcome of a disease.

pruritus itching.

psychopath a person whose behaviour suggests indifference to the rights and feelings of others.

pulse the rhythmic expansion of an artery from the force of the heart beat. In health, the pulse is regular, moderately full and at a rate of between about 50 and 80 beats per minute.

purpura any of a group of bleeding disorders that cause visible haemorrhage into the skin in the form of tiny spots (petechiae), local bruises (ecchymoses) or widespread areas of discolouration.

purulent pertaining to pus.

pus a yellowish or green viscous fluid consisting of dead white blood cells, bacteria, partly destroyed tissue and protein.

pylorus the narrowed outlet of the stomach where it opens into the duodenum.

pyrexia fever.

---

qid four times a day.

quadriceps muscles the bulky muscle group on the front of the thigh.

quinsy an abscess between the tonsil and the underlying wall of the throat.

---

radial nerve one of the main nerves of the arm and hand.

radiologist a doctor who specializes in medical imaging and who is skilled in the interpretation of X-rays, CT scans, MRI, PET scans and radionuclide scanning films.

radius one of the two forearm bones, the other being the ulna.

recovery room a room adjoining an operating theatre, in which patients who have undergone surgical operations are kept under close surveillance until safely recovered from general anaesthesia.

recreational drugs a dubious term that trivialises the dangers and serious social implications of the use of drugs such as cocaine, amphetamine, various hallucinogenic drugs and marijuana.

rectal pertaining to the rectum.

rectum the 12.5 cm long, very distensible terminal segment of the large intestine.

referred pain pain felt in a place other than the site of the causal disorder.

reflex an automatic, involuntary and predictable response to a stimulus applied to the body or arising within it.

regimen any system or course of treatment, especially one involving special diet or exercise.

relapse the reappearance or worsening of a disease after apparent recovery or improvement.

remission a marked reduction in the severity of the symptoms or signs of a disease, or its temporary disappearance.

renal pertaining to the kidneys.

resection surgical removal of any part of the body or of diseased tissue.

retina the complex membranous network of nerve cells, fibres and photoreceptors that lines the inside of the back of the eye and converts optical images formed by the lens system of the eye into nerve impulses.

ribs the flat, curved bones that form a protective cage for the chest organs and provide the means of varying the volume of the chest so as to effect respiration.

rigor a violent attack of shivering causing a rapid rise in body temperature.

roughage dietary fibre, consisting of poly-saccharides such as celluloses, pectins and gums for which no digestive enzymes are present in the intestinal canal.

rupture a popular term for an abdominal hernia.

Sabin vaccine an effective oral vaccine used to immunize against poliomyelitis.

sacrum the large, triangular, wedge-like bone that forms the centre of the back of the pelvis and the lower part of the vertebral column.

sarcoma one of the two general types of cancer, the other being carcinoma. Sarcomas are malignant tumours of connective tissue such as bone, muscle, cartilage, fibrous tissue and blood vessels.

scabies skin infestation with the mite parasite *Sarcoptes scabei* which burrows into the superficial layers, usually of the hands or wrists, to feed on dead epidermal scales and lay eggs.

scalp the soft tissue layers covering the bone of the vault of the skull.

scapula the shoulder blade.

sciatic nerve the main nerve of the leg and the largest nerve in the body.

sclera the white of the eye.

scoliosis a spinal deformity in which the column is bent to one side usually in the chest or lower back regions. This may cause crowding of the ribs on one side.

scotoma a blind spot or area in the field of vision.

screening the routine examination of numbers of apparently healthy people to identify those with a particular disease at an early stage.

scrotum the skin and muscle sac containing the testicles and the start of the spermatic cord.

scurvy a deficiency disease caused by an inadequate intake of vitamin C.

sibling any member of a group of related brothers or sisters.

sibling rivalry strong competition or feelings of resentment between siblings, especially between an older child and a new baby.

sickling test the observation of a blood film, mixed with a solution of sodium metabisulphite, under the microscope. If haemoglobin S is present, the red cells will assume a sickle shape within 20 minutes.

sinus one of the paired mucous membrane-lined air cavities in a bone of the skull.

sinusitis inflammation of the mucous membrane linings of one or more bone cavities (sinuses) of the face.

situs inversus an uncommon mirror-image reversal of the organs of the trunk. The heart points to the right, the liver and appendix are on the left and the stomach and spleen on the right.

skeleton the framework of usually 206 articulated bones that give the body its general shape, and that provides support and attachments for the muscles.

skinfold thickness measurement a method of assessing the amount of fat under the skin by means of special calipers, sprung to exert a standard pressure and fitted with a scale.

skull the bony skeleton of the head and the protective covering for the brain. The part of the skull that encloses the brain is called the cranium.

smegma accumulated, cheesy-white, sebaceous gland secretions occurring under the foreskin of an uncircumcised male with poor standards of personal hygiene.

snake oil an informal term for any fraudulent cure-all.

somatotype the physical build of a person.

speculum an instrument of varying design used to hold open or widen a body orifice such as the ear canal, a nostril, the eyelids, the anus or the vagina, so as to allow examination.

speech therapy treatment designed to help people with a communication difficulty arising from a disturbance of language, a disorder of articulation, difficulty in voice production or defective fluency of speech.

spermatozoa microscopic cells about 0.05 mm long occurring in millions in seminal fluid.

sphincter a muscle ring, or local thickening of the muscle coat, surrounding a tubular passage or opening in the body. When a sphincter contracts it narrows or closes off the passageway.

spinal cord the downward continuation of the brainstem that lies within a canal in the spine (vertebral column).

spinal nerves the 31 pairs of combined motor and sensory nerves that are connected to the spinal cord.

spleen a solid, dark purplish organ, lying high on the left side of the abdomen between the stomach and the left kidney. It is part of the immune system, containing millions of immune cells (lymphocytes) it also helps filter the blood, removing debris and micro-organisms.

spontaneous pneumothorax sudden and unexpected incursion of air into the space between the two layers of the pleura so that the underlying lung collapses.

staging determination of the stage to which a disease, especially a cancer, has progressed.

stenosis narrowing of a duct, orifice or tubular organ such as the intestinal canal or a blood vessel.

sterile free from bacteria or other microorganisms, or incapable of reproduction.

sterilization the process of rendering anything free from living microorganisms, or any procedure that deprives the individual of the ability to reproduce.

sternum the breastbone.

steroid drugs a large group of drugs that are derived from, resemble, or simulate the actions of, the natural corticosteroids or the male sex hormones of the body.

stoma a mouth or orifice.

stomach the bag-like organ lying under the diaphragm in the upper right part of the abdomen into which swallowed food passes, by way of the oesophagus.

storkbites a popular term for the small, harmless, pinkish skin blemishes that commonly occur around the eyes and on the back of the neck in new-born babies.

strabismus squint. The condition in which only one eye is aligned on the object of interest.

superior above, higher than, with reference to the upright body. Compare inferior.

supine lying on the back with the face upwards.

suppuration the production or discharge of pus.

surfactant a substance that reduces surface tension and promotes wetting of surfaces. The lungs contain a surfactant to prevent collapse of the alveoli.

surrogacy an agreement by a woman to undergo pregnancy so as to produce a child which will be surrendered to others.

suture a length of thread-like material used for surgical sewing or the product of surgical sewing, or a fixed joint between bones of the vault of the skull.

symptom a subjective perception suggesting bodily defect or malfunction. Symptoms are never perceptible by others. Objective indications of disease are called signs.

synapse the junctional area between two connected nerves, or between a nerve and the effector organ (a muscle fibre or a gland).

syndrome a unique combination of sometimes apparently unrelated symptoms or signs, forming a distinct clinical entity.

syringe an instrument, consisting of a barrel and a tight-fitting piston with a connecting rod, used to inject or withdraw fluid.

systemic pertaining to something that affects the whole body rather than one part of it.

talipes club foot.

tapeworm a ribbon-like population of joined flatworms, derived from a common head equipped with hooks or suckers by which it is attached to the lining of the intestine.

T cell one of the two broad categories of lymphocyte, the other being the B cell group that produces antibodies.

teething the eruption of the primary teeth.

temperature regulation the process by which body temperature is maintained within narrow limits.

temporal pertaining to the temples.

temporal bone one of two bones forming part of the sides and base of the skull and containing the hearing apparatus.

tenderness pain elicited by touch or pressure.

tendon a strong band of collagen fibres that joins muscle to bone or cartilage and transmits the force of muscle contraction to cause movement.

tendon jerk a reflex contraction of the muscle to which a tendon is attached when the tendon is struck sharply so as to exert a sudden pull on the muscles.

teratogen any agent capable of causing a severe congenital bodily anomaly (monstrosity).

testis one of the male gonads, suspended in the scrotum by the spermatic cord.

test tube baby a popular term for a baby derived from an ovum fertilized outside the body (in vitro fertilization).

therapeutic community a small local population of people of strong antisocial tendency, set up under the supervision of medical staff but in a non-clinical environment, to try to treat personality disorder.

therapy treatment of disease or of conditions supposed to be diseases.

thorax the part of the trunk between the neck and the abdomen.

thrill a coarse vibrating sensation felt with the flat of the hand on the front of the chest.

thrombosis clotting of blood within an artery or vein so that the blood flow is reduced or impeded.

thrombus a blood clot forming especially on the wall of a blood vessel.

thymus a small flat organ of the lymphatic system situated immediately behind the breastbone, that is apparent in children but inconspicuous after puberty.

thyroid gland an endocrine gland, situated in the neck like a bow tie across the front of the upper part of the windpipe (trachea).

tibia the shin bone, the stronger of the two long bones in the lower leg.

ticks small, eight-legged, blood-sucking ectoparasites of the family *Ixodoidea*.

tinea capitis tinea of the scalp. Also known as kerion.

tinea cruris tinea affecting the groin, that tends to spread to the upper thighs and the lower abdomen. Commonly known as crutch rot.

tinea pedis tinea of the skin between the toes and, sometimes, the remainder of the skin of the foot. Known as athelete's foot.

tissue any aggregation of joined cells and their connections that perform a particular function.

tissue typing the identification of particular chemical groups present on the surface of all body cells and specific to the individual.

tongue the muscular, mucous membrane-covered, highly flexible organ that is attached to the lower jaw (mandible) and the hyoid bone in the neck, and forms part of the floor of the mouth.

tonic a mythical remedy commonly prescribed by doctors as a placebo.

tonsil an oval mass of lymphoid tissue, of variable size, situated on the back of the throat on either side of the soft palate.

topical pertaining to something, usually medication, applied to the surface of the body, rather than taken internally or injected.

torsion twisting or rotation, especially of a part that hangs loosely on a narrow support.

toxin any substance produced by a living organism that is poisonous to other organisms.

toxoid a bacterial toxin that has been chemically changed so as to lose its poisonous properties but retain its ability to stimulate antibody production.

trachea the windpipe.

tracheitis inflammation of the lining of the windpipe (trachea), usually from infections originating in the throat or bronchi.

transfusion the replacement of lost blood by blood, or blood products, usually donated by another person.

transplantation the grafting of donated organs or tissues into the body (homograft), or the movement of tissue from one site to another in the same person (autograft).

trapezius muscle a large, triangular back muscle extending from the lower part of the back of the skull (occiput) almost to the lumbar region of the spine on each side.

trocar a sharp-pointed surgical stilette (metal rod) normally used within a cannula to allow its insertion into a body cavity.

tumour a swelling. The term usually refers to any mass of cells resulting from an abnormal degree of multiplication. Tumours may be benign or malignant.

---

ulcer a local loss of surface covering (epithelium) and sometimes deeper tissue in skin or mucous membrane.

ulna one of the pair of forearm long bones.

ulnar nerve one of the main nerves of the arm that supplies some of the muscles of the forearm and all the small muscles of the hand.

umbilical cord the nutritional, hormonal and immunological link between the mother and the fetus during pregnancy.

umbilical hernia protrusion of a loop of bowel through a weakness in the abdominal wall at the navel.

unilateral on or affecting one side only. One-sided.

uniovular originating from one egg, as in the case of monozygotic twins.

uraemia accumulation of the nitrogenous waste products of metabolism in the blood as a result of failure of the kidneys to excrete them (kidney failure).

ureter a tube that carries urine downwards from each kidney to the urinary bladder for temporary storage.

urethra the tube that carries urine from the bladder to the exterior.

urethritis inflammation of the lining of the urethra.

urinary bladder the muscular bag for the temporary storage of urine situated in the midline of the pelvis at the lowest point in the abdomen, immediately behind the pubic bone.

urologist a doctor who specializes in the diagnosis and treatment of disorders of the kidneys, the ureters, the urinary bladder and the urethra.

uterus the female organ in which the fetus grows and is nourished until birth. The womb.

---

vaccine a suspension of microorganisms of one particular type that have been killed or modified so as to be safe, given to promote the production of specific antibodies to the organism for purposes of future protection against infection.

vagina literally a sheath. In the female it acts as a receptacle for the penis in coitus and as the birth canal.

vaginitis inflammation of the vagina from any cause.

varicella chickenpox.

vas a vessel or channel conveying fluid.

vas deferens the fine tube that runs up in the spermatic cord on each side and conveys spermatozoa from the testicle to the seminal vesicle.

vasoconstriction active narrowing of small arteries as a result of contraction of the circular smooth muscle fibres in their walls.

vasodilatation widening of blood vessels as a result of relaxation of the muscles in the walls.

veins thin-walled blood vessels containing blood at low pressure which is being returned to the heart from tissues that have been perfused by arteries.

ventral pertaining to the front of the body.

ventricle a cavity or chamber filled with fluid, especially the two lower pumping chambers of the heart.

vertebra one of the 24 bones of the vertebral column.

vertebral column the bony spine.

virilism masculinization in the female.

virology the study of viruses of medical importance and the diseases they produce.

virulence the capacity of any infective organism to cause disease and to injure or kill a susceptible host.

viscera organs within a body cavity, especially digestive organs.

visual acuity the extent to which an eye is capable of resolving fine detail.

visual fields the area over which some form of visual perception is possible while the subject looks straight ahead.

vital signs indications that a person is still alive.

vitiligo a skin disorder that features white patches, of variable size and shape, especially on the face, the backs of the hands, the armpits and around the anus.

vulva the female external genitalia.

vulvitis inflammation of the vulva.

weaning substitution of solid foods for milk in an infant's diet.

webbing edge-to edge joining of the fingers or toes by flaps of skin.

wet dream a popular term for an erotic dream culminating in a spontaneous orgasm and ejaculation of semen.

wet nurse a woman who breast-feeds another woman's child.

wind a popular term for the result of air swallowing by greedy babies.

wrist the complex, many-boned joint between the hand and the arm.

———

X chromosome the chromosome which, with the Y chromosome, determines the sex of the individual.

xeroderma dryness of the skin.

xerophthalmia dryness of the eyes.

xerostomia dry mouth.

X-linked pertaining to genes, or to the effect of genes, situated on the X chromosome.

———

zinc a metallic element required in small quantities for health.

zoonoses diseases of animals that can affect people.

Z-plasty a plastic surgical technique for relieving skin tension or releasing scar contracture.

zygote an egg (ovum) that has been fertilized but has not yet undergone the first cleavage division. The start of a new individual.

REFERENCES

ABC of Child Abuse (series) – *British Medical Journal* – 18 March 1989 p 727.

Acute viral encephalitis in children – *British Medical Journal* – 21 January 1995 p 139.

Acyclovir for childhood chickenpox – *British Medical Journal* – 14 January 1995 p 108.

Adult outcome of small children – *British Medical Journal* – 18 March 1995 p 696.

Adults, sexually abused, childhood problems of – *British Medical Journal* – 17 March 1990 p 705.

Adults sexually abused as children – *British Medical Journal* – 5 December 1992 p 1375.

Aggression in children – *New Scientist* – 9 April 1994 p 30.

Anogenital warts in children – *British Journal of Hospital Medicine* – 2 November 1994 p 469.

Arthritis in children – *British Medical Journal* – 18 March 1995 p 728.

Asthma in children – *British Medical Journal* – 10 June 1995 p 1522.

Asthma treatment in small children – *British Medical Journal* – 16 July 1988 p 154.

Asthma in childhood, prevalence, severity – *Journal of the American Medical Association* – 18 November 1992 p 2673.

Asthma in childhood – *British Journal of Hospital Medicine* – 20 January 1993 p 127.

Asthma in schoolchildren – *Practitioner* – 8 September 1989 p 1174.

Asthma in children, current concepts – *New England Journal of Medicine* – 4 June 1992 p 1540.

Asthma children, epidemiology – *British Medical Journal* – 18 June 1994 p 1548, 1591, 1596.

Bone turnover in malnourished children – *Lancet* – 19 December 1992 p 1493.

Brain tumours in children – *New England Journal of Medicine* – 1 December 1994 p 1500.

Bronchidilators in pre-school children with asthma – *British Medical Journal* – 6 May 1995 p 1161.

Cancer in children, survival rates – *British Medical Journal* – 14 December 1994 p 1612.

Child abuse – *British Medical Journal* – 7 March 1987

Child abuse – *Journal of the Royal Society of Medicine* – February 1989 p 65.

Child abuse – *Lancet* – 4 October 1986 p 792.

Child abuse, X-ray evidence – *New England Journal of Medicine* – 23 February 1989 p 507.

Child abuse and neglect – current concepts – *New England Journal of Medicine* – 25 May 1995 p 1425.

Child abuse or not? – *British Medical Journal* – 16 February 1991 p 371.

Child cancer treatment – *Lancet* – 23 July 1994 p 210.

Child death, telling parents – *British Medical Journal* – 22 June 1991 p 1524.

Child deaths from guns – *Lancet* – 25 June 1994 p 1642.

Child febrile convulsions – *British Medical Journal* – 26 June 1993 p 1743.

Child hyperactivity – *British Medical Journal* – 24 June 1995 p 1617.

Child hyperactivity and conformity – *New Scientist* – 10 April 1993 p 37.

Child killed by jellyfish – *Journal of the American Medical Association* – 11 September 1991 p 1404.

Child lead screening – *Lancet* – 10 December 1994 p 1587.

Child neglect and obesity – *Lancet* – 5 February 1994 p 324.

Child psychiatry, changing fashions – *Journal of the Royal Society of Medicine* – June 1989 p 324.

Child sexual abuse – *British Medical Journal* – 17 July 1993 p 144.

Child sexual abuse – *Lancet* – 13 April 1991 p 890.

Child sexual abuse and adult mental health – *British Journal of Hospital Medicine* – 17 June 1992 p 9.

Child sexual abuse by women – *British Medical Journal* – 5 May 1990 p 1153.
Child sexual abuse, signs of – *British Journal of Hospital Medicine* – June 1991 p 364.
Childhood blindness – *Eye* – Vol 6 part 2 1992 p 173.
Childhood cholesterol screening – *Journal of the American Medical Association* – 12 June 1991 p 3003.
Childhood cholesterol screening – *Journal of the American Medical Association* – 1 January 1992 p 100, 101.
Childhood drowning – *British Medical Journal* – 30 October 1993 p 1086.
Childhood fever management – *Lancet* – 26 October 1991 p 1049.
Childhood immunization – *New England Journal of Medicine* – 17 December 1992 p 1794.
Childhood leukaemia theories – *Science* – 19 June 1992 p 1633.
Childhood leukaemias review – *New England Journal of Medicine* – 15 June 1995 p 1618.
Childhood origins of antisocial behaviour – *Journal of the Royal Society of Medicine* – January 1993 p 13.
Children and cholesterol, fat streaks, LDL, HDL – *Journal of the American Medical Association* – 5 February 1992
Children and smoking – *British Journal of Hospital Medicine* – August 1991 p 77.
Children coping with death of sibling – *Journal of the Royal Society of Medicine* – August 1995 p 426.
Children deliberately left to die – *Lancet* – 15 September 1990 p 659.
Children shot in Los Angeles – *New England Journal of Medicine* – 1 February 1995 p 324.
Children who witness violence – Journal of the American Medical Association – 13 January 1993 p 262.
Children's dental health and sugary medicines – *British Medical Journal* – 15 July 1995 p 141.
Children's feeding disorders – *British Medical Journal* – 28 January 1995 p 228.
Children's teeth – *British Medical Journal* – 4 February 1989 p 272.
Children's view of health – *British Medical Journal* – 22 April 1995 p 1029.
Chronic cough in children – *Journal of the American Medical Association* – 11 November 1992 p 2572.
Cochlear implants in children – *Journal of the Royal Society of Medicine* – November 1992 p 655.
Constipation in childhood – *British Medical Journal* – 4 November 1989 p 1116.
Cost of children's smoking – *British Medical Journal* – 28 October 1995 p 1152.
Cyanoacrylic superglue in facial wounds in children – *British Medical Journal* – 21 October 1989.
Deafness in children, prevention of – *Journal of the Royal Society of Medicine* – August 1989 p 484.
Dehydration signs in children – *Lancet* – 9 September 1989 p 605.
Delayed speech in children – *British Medical Journal* – 19 November 1988 p 1281.
Depression in childhood, treatment – *British Medical Journal* – 12 May 1990 p 1260.
Diabetes incidence in children rises – *British Medical Journal* – 23 February 1991 p 443.
Diabetes in children under 5 – *British Medical Journal* – 18 March 1995 p 700.
Diagnosing deafness in children – *British Medical Journal* – 13 November 1993 p 1225.
Epilepsy – do fits in childhood affect intellect? – *New England Journal of Medicine* – 24 April 1993 p 1085.
Epilepsy in children, treatment of – *British Medical Journal* – 10 December 1988 p 1528.
Examination of children's eyes – *British Journal of Hospital Medicine* – 3 May 1995 p 454.
Exercise and BP in children – *British Medical Journal* – 21 September 1991 p 682.
Female sexual abuse of children – *Journal of the Royal Society of Medicine* – November 1994 p 691.
Flat feet in children – *British Medical Journal* – 27 October 1990 p 942.

Free radicals vitamin A and child mortality – *Journal of the American Medical Association* – 17 February 1993 p 898.

Diabetic child, denied treatment, dies – *British Medical Journal* – 13 November 1993 p 1232.

Gender identity disorders in children – *British Journal of Hospital Medicine* – 15 March 1995 p 251.

Gifted children – *British Medical Journal* – 30 October 1993 p 1088.

Headache in childhood – *Practitioner* – 8 September 1989 p 1123.

Headaches in schoolchildren – *British Medical Journal* – 24 September 1994 p 765.

Heart disease starts in childhood – *British Medical Journal* – 28 March 1992 p 789, 901.

Helicobacter pylori in childhood effects – *British Medical Journal* – 29 October 1994 p 1119.

Herpes in childhood – *British Journal of Hospital Medicine* – 1 September 1993 p 233 and 15 September 1993 p 301.

HIV, mother child transmission and breast feeding – *Lancet* – 25 April 1992 p 1007.

Injuries to child pedestrians – *British Medical Journal* – 18 February 1995 p 413.

Kidney transplant in children – *British Journal of Hospital Medicine* – October 1990 p 279.

Killed children in cities – *Journal of the American Medical Association* – 3 June 1992 p 2905.

Lead, child intelligence environment pollution – *British Medical Journal* – 5 November 1994 p 1189.

Lethal food allergy in children – *New England Journal of Medicine* – 6 August 1992 p 421.

Life-sustaining in brain-damaged children – *Lancet* – 13 June 1992 p 1472.

Liver transplants in children – *British Medical Journal* – 15 February 1992 p 396, 416.

Long-term AIDS survival in children – *Lancet* – 22 January 1994 p 191.

Management of fever in children at home – *British Medical Journal* – 7 November 1992 p 1134.

Measles vaccine in children allergic to eggs – *New England Journal of Medicine* – 11 May 1995 p 1262.

Melanoma in children – *New England Journal of Medicine* – 9 March 1995 p 656.

Monitoring child growth – *British Medical Journal* – 2 September 1995 p 583.

Mother-to-child transmission of HIV – *New England Journal of Medicine* – 3 August 1995 p 298.

Murder and black children – *British Medical Journal* – 13 June 1992 p 1527.

Murder of street children – *British Medical Journal* – 30 May 1992 p 1423.

Mutation of growth hormone receptor – *New England Journal of Medicine* – 26 October 1995 p 1093, 1145.

Otitis media in children, review – *New England Journal of Medicine* – 8 June 1995 p 1560.

Pain control in infants and children – *New England Journal of Medicine* – 27 August 1994 p 541.

Pain relief in children – *British Medical Journal* – 2 October 1993 p 815.

Paracetamol prescription for children, trends in – *British Medical Journal* – 5 August 1995 p 362.

Parental refusal of children's immunisation – *British Medical Journal* – 28 January 1995 p 227.

Parents' right to allow child to die opposed – *British Medical Journal* – 12 August 1995 p 405.

Passive smoking and child health – *Lancet* – 29 July 1995 p 280.

Paternal radiation and child leukaemia – *British Medical Journal* – 26 June 1993 p 1718.

Peak flow meters in children – *British Medical Journal* – 7 November 1992 p 1128.

Pneumocystis prophylaxis HIV children – *New England Journal of Medicine* – 23 March 1995 p 786.

Predicting adult height of short children – *British Medical Journal* – 7 May 1994 p 1207.

Psychopathology life events in children – *Journal of the Royal Society of Medicine* – June 1994 p 327.

Recurrent suffocation in children – *Lancet* – 11 July 1992 p 87.

Seat belts restraint of children in cars – *British Medical Journal* – 23 November 1991 p 1283.

Seizures, epilepsy in children – *British Journal of Hospital Medicine* July 1992 p 93.

Sex of child not random – *New Scientist* – 3 December 1994 p 28.

Sexual abuse of children, consequences for learning – *British Medical Journal* – 20 July 1991 pp 143–44.

Shaken infant syndrome, child abuse – *British Medical Journal* – 11 February 1995 p 344.

Sleep disorders in children – *British Medical Journal* – 18–25 August 1990 p 351.

Sleep disorders in children – *British Medical Journal* – 6 March 1993 p 640.

STDs and sex abuse of children – *British Journal of Hospital Medicine* – 2 March 1994 p 206.

Stopping artificial feeding child brain damage – *British Medical Journal* – 19 August 1995 p 464.

Sugar and hyperactivity in children – *New England Journal of Medicine* – 1 February 1994 p 301 355.

Sugar, aspartame and children's behaviour – *New England Journal of Medicine* – 30 June 1994 p 1901.

Thalidomide children, obstetric problems of – *British Medical Journal* – 7 January 1989 p 6.

Tobacco selling to children – *British Medical Journal* – 24 November 1990 p 1173.

Traffic volume, curb parking causes child injuries – *British Medical Journal* – 14 January 1995 p 91.

Treating childhood asthma in Singapore – *British Medical Journal* – 14 May 1994 p 1282.

Treatment of children with brain tumours – *British Medical Journal* – 4 November 1995 p 1213.

Tricyclic drugs and child depression – *British Medical Journal* – 8 April 1995 p 897.

TV and children – *New Scientist* – 23 April 1994 p 24.

TV violence and children – *British Medical Journal* – 4 February 1994 p 273.

Urinary tract infection in children – *Lancet* – 28 September 1991 p 767.

Urinary tract infections in childhood – *British Medical Journal* – 25 September 1993 p 761.

Urinary tract infection children, management of – *British Medical Journal* – 10 December 1988 p 1516.

Vaccination saving children's lives – *British Medical Journal* – 23/30 December 1989 p 1544.

Viral diarrhoeas in children – *British Medical Journal* – 7 November 1992 p 1111.

Vitamins and childhood IQ – *British Medical Journal* – 9 March 1991 p 548.

Vitamins and childhood IQ – *Lancet* – 9 March 1991 p 587.

Vitamin K – Lancet 28 January 1995 p 229.

Why children talk to themselves – *Scientific American* – December 1994 p 60.

Zidovudine, effects on mother, fetus, child – *Lancet* – 23 July 1994 p 207.

Zinc supplements for children with diarrhoea – *New England Journal of Medicine* – 28 September 1995 p 839, 873.

USEFUL RESOURCES

Action for the Sick Child,
Argyle House,
29–31 Euston Road,
London, NW1 2SD
Tel: 0171 833 2041

Angel Drugs Project,
33–44 Liverpool Road,
Islington,
London N1
Tel: 0171 226 3113

The Anti-Bullying Campaign,
10 Borough High Street,
London SE 1 9QQ
Tel: 0171 378 1446

Association for all Speech Impaired Children,
347 Central Markets,
London EC1A 9NH
Tel: 0171 236 6487

Association for Spina Bifida and
Hydrocephalus,
Asbah House,
42 Park Road,
Peterborough PE1 2UQ
Tel: 01733 555988
for South-East Region:
123 East Barnet Road,
Barnet EN4 8RF
Tel: 0181 449 0475

British Allergy Foundation,
St Bartholomew's Hospital,
West Smithfield,
London EC1A 7BE
Tel: 0171 600 6127
Helpline Tel: 0171 600 6166

British Association for Early Childhood,
111 City View,
Bethnal Green Road,
London E2 9QH
Tel: 0171 739 7594

British Dyslexia Association,
98 London Road,
Reading,
Berks RG1 5AV
Tel: 01734 668271

British Epilepsy Association,
Anstey House,
Hanover Square,
Leeds LS3 1BE
Linkline Tel: 0345 089599

British Wellness Council,
70 Chancellors Road,
London W6 9RS
Tel: 0181 741 1231

Brook Advisory Services,
Birth Control Clinics,
153A East Street,
London SE17 2SD
Helpline (24 hours): 0171 617 8000

Cancer Relief Macmillan Fund,
Anchor House,
15/19 Britten Street,
London SW3 3TZ
Tel: 0171 351 7811

Centrepoint Night Shelter,
65a Shaftesbury Avenue,
London W1V 5HH
Tel: 0171 434 2861

Clubs for the physically handicapped and
able bodied *see* PHAB

Cerebral Palsy Helpline:
0800 626 216

Cerebral Palsy Sport,
Sycamore Sports Centre,
Hungerhill Road,
St Arms,
Nottingham,
NG3 4NB
Tel: 0115 9401202

Cruse-bereavement Care,
126 Sheen Road,
Richmond,
Surrey TW9 1UR
Tel: 0181 9404818

Department of Health,
Health Information Services
Freephone: 0800 66 55 44

Down's Syndrome Association,
153 Mitcham Road,
London SW17 9PG
Tel: 0181 682 4001

The Eating Disorders Association,
Sackville Place,
44 Magdalen Street,
Norwich NR3 1JU
Helpline (9am to 6.30pm Mon–Fri):
01603 621414

Fragile X Counselling,
Professor SS Segal,
Middlesex University,
Trent Park,
Bramley Road,
London N14 4XS
Tel: 0181 362 5000

Fragile X Society of Great Britain,
53 Winchelsea Lane,
Hastings,
East Sussex,
TN35 4LG
Tel: 0142 813147

Gingerbread Association for One Parent
Families,
16 Clerkenwell Close,
London EC1R OAA
Tel: 0171 336 8183/8184

Health and Safety Executive,
Rose Court
2 Southwark Bridge
London SE1 9HS
Tel: 0171 717 6000

Lifeline for Parents,
101–3 Oldham Street,
Manchester M41 LW
Tel: 0800 716701

London Disability Arts Forum,
34 Osnaburgh Street,
London NW1 3ND
Tel: 0171 916 5419

Mencap (Royal Society for Mentally
Handicapped Children and Adults),
123 Golden Lane,
London EIV 3AT
Tel: 0171 454 0454 and 0171 608 3254

National Assoc. for Child and Family
Mental Health *see* young minds

National Association for the Education of
Sick Children,
18 Victoria Park Square,
London E2 9PF
Tel: 0181 980 8523

The National Association for Gifted Children,
Park Campus,
Boughton Green Road,
Northampton
Tel: 01604 792300

National Association for the Welfare of
Children in Hospital
Argyle House,
29–31 Euston Road,
London NW1 2SD
Tel: 0171 833 2041

The National Asthma Campaign,
Providence Hall,
Providence Place,
London N1 0NT
Helpline (local call rate): Linkline
0345 010203
General enquiries Tel: 0171 226 2260

The National Eczema Society,
Tavistock House North,
Tavistock Square,
London WC1H 9SR
Tel: 0171 388 4097

National Society for Epilepsy,
Chesham Lane,
Chalfont St Peter's,
Gerrards Cross,
Bucks
SL9 ORJ
Tel: 01494 873991

National Toy libraries *see* Play Matters

Network for the Handicapped,
Room 241
2nd Floor
49–51 Bedford Row
London WCIR 4LR
Tel: 0171 831 8031

Outpatients Psychiatric Clinic *see* Tavistock Clinic

PHAB (Clubs for the physically handicapped and able bodied),
Tavistock House North,
Tavistock Square,
London WCIH 9HX
Tel: 0171 388 1963

Play Matters/National Toy Libraries Association,
68 Churchway,
London NW1 1LT
Tel: 0171 387 9592

The Pre-School Playgroups Association,
61–63 King's Cross Road,
London WC1X 9LL
Tel: 0171 833 0991

Release (Criminal Legal Drug Service),
388 Old Street,
London EC1V 9LT
Tel: 0171 729 9904

Royal National Institute for the Blind,
224 Great Portland Street,
London WIN 6AA
Tel: 0171 388 1266

Royal National Institute for Deaf People,
19–23 Featherstone Street
London
ECIY 85L
Tel: 0171 296 8000

Samaritans (Headquarters),
10 The Grove,
Slough SL1 1QP
Tel: 01753 532713
Check phone book for local branches
Tel: 0171 734 2800 (Helpline Central London)
Deaf callers 0181 780 2521

SCOPE
Shackleton Square,
Priestly Way,
Crawley,
West Sussex RH10 2GZ
Tel: 01293 522655
 Cerebral Palsy Helpline: 0800 626 216

The Standing Conference on Drug Abuse (SCODA),
1–4 Hatton Place,
Hatton Garden,
London EC1 8ND
Tel: 0171 430 2341
Freephone 100 and ask for Freephone Drug Problems

The Tavistock Clinic (outpatient psychiatric clinic),
120 Belsize Lane,
London NW3 5BA
Tel: 0171 435 7111

Toxoplasmosis Trust,
61 Collier Street,
London N1 9BE
Tel: 0171 713 0663
Helpline: 0171 713 0599

Turning Point,
101 Backcurch Lane,
London E1 1LU
Tel: 0171 702 2300

Under-Fives Counselling Service,
Tavistock clinic,
120 Belsize Lane,
London NW3 5BA
Tel: 0171 435 7111

Voluntary Reading Help,
Ebury Building Centre,
London SW1V 4LH
Tel: 0171 834 6918

Young Minds/The National Association for Child and Family Mental Health,
22A Boston Place,
London NW1 6ER
Tel: 0171 724 7262

Young People's Counselling Service,
Tavistock Clinic,
120 Belsize Lane,
London NW3 5BA
Tel: 0171 435 7111 ext. 2337

Youth Helpline (4–6pm Monday, Tuesday, Wednesday):
Tel: 01603 765050

INDEX